AF437226

This symposium was organized jointly by

CEC
Commission of the European Communities,
Directorate General for Employment and Social Affairs
Health and Safety Directorate

EPA
United States Environmental Protection Agency

and

WHO
World Health Organization

Organizing Committee

Chairmen:
D. Barth, EPA
B.H. Dieterich, WHO
P. Recht, CEC

Scientific Advisors (Rapporteurs):
P. Lafleur, U.S. National Bureau of Standards
R. Lauwerys, University of Louvain
G. Nordberg, Karolinska Institute

Vice Chairmen:
F.G. Hueter, EPA
J. Smeets, CEC
V.B. Vouk, WHO

Technical Secretariat:
A. Bonini, CEC
S. Braman, WHO

Scientific Secretariat:
A. Berlin, CEC
A.H. Wolf, University of Illinois
Y. Hasegawa, WHO

Luxembourg, 18-22 April 1977

The Use of Biological Specimens for the Assessment of Human Exposure to Environmental Pollutants

Proceedings of the International Workshop at Luxembourg, 18-22 April 1977

Editors

A. Berlin
EEC, Luxembourg

A.H. Wolff
University of Illinois, Chicago

and

Y. Hasegawa
WHO, Geneva

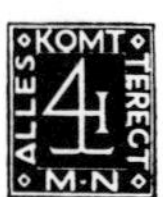

Martinus Nijhoff Publishers - The Hague/Boston/London 1979
for
The Commission of the European Communities

Publication arranged by

Commission of the European Communities,
Directorate-General Scientific and Technical Information
and Information Management, Luxembourg

EUR 5824 EN

ISBN 90 247 2168 7

EDITORIAL NOTE

For the preparation of this Workshop, a number of background contributions have been requested by the Organizing Committee. These have been used by the rapporteurs:

P. LAFLEUR
R. LAUWERYS
G. NORDBERG

and the coordinator:

A.H. WOLFF

to prepare a draft report which has been used as the basic discussion document during the Workshop.

Both the final approved general report and the background documents are published in these proceedings.

A. BERLIN   -   A.H. WOLFF   -   Y. HASEGAWA

CONTENTS

PREFACE

This International Workshop on the use of biological specimens for the assessment of human exposure to environmental pollutants, has been organized jointly by the Commission of the European Communities, the World Health Organization and the Environmental Protection Agency of the United States.

The objectives of this Workshop were to assess types of pollutants and 'human samples' best amenable for 'biological monitoring' and 'collection for future reference' and to examine the technical feasibility of such programmes.

A number of recommendations have been developed regarding both implementation and research activities, and are incorporated in a general report.

The implementation of biological monitoring programmes should be considered at once, whereas in the present state of knowledge, tissue banking needs some more study; however, some programmes should be initiated in this field at a pilot-scale level.

The three sponsoring organizations are taking note of these recommendations in their respective programmes.

on behalf of the Organizing Committee,

D. BARTH   -   B.H. DIETERICH   -   P. RECHT

INTERNATIONAL WORKSHOP

ON

THE USE OF BIOLOGICAL SPECIMENS FOR THE ASSESSMENT OF

HUMAN EXPOSURE TO ENVIRONMENTAL POLLUTANTS

REPORT

LUXEMBOURG
18-22 April 1977

FOREWORD

TERMINOLOGY AND DEFINITIONS

The terminology used in this report takes very careful account of the terminology and definitions accepted and widely used by the three sponsoring organisations. However in a few specific cases the terms and definitions had to be adapted to the special needs of this report. Although man and his environment form an integral whole, an arbitrary distinction is being made in this report for technical reasons between human biological specimens and other environmental biological specimens.

The following terms with their definitions are used in the present report :

human biological specimens — organs, tissues (including blood), secreta and excreta from man ;

other biological specimens — organs, tissues, secreta and excreta from living organisms other than man ;

biological monitoring — systematic collection of human or other biological specimens for which analysis of pollutant concentrations, metabolites and biotransformation products, is of immediate application ; analysis and evaluation will generally be performed within a period of weeks after collection. Unless qualified, 'biological monitoring' will refer in this document to human specimens ;

biological specimen banking — the systematic collection and storage of samples for deferred examination, analysis and evaluation. These activities generally will be deferred for a period of years or even decades following collection. In the context of the present document these collections will refer only to human specimens. 'Collections for future reference' may be used as an alternative.

indicator specimen — the sample most appropriate for biological monitoring and/or biological specimen banking ; 'index specimen' may be used as an alternative ;

environmental monitoring — the systematic collection, analysis and evaluation of environmental samples, such as air, water or food for pollutants ;

body burden — in general refers to the total amount of a specific pollutant in the body of an individual at the time of sampling, but in the context of this report the term is used to reflect the amount of a pollutant in a given tissue ;

exposure to a given pollutant is a measure of contact between the pollutant and the outer or inner (e.g. alveolar or gut) surface of the human body, usually expressed in terms of concentrations and the amount of time the pollutant in the medium (e.g. ambient air and food) interfaces with the body surfaces. Once absorbed through the body surfaces, the pollutant gives rise to 'doses' in various organs and tissues ;

dose — the amount of a pollutant absorbed or retained in an organism during a specific time interval. Dose is generally assessed in terms of concentration in the tissues. Any record of exposure and dose should include an indication of the time and frequency at which an individual is subjected to them ;

critical organ — the organ which under specified conditions of exposure exhibits the first or the most serious effect. This effect is the 'critical effect'. The mean concentration of pollutant in the critical organ at this point is the 'critical organ concentration' ;

biological effect is any measured (biochemical, functional or structural) change which is the result of a reaction of the organism to exposure. For the purpose of this report, an effect will be termed 'adverse' if there exists an impairment of functional capacity, a decreased ability to compensate for additional stress, a decreased ability to maintain homeostasis, an enhanced susceptibility to other environmental influences — or if such impairments are likely to become manifest in the near future.

1. SUMMARY

1.1. INTRODUCTION

This document is the report of the International Workshop " **The Use of Biological Specimens for the Assessment of Human Exposure to Environmental Pollutants**" that was sponsored by the Commission of the European Communities, the United States Environmental Protection Agency and the World Health Organization.   The Workshop was held at Luxembourg City, Luxembourg, April 18 – 22, 1977.

Conceptual and operational aspects of the systematic sample collection, preparation, analysis and storage of biological specimens are presented, with the aim to contribute towards discerning potential risks of pollution to man.

1.1.1. Objectives

The main objectives of the Workshop were :
-- to assess the types of environmental pollutants and human specimens most suitable for 'biological monitoring' and to evaluate the probable usefulness of biological specimen banking ;
-- to examine the state of the art and the technical feasability of programmes designed to collect, analyse and store samples relative to biological monitoring and biological specimen banking ;
-- to develop guidelines for sampling, sample preparation, analytical requirements and storage ;
-- to draw up recommendations for further research and development.

1.1.2. Biological Monitoring

Systematic sampling and prompt analysis of human or other biological specimens may help greatly in understanding the relationship between exposure to pollution and health hazards. Biological monitoring can establish reference baselines of pollutant concentrations in human beings and provide early warning of increasing levels.

In addition biological monitoring can make existing environmental (physical and chemical) monitoring systems more cost-effective by establishing direct or indirect links to humans ; pollutant concentrations at the point of impact, the human being, can be related to sources of environmental contamination, and the populations at risk can be defined. The effectiveness of control measures may be assessed through subsequent periodical biological monitoring which will detect changes in levels of pollutants in man.

1.1.3. Biological Specimen Banks

The systematic collection and storage of samples for future analysis have several advantages :
-- specimens can be analysed some time after collection to validate, or resolve discrepancies in, previously obtained data or to take advantage of major improvements in methods of analysis ;
-- retrospective estimation of exposure can be made where chronic or latent health effects are involved ;
-- long-term trends can be retrospectively determined to show changes in levels of pollutants relative to the effectiveness of control measures ;
-- warning of increasing pollutant levels can be obtained, and new or previously unrecognized pollutants can also be assessed.

1.2. SELECTION OF POLLUTANTS AND BIOLOGICAL SPECIMENS OF INTEREST

A brief review of past and current programmes in biological monitoring is given. Relevant parts of present knowledge concerning existing exposure to various pollutants and the biological specimen (indicator tissue) best amenable for use in biological monitoring programmes are given in more detail and include : elements (As, Be, Cd, Co, Cr, Cu, F, Hg, Mn, Mo, Ni, Pb, Pd, Pt, Se, Sn, V, Zn), organometallic compounds, minerals, organochlorine pesticides, polychorinated biphenyls, dioxin and related compounds, halogenated solvents, propellants, aliphatic and aromatic hydrocarbons, polycyclic hydrocarbons, amino and nitro derivatives and some other organic compounds.

Based on present scientific knowledge the most useful indicator specimens are tabulated for each pollutant. From this and other available information, pollutants are suggested for which biological monitoring programmes could now be implemented. More information is needed before any monitoring activity can be initiated for other pollutants of interest.

1.3. TECHNICAL CONSIDERATIONS

1.3.1. Specimen Collection, Preparation and Storage

In excising tissue and collecting body fluids for biological monitoring or biological specimen banking, necessary precautions must be taken to obtain adequate information relative to the purpose of the study and the substance to be analysed. Contamination of the sample during collection and preparation may be more of a problem in some cases than others, and specific risks of contamination are reviewed in the document.

Current methods of sample storage include freeze drying, rapid freezing, chemical preservation and ashing. Appropriate applications for each method are reviewed in the document.

1.3.2. Analytical Aspects

Analytical procedures for a variety of pollutants have been reviewed. Where appropriate, specific techniques have been listed, and special problems and cautions considered.

1.3.3. Standards and Quality Control

Assessment of exposure to pollutants almost always involves analytical procedures for very small quantities of the substances of interest and may result in relatively large experimental errors. In order to minimize contamination it is of prime importance that laboratories maintain strict control of the environment in which the analyses are performed.

A reliable system for maintaining a high quality of analytical performance is essential. The procedures used to ensure quality control, along with estimates of the accuracy and the precision of data, should be included when reporting results. Some specific considerations have been discussed.

1.3.4. Feasibility of Collection and Storage of Samples

Sampling in areas remote from laboratories requires special precautions with regard to preservation and transportation. Storage of samples for trace metal analysis may be relatively easy compared to the storage of samples containing substances which may undergo changes in composition, e.g. organic compounds.

1.4. DESIGN AND ORGANIZATION OF PROGRAMMES

1.4.1. Programme Design

The design of individual programmes will depend on the type of programme to be undertaken, the types of samples to be collected and the pollutants considered. Several types of programmes are described in the document. General guidelines and requirements for establishing programmes are presented in tabular form. Some requirements deemed especially important are highlighted and discussed.

6

1.4.2. Practical considerations

Various operational aspects were discussed. These include :
-- the number of samples required to provide statistically meaningful results ;
-- selection of population groups and biological specimens ;
-- information required on donor and specimens ;
-- handling, storage and presentation of data ;
-- evaluation of results ;
-- follow-up action ;
-- management and training.

1.4.3. Cost Estimations

Although the costing of biological monitoring programmes is dependent on the size of the programme undertaken, it can be estimated that analytical costs account for about 50 % of the total operating budget. Personnel services are another large portion of the total. While information is lacking on cost estimation for tissue banking, the cost of storing samples is expected to be a large fraction of the total budget for such programmes.

1.4.4. Ethical and Legal Considerations

There are differences among various countries and among states within the same country regarding regulations, customs, and restrictions that must be considered in collecting, analysing and storing human samples. All investigators must be cognizant of the customs and legal restrictions applicable to their countries and/or any collaborating countries.

1.4.5. Collaborative programmes

Because pollution occurs independently of national boundaries, collaborative programmes between countries are needed to discern the distribution patterns of pollutant exposure. It was recognized that such programmes can provide a degree of economy and effectiveness not possible in cases of independent investigations.

2. CONCLUSIONS

The Workshop's main conclusions were as follows :

Human populations are increasingly exposed to substances that are potentially detrimental to health. Many of these substances are already found in human tissues, fluids, secreta and excreta, and some tend to concentrate in specific parts of the human body. Biological monitoring programmes can provide direct evidence of exposure and must therefore be implemented to supplement physical and chemical monitoring programmes in areas where these exist already.

In areas where no monitoring efforts are conducted, should the need arise, biological monitoring might be considered first.

Environmental specimens other than human may also be useful, and in some instances particularly appropriate, for evaluating human exposure to certain pollutants.

Based on the knowledge currently available, it is feasible to conduct biological monitoring programmes for the compounds (pollutants) and human tissues listed in the following table (Table I). The biological specimens to be studied will depend upon the specific objectives and design of the programme considered.

'Biological tissue banking' will be of great importance in analysing trends in exposure to previously unrecognized harmful pollutants or pollutants for which current measurement techniques are inadequate. Biological monitoring and analysis of stored specimens can provide a warning for the initiation of remedial measures.

TABLE I

POLLUTANTS AND HUMAN BIOLOGICAL TISSUES

AMENABLE AT PRESENT TO BIOLOGICAL MONITORING

Pollutants / Tissues	Arsenic	Cadmium	Chromium	Lead	Inorganic Mercury	Methyl Mercury	Carbon Monoxide	Organochlorine Pesticides	Pentachlorophenol	Polychlorinated biphenyls	Chlorinated solvents	Benzene
Adipose tissue								X		X		
Blood	X	X		X	X	X	X	X		X	X	X
Bone				X								
Brain					X	X						
Expired air							X				X	X
Faeces		X										
Hair	X			X		X						
Kidney		X		X	X							
Liver		X		X		X						
Milk								X		X		
Placenta		X		X								
Teeth				X								
Urine	X	X	X	X	X				X		X	X

Measurement of the concentrations of certain elements in human body fluids is a valuable tool in clinical medicine.   It is likely that biological monitoring programmes for various pollutants will play an equally important role in the future of environmental medicine.   More reliable dose—response relationships are expected to emerge for compounds measured in biological specimens when simultaneous evaluations of biological effects are available.

Standards and quality control are essential in biological monitoring programmes and in establishing collections for future reference.   The Workshop concluded that a reliable system of checking and maintaining a high quality of analytical performance demands :
-- 	availability of experienced analytical personnel,
-- 	interlaboratory quality control programmes for participating laboratories,
-- 	use of certified reference material and/or reference laboratories for the validation of analytical techniques.

Present knowledge indicates that the substances listed in Table II are important from the environmental health point of view and that the associated tissues are potentially useful indicator specimens.   However, increased knowledge is essential for the optimum design and efficiency of current and future biological monitoring programmes related to these substances.

Developing countries can present special environmental health problems largely because of greater exposure to certain chemicals such as pesticides which tend to be used there more intensively than in industrialized countries.   But often the problems posed by environmental contaminants are not well defined in these countries for lack of adequate environmental monitoring programmes.

3. RECOMMENDATIONS

In several of the recommendations covering both implementation and research aspects, reference is made to the sponsoring organizations of this Workshop, but it is clear that some will apply equally to other international and national bodies.

3.1.   RECOMMENDATIONS FOR IMPLEMENTATION

When developing programmes to collect and analyse human specimens for evaluating exposure to environmental pollutants, emphasis should be placed on public health objectives.

The Workshop estimated that for a number of the pollutants indicated in paragraph 5.3. the starting of biological monitoring programmes should be considered.   Priorities should be established on the basis of current and predicted exposure, the size of population at risk and the severity of health effects.   It is recommended that the sponsors of this Workshop convene a series of subsequent meetings for the detailed planning and implementation of programmes for some of the pollutants listed in Table I.

Present knowledge concerning the stability of elements, minerals and some organohalogenated compounds in biological tissues (taking into account sample preparation and storage methods) is sufficient to initiate some pilot-scale biological specimen banks for future reference. It is recommended that such banks be set up as soon as practicable in order to establish base-line levels for the future and to facilitate the collection of further information on the methodology needed for full scale banks.

Careful planning for biological specimen banks is recommended because of the long time periods involved for implementation.   This planning should take account of the biological monitoring programmes and existing research related to the development of specimen banks.

The importance of the collection of environmental samples (air, water) and biological samples other than human specimens for the assessment of pollutant levels and sources, as well as for the evaluation of human exposure, has also been stressed.   It is recommended that an international workshop similar to the present one be convened to discuss the operational aspects of biological monitoring and the feasibility of establishing a specimen bank for environmental and biological materials other than human tissues.

TABLE II

SUBSTANCES AND INDICATOR SPECIMENS REQUIRING FURTHER RESEARCH

Nickel	:	blood, brain, hair and nails, kidney, liver, lung and adjacent tissues.
Asbestos	:	faeces, intestine - G.I. tract, lung and adjacent tissues, lung washings, lymphs nodes, pleura and peritoneum, sputum.
Phenoxy-herbicides	:	blood, liver, umbilical cord blood, urine.
Tetrachloro-dioxin, benzofurane and azobenzene	:	adipose tissue, bile, blood, brain, foetal tissue, liver, milk, placenta, skin, umbilical cord blood.
Chlorinated solvents and plastic monomers	:	adipose tissue, bile, brain, liver, milk, peripheral nerves, placenta, spinal cord, umbilical cord blood, urine.
Polycyclic hydrocarbons	:	adipose tissue, bile, blood, liver, lung and adjacent tissues, lung washings, placenta, sputum umbilical cord blood, urine.
Amino and nitro derivatives	:	adipose tissue, bile, blood, umbilical cord, blood, urine.
Nitroso derivatives	:	blood, intestine - G.I. tract, kidney, liver, urine.
Organo phosphorus esters	:	cerebrospinal fluid, milk, umbilical cord blood.
Mycotoxins	:	adipose tissue, bile, blood, intestine – G.I. tract, kidney, liver, milk, umbilical cord blood, urine.
Antibiotics	:	bile, blood, bone, liver, muscles, saliva, teeth, umbilical cord blood, urine.

10

Biological monitoring and specimen banking programmes should utilize the resources and experience of closely related programmes where they exist. Special attention is drawn to the existing biological monitoring programmes in the occupational health field.

Multi-national collaborative programmes should be encouraged since environmental problems are quite independent of national boundaries. It is recommended that the sponsoring organizations encourage biological monitoring and biological specimen bank programmes in the future and develop harmonized systems for data acquisition and evaluation.

In planning any study involving human specimens, ethical and legal constraints must be taken into account.

It is recommended that foremost attention be paid to maintaining a high quality of analytical performance in implementing biological monitoring programmes and establishing biological specimen banks. Special attention must be paid to the use of standards and to the participation in interlaboratory quality control programmes.

A biological monitoring and biological specimen bank programme should take into consideration pre-screening and other available data on new chemicals as well as new technological developments.

When selecting samples for both biological monitoring and biological specimen banks, the medical history and health status of the donor must be considered.

Results from specific individuals (living or dead) must be confidential. However, in the case of a living donor, the individual in question and/or his physician will be informed if the subject so wishes. In that case the results should be accompanied by an explanation regarding their health significance. Whenever appropriate, the public should also be informed by the proper authority of the significance of the evaluated data on a population basis.

Biological monitoring programmes and specimen banks should be planned in consultation with medical experts, statisticians, analytical chemists and others concerned, to ensure adequate design, sampling and analytical methodology.

It is recommended that, in developing criteria documents* for pollutants for which indicator specimens have been identified, careful consideration be given to the relationship between environmental exposure and the concentrations in biological indicator specimens. 'Normal' concentrations and those associated with an unaccceptable risk of adverse effects should also be defined. Such information will assist in data evaluation and initiation of appropriate action whenever necessary. If such information is not included in the criteria documents already available for some pollutants, efforts should be made to fill this gap.

In order to ensure efficient and economic operation of specimen banks, sample collection, storage, analysis and quality control of data should be performed or coordinated centrally for each programme. The number of storage sites should be kept to a minimum.

It is recommended that in planning future specimen banking programmes, careful attention be given to the qualifications of the persons having access to the stored specimens.

3.2. RESEARCH RECOMMENDATIONS

For a number of pollutants the identification of appropriate indicator specimens is urgently needed. It is recommended that research be undertaken on the metabolism of these pollutants in mammalian systems to determine the relationship between environmental exposure and pollutant levels in accessible indicator specimens. It is recommended that research be carried out to determine the concentrations in the critical tissues (or body fluids) at which adverse effects begin to occur.

Among the substances listed in Table II it is recommended that a special research effort should be directed towards those substances for which the current or predicted exposure is the highest, and the size of the population at risk and the severity of health effects greatest.

---

*   Criteria documents are critical reviews of the existing knowledge, ready for application and expressed, as far as possible, in quantitative terms, on the relations between the exposure to a pollutant and the risk of magnitude of an undesirable effect on a target under specified circumstances.

Further research on storage technology is recommended since present knowledge is large-ly limited to low-temperature storage of samples, for the determination of trace metals. Factors that may inactivate, and thus inhibit degradation of organic compounds should be investigated.

Research is needed to identify non-human environmental substrates which can serve as useful indicator specimens both for non-human biological monitoring and environmental speci-men banking. The analysis of such specimens can also be useful in assessing human exposure to pollutants.

Further research in sampling, sample transport techniques, and analytical methodology is required for the effective implementation of both biological monitoring programmes and tissue banks.

It is recommended that a wide variety of certified reference materials be developed for the validation of analytical techniques.

4. INTRODUCTION

4.1. RATIONALE AND OBJECTIVES

Human populations are being increasingly exposed to substances potentially noxious to man. In recent years it has been shown that several of the pollutants in concentrations found in the environment can adversely affect man's health. However, there is relatively little know-ledge of the potential risks that the majority of these pollutants present to man and his environ-ment. Since a number of substances (pollutants, metabolites and bio-transformation products) are known to occur and/or concentrate in various human tissues and organs, there is a need to carry out programmes for biological monitoring and/or collections for future reference.

The objectives of the Workshop were :
-- to assess the types of environmental pollutants and human specimens most suitable for biological monitoring and to evaluate the probable usefulness of biological specimen banking ;
-- to examine the state of the art and the technical feasibility of programmes designed to collect 'human biological specimens' for 'biological monitoring' and 'biological specimen banking' ;
-- to develop guidelines on sampling, sample preparation, storage and analytical require-ments ;
-- to draw up recommendations for further research and development.

4.2. POTENTIAL USES OF 'BIOLOGICAL MONITORING' PROGRAMMES AND OF 'BIOLOGICAL SPECIMEN BANKS'

4.2.1. Biological monitoring in given situations may be valuable for :

-- determining the presence and extent of human health hazards from environmental expo-sure to pollutants ;
-- establishing reference base-lines of pollutant concentration ranges in human beings ;
-- correlating levels of pollutants in humans with sources of contamination and environmen-tal levels, and determining risks to defined target populations ;
-- determining trends of pollutant levels in humans :
    i   to ascertain needs for pollution control programmes
    ii   to help evaluate the efficacy of pollution control programmes and standards
    iii   to help predict future human health problems and risks, and provide early warning ;

--   assisting in the elucidation of dose—response relationships ;
--   complementing existing environmental monitoring systems to make them more cost-effective and, at the same time, more relevant by establishing a direct or indirect link with humans, thus providing a better basis for developing public health indices with respect to environmental pollution ;
--   for establishing priorities as regards research related to human health.

4.2.2. 'Biological specimen banks' are needed to provide biological samples for retrospective analyses and may present the following advantages :

--   re-analysis of indicator specimens to validate data or to resolve discrepancies ;
--   re-analysis of specimens to take advantage of major improvements in analytical methodology and instrumentation with respect to sensitivity and selectivity ;
--   use of stored organs and tissues that are found to be more indicative of exposure than those formerly analysed ;
--   analysis of stored specimens following the discovery or elucidation of relationships between dose from one or more pollutants and biological effects ;
--   possibility of determining trends in pollutant levels in relation to the efficiency of control programmes and standards, or to giving warning of increasing levels ;
--   re-analysis of samples using reference standards as soon as available, and assistance in international comparability of analyses.

4.3.   CLASSIFICATION OF POLLUTANT CATEGORIES

Within the context of this document the Workshop agreed to the following three broad classifications of present and potential environmental pollutants :

--   inorganic substances ;
--   organo-halogenated compounds ;
--   other organic compounds.

For the purpose of detailed discussions the three broad categories have been further subdivided as follows :

--   inorganic compounds of Al, As, Be, Cd, Co, Cr, Cu, F, Hg, Mn, Mo, Ni, Pb, Pt/Pd, Se, Sn, V, Zn, organo-metallic compounds and minerals ;
--   organochlorine pesticides, polychlorinated biphenyls, dioxin and related compounds, halogenated solvents and propellants ;
--   non-substituted aliphatic and aromatic hydrocarbons, polycyclic hydrocarbons, amino and nitro derivatives, alcohols, glycols, ethers, ketones, aldehydes, acids, amides, phenol and derivatives, esters and some other organic compounds of interest.

Given the scope of the Workshop, pollutants such as sulphur dioxide, ozone, nitrogen dioxide, etc., whose direct presence, or that of their metabolites, cannot be measured in the human body, have not been considered.

Study on radionuclides in human tissues and excreta from the view-point of environmental hazards started very early and have been used as models for programmes on other environmental pollutants. Such programmes have been reviewed in a working paper for this Workshop and will not be further discussed in this document, as radioactive substances are considered outside the scope of the Workshop.

4.4. REVIEW OF PAST AND CURRENT PROGRAMMES

Any review of current and past human monitoring programmes is beset by a number of difficulties :

-- the aim, scope and presentation differ widely from one investigation to another, so that data should only be compared with caution ;

-- data are often not comparable because of the use of non-standardized analytical methods, the poor descriptions of the methods employed or because of the lack of information on the quality control procedures.

Useful data have, however, been reported from a small number of studies performed for limited purposes. For some compounds approximate estimates of the degree of exposure have thus been obtained as regards countries with varying geographical, social, ethnic and racial backgrounds. In the following sections, a broad overview of past and current programmes will be given. Guidance regarding specific data from past experience, that can be used as a basis for future programmes for the various compounds under consideration, will be given.

Numerous programmes on biological monitoring for various compounds have been conducted and are at present in progress. It is not possible to enumerate all the occupational related programmes here, nor even the less numerous programmes for environmental exposure, but some general comments, particularly regarding the latter category, will be given. However a few programmes will be mentioned as examples in order to illustrate various approaches.

4.4.1. Inorganic substances

4.4.1.1. Inorganic compounds

For certain toxic metals, e.g. lead and cadmium, biological monitoring programmes in conjunction with evaluation of health effects have given valuable information on dose-response relationships and have thus provided a basis for preventive measures to avoid adverse health effects from these metals. Biological monitoring of certain population groups has been carried out following demonstration of the existence of exposure and subsequent concern about possible adverse health effects. For comparison, biological monitoring has been carried out in reference areas, where the specific exposure situation was not present.

In occupational health, the blood concentrations of certain toxic elements, e.g. lead, are monitored on a fixed schedule to ensure that workers' tissue concentrations maintain non-toxic levels. Biological monitoring for lead has also been used to prevent adverse effects from lead exposure in the non-industrial population. These programmes have been of great practical value.

A study concerning cadmium concentrations in human samples from non-occupationally exposed persons in three countries, (USA, Japan and Sweden) provides an example of another programme in which a great effort has been made to ensure accuracy in analysis and make possible a comparison of body burdens of this particular metal.

Deviations from 'normal' trace element levels have been found in persons with certain diseases. It is not known from these studies whether the abnormal trace element distribution was a contributing factor in the disease development or whether it was simply a secondary result of the tissue damage from the disease. However, some very elaborate programmes in this field of research are still underway, and definite conclusions as regards the suitability of this approach for identifying risk factors operative in various diseases cannot yet be drawn.

14

Some studies have been carried out to establish the 'normal' concentration ranges of trace elements in human tissues in defined populations. Deviations from these concentration ranges may be used to indicate the existence of environmental exposures above natural background levels. However, as mentioned above, similar deviations have been found in persons with certain diseases. It must therefore be recognized that medical histories as well as health status have inevitably to be considered in selecting samples when biological monitoring is used for human pollution exposure estimation.

Measurement of concentrations of certain elements is a valuable tool in clinical medicine. It is likely that biological monitoring programmes for trace elements will play an equally important role in environmental medicine in the future.

4.4.1.2. Organometallic compounds

Programmes based on the analysis of total mercury or methylmercury in indicator specimen, such as blood and hair, have been successfully conducted in areas where epidemics of poisoning have occurred (Iraq, Japan), and in areas where consumption of contamined food items has caused increased, but not clearly toxic, body burdens, as well as in reference areas. The results of these programmes make it possible to draw rather detailed conclusions regarding dose-response relationships and adequate preventive measures with regard to methylmercury.

4.4.1.3. Minerals

In the present document the classification of minerals is a broad one. The physiological effects of many man-made materials are often similar to those of naturally occurring minerals ; for example it has been suggested that fly-ash may have a similar action to free SiO_2 , while data from animal experiments indicate that many types of fibrous materials may have a quantitatively similar action to that of asbestos. Therefore, the class of minerals will include pollutants of inorganic origin that are biologically important owing to their physical, and possibly chemical, characteristics. At present time, dose-response relationships have not been established for minerals, except for some occupational exposure situations such as in the case of asbestos workers or cotton workers (bysionosis).

4.4.2. Organo-halogenated compounds

The occurrence of organochlorine pesticides (OCPs) and related compounds in human samples is still a matter of concern in many countries. Many monitoring programmes are being, or have been, carried out throughout the world. This is the case not only in countries where spraying with organochlorine pesticides is still practiced, but also in countries where the pesticides are manufactured or formulated and where — even if the use of persistent organochlorine pesticides has been banned or largely reduced — the populations are still environmentally, or via the food chain, exposed to such pesticides. Systematic monitoring programmes for pesticide residues in human subjects started as early as 1967. A sampling programme for poly-chlorinated biphenyls was introduced in the USA in 1969 and analysis for these compounds has been made since 1971. Through periodic evaluation of the results from the monitoring programmes, definite trends towards decreasing levels have been revealed. Another programme in the United Kingdom has also shown a downward trend for the past 5 - 7 years. Programmes dealing with pesticides in samples of human adipose tissues, blood and maternal milk are being carried out in various countries.

4.4.3. Other organic compounds

To date, experience regarding biological monitoring of the populations and the banking of tissues for organic chemicals, other than organo-halogenated compounds, is very limited. Only preliminary trials have been carried out to evaluate intensity of exposure to organophosphorus pesticides. However, during the last 30 years some experience in biological monitoring for organic chemicals has been gained in the field of occupational health. Such programmes have been concerned mainly with solvents and organophosphorus pesticides.

Biological monitoring for organic compounds (which are metabolized in the human body) have been carried out using urine samples for the detection of their metabolites. For example, promising analytical procedures for the metabolites of certain organic compounds, such as organophosphorus, carbamates and chlorophenoxy pesticides, have been reported. These programmes indicate that the concentration of pesticide residues correlate to exposure, and thus hold out promise of a satisfactory monitoring method. This type of biological monitoring may also be applicable to other organic compounds such as benzene and various solvents.

5. RATIONALE FOR INTEREST OR CONCERN AND CONSIDERATIONS FOR SPECIMEN COLLECTION

In this chapter the pollutants of interest and concern have been selected on the basis of knowledge regarding their health and environmental importance. The indicator specimens (biological tissues) have been selected on the basis of currently available scientific knowledge regarding exposure/effect relationships and accumulation of certain pollutants in specific organs. Most of the human data have come from occupational exposures at relatively high levels. Considerations with respect to the feasibility of sampling, storage and analysis for the various indicator specimens and pollutants are set out in Chapter 6.

5.1. INORGANIC SUBSTANCES

5.1.1. Inorganic compounds

Unlike many man-made substances, virtually all elements are normally present in most human tissues. Some elements (the so-called essential elements) are necessary for normal biological development and function, whereas others are not known to have any useful function in the body.

For non-essential elements, concentrations are usually low and, in many cases, there is a large safety margin between 'normal' concentrations and those which cause adverse effects. For some elements, this margin is less wide, whilst for others the margin is unknown, since 'normal' and/or 'toxic tissue concentrations' have not been adequately established.

Since the body is usually able to regulate the tissue levels of the essential elements, non essential elements are more likely to cause environmental pollution problems. However, there are exceptions to this rule and the following discussion, therefore, does not relate to essentiality of elements.

The general philosophy for obtaining and using data on tissue concentrations of toxic metals in the prevention of related adverse health effects has been stated by various international task groups.

While it is difficult to decide which elements should be given priority for study, summing up the present state of knowledge, the elements of greatest interest as environmental pollutants are : arsenic, cadmium, chromium, lead and mercury. These, together with a number of other elements of potential environmental significance, will be reviewed in the following paragraphs.

5.1.1.1. Arsenic

Arsenic in inorganic form may be discharged in large quantities into the ambient air and water from refining and smelting operations which use certain sulfide ores and from coal combustion. Populations living around the sites of such operations may be directly exposed. Exposure to arsenic may also occur through drinking water obtained from wells drilled in geological formations rich in arsenic, and from some food products and beverages.

Occupational exposure in industry and agriculture to dusts containing inorganic arsenic compounds has been associated with lung cancer. Perforation of the nasal septum, peripheral nervous system symptoms and certain skin lesions have also occurred. Exposure through the oral route may be associated with skin cancer and circulatory disturbances (Blackfoot disease).

After intake, arsenic compounds undergo metabolic changes in the human body that are not yet fully understood. These transformations include the formation of methylated organo-arsenical compounds that have a short biological half-life (hours to a few days) ; such changes also take place in the environment. Urine has been used as an indicator specimen in several occupational programmes ; however, great fluctuations can occur depending on the dietary intake of arsenic. Blood is also an indicator specimen but presents similar fluctuation in relation to dietary arsenic intake. Hair is a useful indicator specimen for the oral intake and the inhalation of inorganic arsenic as a pollutant in the general environment. However it is less reliable for airborne occupational exposures because of external contamination of hair. There is also some uncertainty about the interpretation of data from biological monitoring programmes related to the ingestion of organic arsenicals in food and more information is needed on the metabolism of such compounds.

To sum up, biological samples useful for arsenic bioassay are blood, hair and urine. Skin, kidney, lung and liver could also be of interest.

5.1.1.2. Cadmium

Cadmium pollution of the environment may result from a number of industrial and agricultural activities. The most important sources are mining, refining and smelting operations utilizing ores rich in cadmium (particularly some sulfide ores primarily used for zinc and lead production), and manufacturing of cadmium batteries and pigments. Coal may contain traces of cadmium which will be emitted during combustion, while the soil may be contamined from the use of cadmium-rich sewage sludge or phosphate as fertilizers in agriculture. Once soil has been contamined, it may remain so for decades and the cadmium may be taken up by the crops grown in that soil. Tobacco smoke is an important source of human exposure through inhalation ; with the exception of areas immediately surrounding cadmium emitting industries, smoking is the dominant source of cadmium inhalation for the general public.

Upon ingestion, only a small proportion (approximately 5 %) is absorbed and even a smaller proportion is retained in the human body. However, once absorbed, cadmium is stored in the organism for many years. The renal cortex, which is the critical organ, shows the highest concentration of cadmium. Proteinuria, pulmonary effects, mild anaemia and osteomalacia have been reported in occupationally exposed workers. There are also reports from Japan indicating that an outbreak of osteomalacia and increased prevalence of proteinuria occurred in an area polluted by cadmium through mining activities. An issue of current concern is the possible carcinogenicity of cadmium, as lung and prostate cancer have been reported in cadmium-exposed industrial workers. Although there is no definite human evidence showing an association between cadmium and hypertension, experiments in rats have indicated that cadmium can induce hypertension in that species. Programmes based on cadmium analysis of indicator specimens have been of great value and should be continued on a broader scale. Both selective programmes focused on specific areas and more general programmes are useful. Useful indicator specimens are blood, urine, faeces, liver and kidney cortex. Hair, lung, placenta and pancreas might also be of value.

5.1.1.3. Chromium

Concern regarding chromium pollution is currently focused on population groups around smelting and ferrous alloy manufacturing plants, electroplating factories, as well as around chromate industries. Hexavalent chromium has been recognized as a cause of lung cancer in human for some time, but it is at present not clear whether trivalent chromium should also be regarded as a less potent carcinogen, or as entirely innocuous. It should be noted however, that the differentiation between trivalent and hexavalent chromium is very difficult in routine biological monitoring. No body-burden/effect relationships for chromium have as yet been established ; biological monitoring programmes may be of value in this respect. Indicator specimens include urine and possibly blood and lung.

5.1.1.4. Lead

The sources of environmental lead contamination are manifold, an important one being the tetraethyl-lead used as a fuel additive which results in the discharge of inorganic lead compounds into the atmosphere. Other sources are non-ferrous smelting operations, the manufacture of lead batteries, lead-containing paints, lead-coated cables, etc. The widespread use of lead in paint has led to the exposure of children who may ingest paint chips. The use of lead in sealing wine bottles and the use of lead piping for drinking water are other sources of exposure for the general public.

The absorption of inorganic lead compounds in the gastrointestinal tract depends on age and nutritional factors. For adults this absorption is of the order of 10 %, but it can reach 50 % for children. Pulmonary absorption of inhaled lead is of the order of 35 %. Absorbed lead is distributed to various soft tissue compartments of the body and is finally incorporated in bone in a biologically inactive form.

A number of the effects of lead exposure have been studied in some detail, particularly in occupationally exposed subjects. Such effects include : alterations in the enzymes involved in haematopoiesis (decrease of ALA-D in blood and bone marrow, increase in erythrocyte protoporphyrin, ALA and coproporphyrin in urine, and anaemia) ; impairment of peripheral nerve function (ranging from decreased nerve conduction velocity to clinical neuropathy) ; effects on the central nervous system and renal dysfunction. In addition, there are some incomplete data that suggest pre- and post-natal (infants and pre-school children) effects on the central nervous system from relatively low exposures. Biological monitoring programmes using blood lead determinations are useful and are routinely applied in many occupational settings. Such programmes are also of value in assessing the general environmental exposure of the population and should be encouraged. Suitable indicator specimens are blood, bone, hair, kidney, liver and urine, with teeth being of interest in special cases.

5.1.1.5. Mercury

The mercury compounds that are of concern as environmental contaminants include methylmercury compounds (see Section 5.1.2.2.). Other forms of mercury of toxicological importance are mercury vapour and mercuric (Hg^{2+}) compounds ; when mercuric compounds are released into the aquatic environment, they can be converted to methylmercuric compounds.

5.1.1.5.1. Mercury vapour

Mercury vapour is efficiently absorbed (80 %) via inhalation. The mercury is carried by the blood to the brain and other tissues, e.g. liver and kidney cortex. Predominant symptoms in chronic mercury vapour poisoning are effects on the nervous system ; loss of weight and teeth, salivation and kidney damage may also occur. There is some controversy as to the dose-response relationships for some of these symptoms. Toxic tissue levels are not known in any detail. Biological monitoring of urine or blood samples in occupationally exposed persons has been valuable and is routinely used in some occupational health programmes. Autopsy programmes may use brain and kidney specimens.

5.1.1.5.2. Inorganic mercuric compounds

Inorganic mercuric compounds are absorbed (10 %) via the gastrointestinal tract. Inhalation of dust containing these compounds may (depending on particle size) show higher absorption. This form of mercury accumulates in the kidney and causes renal disease.

Blood, urine and kidney may be useful indicator specimens.

5.1.1.6. Nickel

Exposure to nickel can occur inside and around industrial operations dealing with this element (steel plants, plants manufacturing goods and equipment containing nickel). Nickel may also appear in the environment as a product of oil combustion. Exposure through tobacco smoke may also be significant. Background environmental levels are fairly high but human exposure to nickel through food has not been considered a problem.

Industrial exposure to certain types of insoluble inorganic nickel compounds and nickel carbonyl has given rise to an increased incidence of sinus and lung cancer. There is no current evidence of significant population exposure, but some monitoring is desirable. The monitoring of workers in nickel industries by the determination of nickel concentrations in urine is already in progress, but the interpretation of results is complicated and requires further study. On the other hand autopsy studies should take advantage of the possibility of obtaining specimens from nasal mucosa and lung (including bronchial) tissue. Such programmes have not yet been reported but could prove valuable.

Urine should be a useful indicator specimen.

5.1.1.7. Beryllium

Beryllium is used in certain space-vehicle components and in various apparatuses such as electrical relays and X-ray windows. Its major use is in copper alloys.

Freshly-produced beryllium oxides are extremely toxic and the main lesions produced by chronic exposure are granulomatosis or fibrosis of the lung. The question of beryllium-induced lung cancer in humans is currently being studied. Cases of beryllosis have occurred not only in workers occupationally exposed but also in persons working or residing in the vicinity of industries using beryllium. Body-burden or lung-burden/effect relationships have not been established, and since granulomatosis involves several immunological factors, an extremely large individual variability is to be expected, which is probably why dose-response relationships are less evident. The use of a biological monitoring programme might help to elucidate these relationships.

Bone and lung might be of interest as indicator specimens.

5.1.1.8. Fluorine

Excessive exposure to fluorine may occur from airborne dust in the vicinity of aluminium refineries, steel-works and plants producing phosphate fertilizers, glass and ceramics. The most conspicuous effects from such airborne exposure are those seen in vegetation and cattle around the factories. Many trees and other plants exhibit a sensitivity that is higher by several orders of magnitude compared to that of humans.

Since fluorides are generally soluble in human tissues and fluids, a major part of the absorbed element has a short biological half-life, excretion being mainly by the urinary route. Human intakes may be evaluated through analysis of urine samples. The exposure of children to high levels of fluoride in water produces mottled teeth, while osteoporosis and osteosclerosis have been seen in industrially exposed individuals and even in some groups of the general population.

Useful biological indicator specimens might be urine, bone and teeth. It should be noted that osteoporosis and osteosclerosis may also be observed by X-ray examination.

5.1.1.9. Manganese

Manganese is an essential element but excessive exposure by inhalation has caused acute pulmonary disease (pneumonitis) and a chronic Parkinson-like syndrome. Exposure can occur in and around steel-works and ferrous alloy manufacturing plants. Biological monitoring programmes are difficult to perform because of interference from normal oral intakes of dietary manganese with blood and urine levels.

Blood, kidney , lung and brain may be useful indicator specimens.

5.1.1.10 Vanadium

This element occurs in oil used for energy production, domestic heating, etc., and is emitted into the air in fly-ash particles when oil is burned. No specific disease has as yet been related to vanadium.

Biological monitoring may be possible on urine and blood, and autopsy studies using lung tissues may also be of value.

5.1.1.11 Molybdenum

Molybdenum is an essential element but in some areas where high natural concentrations occur in the soil, widespread excessive exposure may occur. In such areas epidemiological studies have indicated an excess frequency of a gout-like disease. Molybdenum may thus be a metal of concern for biological monitoring.

Indicator specimens that should be further investigated are : blood, urine, liver, kidney, hair and nails.

5.1.1.12 Aluminium

Aluminium as Al_2O_3 is known to produce lung damage and has been found in the arterial walls of the brain in association with a Parkinson-like syndrome.

Indicator specimens might be lung and brain.

5.1.1.13 Copper, Selenium and Zinc

No appreciable health problem is known to occur as a result of discharges of zinc and copper into the environment. Selenium may cause selenium-toxicity in cattle grazing on pastures rich in selenium, but consequent human toxicity has not been reported. The main reason for including a discussion of these elements here is that they are known (mainly through animals experiments) to influence the toxicity of some of the previously mentioned metals. Thus selenium has been shown to influence the toxicity of mercury, cadmium, lead and arsenic, while zinc and copper have been shown to influence cadmium toxicity. However, it is not yet clear how these interactions influence the toxic tissue levels of metals in quantitative terms.

Copper, selenium and zinc may preferably be determined in indicator specimens such as hair and nails, urine, blood, kidney and liver, along with the appropriate measurements of cadmium or mercury.

5.1.1.14 Other elements

Some possible human exposures to other metals include cobalt in beer, tin in canned foods, and platinum or palladium from automobile emission control devices in the USA, but no complete data are available on health effects.

5.1.2. Organometallic compounds

Organometallic compounds have been described for more than 35 elements. Some of these compounds have industrial and agricultural uses, but only a few are known as environmental contaminants. Those of greatest concern at present are alkyl-lead and alkyl-mercury compounds. Nickel carbonyl, alkyl-tin and some organoarsenical compounds are also under study. If high local pollution occurs, each of these compounds may create problems of toxicological importance.

5.1.2.1. Alkyl-lead compounds

Alkyl-lead compounds can cause central nervous system symptoms when workers producing these compounds and preparing leaded petrol are exposed to high levels. After combustion of petrol, however, the lead will be converted to an inorganic form, which has been already considered. Biological monitoring programmes, including specific analysis of organic lead compounds in human tissues, have not yet been carried out to any extent and their usefulness cannot be evaluated at the present time. Workers exposed to alkyl-lead compounds can be monitored by measuring total lead in urine.

5.1.2.2. Alkyl-mercury

The organomercurials, particularly monomethylmercuric compounds, have given rise to great concern, since these compounds may be formed in the environment from other mercury compounds and accumulate there. In addition, such compounds have a tendency to concentrate along man's food chain. Contamination of the environment by any mercury compound will therefore be of concern to populations whose diet is based on food items that concentrate methylmercury, particularly fish.

Following ingestion by man, methylmercury is efficiently absorbed (more than 95%) and distributed to various parts of the body. Particularly high concentrations are found in the central nervous system, kidney, liver and hair. The blood concentration is also relatively high and in equilibrium with the afore-mentioned tissues. The biological half-life is of the order of 70 days in man and 44 days in lactating females. This relatively long biological half-life means that methylmercury levels in human organs rise continuously, and only reach a steady state within one year from the start of a countinuous daily intake. These facts, as well as the time taken for biomagnification to occur, explain why a considerable time can be expected to pass before symptoms of toxicity (mainly neurological) occur as a result of the release of mercury in the environment.

'Normal' and 'toxic' tissue levels of methylmercury are relatively well-known from the biological monitoring investigations of human poisoning that have occurred in Japan and Iraq. The outbreaks in Japan were caused by contaminated fish, whereas in Iraq the cause was from bread made from cereals that had been treated with methylmercury used as a fungicide. For populations with a relatively high dietary intake of fish products (e.g. Japan and Sweden), restricted consumption of certain species of fish has been officially recommended.

Biological monitoring of such populations for tissue levels of methylmercury thus seems appropriate. For the biological monitoring of living persons, blood or hair samples can be used since these will reflect the concentration of methylmercury in the central nervous system, which is the critical organ. Urine samples are not useful. Hair samples have an advantage over blood in that it is possible, by analysing segments of a sample, to assess recent fluctuations in body burden. In autopsy samples, the critical organ, brain, is of interest, and other internal organs such as liver and kidney cortex may be considered. Methylmercury is not distributed uniformly throughout the brain, so that if a whole hemisphere cannot be sampled, it is of great importance to define precisely which part of the brain is sampled.

5.1.3. Minerals

Some minerals, when brought into contact with human tissues by inhalation, give rise to adverse effects on account of their chemical and/or physical properties. Present experience from occupationally-exposed individuals has drawn attention to several of such minerals — silica (alone or mixed), coal dust, iron ore dust, asbestos fibres and talc. Glass fibres which have similar physical characteristics may also have to be considered. Detailed information has been obtained for asbestos as an environmental pollutant because of its carcinogenic effect.

5.1.3.1. Asbestos

Exposure to asbestos has been associated with fibrosis of the lung, pleural plaques, lung cancer, mesothelioma, laryngeal cancer and probably gastrointestinal cancer. High concentrations of asbestos fibres occur in the air of industrial areas where asbestos is used in the manufacturing process or for insulation. However increased concentrations of asbestos fibres have also been demonstrated in the general environment : in the homes of asbestos workmen, in buildings fireproofed with asbestos, in the vicinity of asbestos plants, wherever asbestos spray operations are being carried out, and in some city centres. Drinking water and certain beverages have also been reported to contain increased concentrations of asbestos fibres in certain cases.

Since it is not known whether there is a threshold for the carcinogenic effect of asbestos fibres, there is considerable public concern about exposure to asbestos. The kinetics of alveolar retention of asbestos fibres in the human lung follow the same general mechanism for deposition and clearance as that of insoluble particulates, but will also be affected by the shape and size of the fibres. Some inhaled asbestos fibres may be swallowed as a result of the clearance mechanism. Because of the difficulties in performing quantitative analysis on a sufficient number of human tissue samples for asbestos, no quantitative relationship has been established between body burden and effects.

Critical organs or tissues are the lung, the mediastinal lymph nodes, the pleura and peritoneum ; these tissues should be sampled in autopsy cases. For living subjects, biological monitoring based on samples related to the clearance process (sputum, bronchial aspirate, gastric juice and faeces) may be used, although the relationship of the concentration in these media to pulmonary burden is not well established. Biopsy material from lung parenchyma, pleura, gastric mucosa or peritoneum may also be used, but on a more limited scale. The small samples obtained by this method present problems with regard to representiveness and analysis.

5.1.3.2. Other Minerals

Ther are many other types of solid particles in the lungs of urban residents : sheet silicates, fly-ash and carbon black with its associated organic pollutants. Some of these, together with glass fibres and the metal oxides mentioned earlier, may be of environmental concern. To date, however, no significant health problems have been associated with the lung burden of these particles.

5.2. ORGANIC COMPOUNDS

There are tens of thousands of organic compounds which may be of importance in environmental pollution studies ; in many cases the effects on human subjects of organic compounds currently on the market are unknown, and often the presence of some compounds may not even be suspected. This situation is aggravated by the fact that organic compounds can be metabolized readily in the body and thus the presence of parent compounds can be inferred only indirectly.

Residues of pesticides and their metabolites in various human tissues and body fluids have been reported by numerous investigators. Pesticides may gain entrance to the human body through the intestine subsequent to ingestion, through the lungs as a result of inhalation of airborne pesticide-laden dusts, vapours and aerosols, by penetration through the intact skin, and sometimes by absorption directly into the bloodstream through broken skin.

Once within the human body, the residue is submitted to numerous metabolic pathways and other processes. In the case of certain lipophilic organochlorine pesticides, residues of the parent compound or metabolites accumulate and are stored in the lipid portion of various tissues. Residues of these chemicals may also be detected in the lipid portion of such fluids as milk or serum. Some other pesticides are rapidly metabolized in the human body and excreted. Certain of the organophosphorus and carbamate pesticides undergo such dynamic metabolic changes. Other chemicals are capable of passing through the human body virtually unmetabolized (certain organochlorine and chlorophenoxy herbicides).

From a regulatory perspective, the detection of pesticide residues in human subjects representative of the general population or in certain groups considered 'at risk' (foeti, neonates, lactating women) provide a major element in pesticide policy decision-making. These residues are demonstrative of the extent of environmental distribution of the particular pesticide and are useful in the evaluation of any potential public health hazard.

5.2.1. Organo-halogenated compounds

5.2.1.1. Persistent organochlorine pesticides

The persistent organochlorine pesticides (OCP) such as hexachlorocyclohexane (HCH), hexachlorobenzene (HCB), dichlorodiphenyltrichloroctane (DDT), polychlorinated cyclodiene compounds (aldrin, dieldrin), have been the primary cause of concern for well over 15 years, mainly because of their resistance to biodegradation in the environment and their capacity for bioaccumulation in the biological chains. These organochlorine compounds are resistant to the effects of oxygen or acid, but less so to the effect of alkali and light. Some of them have a relatively high vapour pressure. Most of them are sparingly soluble in water and partition into the lipoid phases of biological structures. These properties lead to build up and storage of OCPs in plants and animals ; elimination by mammals occurs partly in an unchanged state in the faeces and milk, and partly by means of biochemical transformation processes, through the urine and milk.

Human beings store OCPs for relatively long periods in their fatty tissues and some animal experiments do not rule out DDT as a potential carcinogen. Dramatic restrictions and, in some instances, a total ban on the agricultural application of DDT have been introduced in many countries in recent years, with a corresponding fall in contamination levels in the environment. In many samples, however, a levelling off of the concentration is observed and, taking into consideration the slow rate of elimination of the main metabolite of DDT - DDE - from the human organism, its residues in human subjects are expected to remain for a long period. In addition, some countries still use sizable quantities of DDT in their public health programmes. Thus, further inputs of DDT into the environment should be expected at least for the next 5 to 10 years. Indeed, some data indicate that DDT residues in human milk in the rural areas of developing countries are one to two orders of magnitude greater than those in the industrialized countries, and it has been suggested that the house-spraying of DDT in anti-malarial campaigns is a relatively greater contributor to this accumulation than agricultural spraying. In one country, it has been observed that the interruption of indoor spraying of DDT, on account of vector resistance, was followed by a significant lowering of DDT levels in human milk. There are also indications that the levels of other OCPs in body fat and human milk may be highest in the developing countries. The health significance of this observation should be carefully evaluated, since animal experiments have demonstrated that OCP toxicity may increase under conditions of protein deficiency. It is not known whether these substances are chronically toxic to mammals, or what form any deleterious effects may take ; there is thus no basis at present for risk assessment and it might therefore be useful to store samples for future examination.

Some indications of the possible hazards accompanying exposure to organochlorine compounds over a number of years are provided by findings concerning the central nervous system and the liver ; practically all insecticidal organochlorine compounds are acutely neurotoxic. The build-up of organochlorine compounds in the central nervous system begins at a very early stage of its complex ontogeny. So far it has not been discovered whether this phenomenon can impair the normal development and functioning of the nervous system. One reason for this uncertainty is that at present many of the numerous functions of the central nervous system can be measured only very imprecisely, and in some cases not at all, since neither the psychometric methods nor the biophysical or biochemical techniques available at present are sufficiently specific. However, the important functions of the liver, unlike those of the central nervous system, can be measured with a sufficient degree of accuracy, and it is known that a number of the functions of this organ are affected by organo-halogen compounds.

Most of the chlorinated hydrocarbons mentioned above cause an increase in the activity of microsomal enzymes, both in the liver and in a number of other organs. These enzymes play an important role in the endogenous metabolism, e.g. regulating the metabolism of steroid hormones. Enzyme induction for instance, can cause imbalance in the sexual hormones, the mineralo- and glucocorticoid hormones, which cause permanent damage, such as fertility impairment. There are also important indications of shifts in the triglyceride and cholesterol levels, caused by the inductive effect of chlorinated hydrocarbons. Increased activity of the oxidizing, reducing, hydrolizing and conjugating enzymes of the liver and other organs, caused by chlorinated hydrocarbons, accelerate the metabolism of drugs and many other foreign substances, and can also cause shifts between toxifying and detoxifying reactions to foreign substances.

A number of the organo-halogen compounds, such as hexachlorobenzene, impair metabolism and heme synthesis, at least when present in large quantities. Some produce enlargement of the liver and possibly of a number of other organs, a condition which occurs through hyperplasia, hypertrophy, and polyploidy. This process seems to be only partly reversible, but so far it has not caused any recognizable functional impairment of the organ.

The most suitable indicator specimen for monitoring the levels of OCPs in humans is adipose tissue ; data are available showing remarkably uniform distribution of OCPs in the fat from different sites of the body. However blood has been also used extensively to assess exposure to, and the body burden of OCPs. Several studies have established varying, but generally high, degrees of correlation between blood and fat levels of OCPs and particularly of total DDT ; there are, however, some differences in the interpretation of the results.

Blood DDT levels seem to be indicative of only very recent exposure in contrast to DDE which reflects chronic exposure to DDT.   There is enough consistency in the DDE levels of individuals from the general population to consider blood as a tissue with a high potential for measuring long-term exposure to DDT.   Milk, due to its fat content, can also be used to monitor OCP contamination and is a good indicator specimen of exposure of young children, particularly in the rural areas of developing countries where children depend mainly on mothers' milk for their nourishment during the first six to eighteen months of their life.

5.2.1.2. Other polychlorinated hydrocarbons of low volatility

Polychlorinated byphenyls substances are widely used in electrical capacitors and transformers, in plasticizers for waxes, heat transfer liquids, hydraulic liquids for mining equipment, flame retardants, etc.   Voluntary restrictive action has been undertaken by some producers, and some countries have restricted or banned their production.   However, further pollution by PCBs and exposure of human subjects by the routes already established can be expected.

Much of what was stated earlier concerning the acute and medium-term effects of organochlorine pesticides applies also to PCBs.   At the present time, the long-term chronic effects on human subjects at typical environmental concentrations are not fully known. The considerations already set out regarding indicator specimens for chlorinated organic pesticides also apply here.

2,3,7,8-tetrachlorodibenzo-p-dioxin (TCDD) is a by-product in the manufacture of trichlorophenol, an intermediate in the production of both 2,4,5-T and hexachlorophene (an antibacterial agent often used in cosmetics and soap).   It is highly toxic causing severe impairment of the nervous system and the liver, porphyria and chloracne in humans.   It has also been shown to be teratogenic, mutagenic and carcinogenic in some animal species.   Most manufacturers of 2,4,5-T and hexachlorophene have now taken steps in order to reduce or eliminate TCDD in the final product.   2,3,7,8-tetrachlorodibenzofuran (TCDBF) occurs as a contaminant of PCB and has toxic properties similar to those of TCDD.   3,4,3'4', tetrachloroazobenzene (TCAB) occurs as a by-product during the manufacture of several herbicides derived from 3,4-dichloroaniline ; it can also be formed by the degradation of these herbicides in the soil.

Because of the potential for long-term environmental effects from these compounds, the storage of indicator specimens (adipose tissue) for later analysis may be useful.

Pentachlorophenol is widely used as a wood preservative.   Potential problems may arise from the relatively high concentrations of pentachlorophenol which may be present in wooden buildings (particularly farms) ; farm animals lick the wood, concentrate the pentachlorophenol in the flesh and milk which may be ingested by humans.   Pentachlorophenol itself has at present no known long-term deleterious effects on humans at typical environmental concentrations.   Urine is a good indicator specimen for this compound, however, pentachlorophenol in urine may also arise from exposure to other chlorinated chemicals (e.g. hexachlorobenzene).

Hexa-, hepta- and octochlorodibenzo-p-dioxins are formed in the manufacture of pentachlorophenol.   These have not been widely studied.   Possible indicator specimens to be investigated are adipose tissue, blood, skin and foetus.

5.2.1.3. Volatile halogenated hydrocarbons

A number of volatile halogenated hydrocarbons are used in industry and dry-cleaning as solvents and in agriculture as pesticides.   They are neurotoxic and some of them are hepatotoxic, but their effects, at environmental concentrations, are not well known. Monitoring programmes for these substances are very few at present.

Carbon tetrachloride, for years a commonly used household cleaner, is now known to produce extensive liver damage.   For this reason, many governments have placed restrictions on its sale except for recognized industrial processes.   Traces of carbon tetrachloride, trichlorethylene, chloroform and other halogenated hydrocarbon have been demonstrated in the water supplies of some cities of the United States.   Trichlorethylene, used as a degreaser in industry and in household products, has been reported to be carcinogenic in mice.

Biological monitoring for trichloroacetic acid and trichlorethanol in urine has been in progress for many years for occupationally exposed persons. The long-term chronic effects need to be studied and the storage of indicator specimens (adipose tissue and blood) for future reference may be of great assistance.

The extensive use of polyvinyl chloride (PVC) for food wraps, furniture, domestic water piping, etc. is of considerable concern in the light of the demonstrated effect of vinyl chloride monomer (VCM) in producing angiosarcoma of the liver. The use of vinyl chloride as a propellant in aerosol spray cans has been discontinued, but the long-term effects of traces of VCM trapped in PVC materials need careful study. Chloroprene used for the production of synthetic rubber exhibits mutagenic properties and has also caused lung and skin cancer in workers.

It may be relevant to consider whether direct monitoring of the intensity of exposure of the general population (by blood, urine or tissue analysis) is feasible. It has been demonstrated that vinylchoride metabolites can be detected in the urine of exposed animals but the limit of detection in such analyses and the possibility of extrapolating this information to man have not yet been ascertained.

Methylbromide, used as a soil disinfectant, has given rise to many cases of acute intoxication in man. Accumulation of bromide have been found in vegetables grown on treated soil. Compounds such as tris (2,3-dibromopropyl) phosphate are used as flame retardants in clothing. They can be absorbed through the skin. Tris (2,3-dibromopropyl) phosphate and impurities present in commercial preparations such as 1,2 dibromo-3-chloropropane, 1,2,3-tribromopropane and dibromopropanol have been reported to be mutagenic. The possibility of evaluating exposure to tris (2,3 dibromopropyl) phosphate by monitoring the presence of its metabolites (e.g. dibromopropanol) in urine should be evaluated.

At the present time there is incomplete knowledge about the chronic toxicity of fluorinated hydrocarbons. Dichlorodifluoro methane and trichlorofluoro methane may have considerable long-range environmental impact owing to their possible effects on the ozone layer in the stratosphere. Toxic effects on humans, animals or plants can only be determined by careful, long-term studies. Blood and expired air may be used as indicator specimens. Expired air may be used as an indicator specimen for all halogenated hydrocarbons.

5.2.2. Other organic compounds

5.2.2.1. Aliphatic and aromatic hydrocarbons

The general population is exposed to a range of saturated or unsaturated aliphatic and aromatic hydrocarbons such as benzene, toluene, xylene, cumene, ethylbenzene, styrene, butadiene and diphenyl, e.g. from the volatilization of petroleum spirit.

These volatile chemicals are probably rapidly eliminated, either unchanged with expired air or as polar metabolites in the urine (e.g. n-hexanol, phenol, hippuric acid, methylhippuric acid, mandelic acid, phenylglyoxylic acid, etc.). Since these volatile chemicals are not extensively stored in tissues, monitoring of the population (analysis of blood, urine or expired air) is probably the most practical approach when it is considered desirable to evaluate current exposure, as the storage of biological fluids or tissues for future analysis may raise important technical difficulties. Among these hydrocarbons benzene may be a pollutant that will raise some concern. Its concentration in petrol may reach several percent, and because of its volatility it may contaminate the general environment. Its long-term toxicity is well established (aplastic anaemia, leukaemia) and since the no-effect level is unknown, it is desirable to keep the degree of exposure of the general population as low as possible.

Recently benzene was found to be present in the expired air of men not occupationally exposed to aromatic hydrocarbons. It may thus be relevant to follow-up the intensity of exposure to benzene by measuring regularly its concentration in expired air or blood in representative target groups of the general population.

5.2.2.2. Polycyclic hydrocarbons

The general population is exposed to various polycyclic hydrocarbons, some of which are carcinogenic, either through the diet (e.g. consumption of smoked fish or meat) or through the inhalation of contaminated air (in urban and industrialized areas) and tobacco smoke. The atmospheric concentration of benzpyrene has been reported to be from 100 to 200 times higher in the vicinity of coke ovens and generally somewhat higher in urban areas than in rural areas. In man, the main sites of action of polycyclic hydrocarbons are the skin and the lungs ; in animals they can induce cancer at other sites. Although the fate of polycyclic hydrocarbons in the human organism has not been fully established, it is known that some of them can give rise to active intermediates (epoxy derivatives) which are probably responsible for their carcinogenic activity. Concomitant inhalation of solid aerosols may increase their persistence in the lungs.

Measurement of polycyclic hydrocarbon concentrations in the lungs might provide a useful method of evaluating intensity of exposure, however, no data are at present available. The 'activation' of polycyclic hydrocarbons by human leucocytes can be determined **in vitro**, and this method of monitoring should be investigated to determine its usefulness for detecting those at risk (higher activation rate) if exposed to polycyclic hydrocarbons.

5.2.2.3. Amino and nitro derivatives

These chemicals exhibit a large range of toxic manifestations (methaemoglobinaemia, allergic reactions, hepatotoxicity, uncoupling of oxidative phosphorylation, aplastic anaemia, carcinogenicity, etc.). Epidemiological surveys among workers in the rubber and dyestuff industries have demonstrated that several aromatic amines (benzidine, beta-naphtylamine, auramine, magenta) are carcinogenic (bladder cancer) for man. Alpha-naphtylamine is also present in coke-oven emissions and in cigarette smoke. Other aromatic amines have been shown to be carcinogenic in animals (e.g. 3,3 dichloro-4,4' diaminodiphenylmethane or methylene-bis-0-chloroanile (MOCA) used in the production of polyurethane resin). The general population may also be exposed to some amino and nitro derivatives (cigarette smoke, hair dyes, drugs, food additives). Some derivatives of p-phenylenediamine used as hair dyes have caused cancer in man and are mutagenic in microorganisms. Secondary amines may give rise to toxic derivatives **in vivo** (nitrosamines).

The main metabolic biotransformations undergone by various amino and nitro-derivatives **in vivo** have been studied, and in a number of cases the main urinary metabolites have been characterized (e.g. p—nitrophenol, p-aminophenol). Some aromatic amines can also be detected in the urine of exposed persons. However, insufficient data are available to determine whether blood and urine analysis could be useful for biological monitoring of the population. Although some of these chemicals probably accumulate in lipids, it is not known whether analysis of such fatty tissues would permit an evaluation of the body burden.

5.2.2.4. Alcohols

They are extensively used. Methanol has a relatively high acute toxicity but the toxicity of the longer chain (C8 to C18) aliphatic non-substituted alcohols is usually more moderate ; some halogenated derivatives appear to be mutagenic (e.g. ethylene chlorohydrine and chloropropanol) and may arise as residues in products sterilized with propylene oxide. Knowledge regarding the chronic toxicity of alcohols is still speculative. Exposure to the volatile alcohols can be monitored by analysis of expired air, blood or urine. Since these chemicals are quickly metabolized, they do not accumulate in the organism, so that it is impossible to evaluate a time-integrated cumulative exposure by tissue analysis. The long-chain alcohols may be more stable **in vivo**, but no data are available to suggest accumulation in tissues.

5.2.2.5. Glycols

The metabolism of some glycols in the organism has been established (e.g. ethyleneglycol gives rise to glycoaldehyde, glycolic acid, glyoxylic acid and oxalic acid). No data are available to suggest the usefulness of biological monitoring, nor is there any information regarding the possible accumulation of some glycols or their metabolites in vivo , and it is not known whether these chemicals represent an environmental or public health hazard.

It is known that acute over-exposure to short-chain glycols (e.g. methyl-cellosolve) can induce nervous system effects and renal damage (e.g. following ingestion of antifreeze agents), but these chemicals do not appear to possess a high degree of chronic toxicity. Longer chain glycols have low toxicity and some are used as food additives.

5.2.2.6. Ethers

Some ethers are highly reactive (e.g. induction of lung cancer by bischloromethylether). Their volatility makes their detection in tissues unlikely once exposure has ceased. Octochlordipropylether is present in some household pesticide preparations to increase pyrethrin activity. Some cyclic ethers (e.g. ethylene oxide) are suspected of being mutagenic and/or carcinogenic. Some ethers are easily analysed in expired air.

5.2.2.7. Ketones

Some ketones are extensively used as solvents (even in various household preparations). They are volatile and the general population may therefore be easily exposed to some of them. Following an outbreak of peripheral neuropathy reported recently among workers exposed to methyl-n-butylketone, the metabolism of various ketones has been investigated. The information is still too limited to suggest whether biological monitoring (urine or blood analysis) would be of practical value. Volatile ketones can easily be detected in expired air. No long-term accumulation of the most widely used ketones seems to occur in human tissues.

5.2.2.8. Aldehydes, acids and amides

Several of these chemicals are highly reactive (e.g. formaldehyde, acrolein) and act mainly locally, without entering the organism. Others can be absorbed by the oral route (e.g. oxalic acid, fluoroacetic acid, chloral). The metabolism and/or the mechanism of action of some of these compounds had been investigated (e.g. chloroacetaldehyde, oxalic acid, fluoroacetic acid, acrylamid, dimethylamides). This has led to the development of biological tests for controlling persons exposed to these chemicals (e.g. monomethylamide determination in blood or urine for evaluating exposure to the corresponding dimethylamide). At the present time there is no information on the extent of exposure of the general population to these chemicals or on the practicability of monitoring potential exposure.

5.2.2.9. Phenol and derivatives

Some phenols are extensively used and animal investigations have demonstrated that they can be formed in the organism from aromatic or cyclo-aliphatic precursors. They are excreted as free phenol or conjugated with sulfuric and glucuronic acids. The formation of mercapturic acids has also been observed ; they are excreted as such, or after hydrolysis to thiophenols, in urine and faeces. Urine and faeces may therefore be useful as indicator specimens.

5.2.2.10 Esters

It has been demonstrated that some esters of phthalic acid [e.g. bis (2-ethylhexyl) phthalate, diethylphthalate] present in PVC resins can be found in the tissues (liver) and blood of patients who have received a blood transfusion, owing to migration from the plastic pack to the stored blood. Since PVC containing phthalate ester plasticizers [mainly bis (2-ethylhexyl) phthalate] are extensively used in food packaging, the general population is certainly exposed to these phtalate esters. At high doses, bis (2-ethylhexyl) phthalate is hepatotoxic, and in animals it can induce testicular atrophy. Phthalate esters can also cross the placenta. Although animal investigations do not indicate a tendency for phthalate esters to accumulate in tissues, it may be relevant to monitor their presence in human tissues (e.g. liver).
The mechanism of toxicity of some organophosphorus esters and carbamates used as pesticides is well known (e.g. inhibition of the enzyme acetylcholinesterase). However, recent experience suggests that subclinical changes in the nervous system may occur in the absence of measurable enzyme inhibition. Enzymes other than acetylcholinesterase are also inhibited **in vivo** (e.g. plasma pseudocholinesterase, aliesterases).

It is possible to evaluate the intensity of exposure to these chemicals by determining blood enzyme RBC acetyl cholinesterase or plasma pseudocholinesterase activity, and in some circumstances by measuring the concentration of their main urinary metabolites. These pesticides are rapidly metabolized in the organism and do not therefore accumulate in tissues.

5.2.2.11 Asphyxiants

Methods are available to evaluate the intensity of exposure to the main chemical asphyxiants : carboxyhaemoglobin level and breath analysis for carbon monoxide, methaemoglobin-forming agents such as nitrites. Determination of thiocyanate in blood and/or in urine might also be useful for CN-liberating substances (cyanide, aliphatic nitriles). Since these chemicals are not cumulative toxicants, the time of blood or urine sampling is critical.

5.2.2.12 Other organic carcinogenic and/or mutagenic chemicals

Some of the carcinogenic and mutagenic chemicals have already been discussed in the previous paragraphs (e.g. polycyclic hydrocarbons). The highly carcinogenic nitrosamines can be found in some food products. For some compounds the ultimate carcinogens are formed in the organisms. It is believed that most mutagenic and carcinogenic chemicals act as alkylating agents (e.g. compounds with reactive halogens, epoxides, epochlorhydrin, dimethyl sulfate). The possibility of detecting them in urine and human tissues should be further investigated in order to identify the groups potentially at risk.

5.2.2.13 Toxins, hormones and antimicrobial agents

In some areas the monitoring of human tissues for the presence of naturally-occurring toxins (e.g. aflatoxins) may be indicated. Whether steroid hormones and antimicrobial agents consumed with food could be monitored by analysing human tissues is still unknown. Yet this area deserves much attention since it has been demonstrated that exposure to diethylstilboestrol during foetal life may have severe delayed effects (cancer) on the female descendants.

5.3. COMMENTS AND CONCLUSIONS

Based on the discussion in this chapter and on other available information, including the working papers, Table III has been prepared showing the major environmental pollutants (actual or potential) of concern from the public health viewpoint, and the various human tissues, organs and fluids that might be considered for collection, either for 'biological monitoring', or for 'collections for future reference'.

The following conventions have been used for the notations in the table :

÷   correlation with body burden or exposure and sufficient practical experience

?   possibly useful as an indicator specimen but further research is required to confirm

0   known as not useful

blank - no information available.

It is felt that for entries with ÷ , there is sufficient information available at the present time to suggest a valid method for monitoring, should programmes be initiated. The practical feasibility aspects are discussed in Chapter 6 and therefore no distinction has been made in Table III between indicator specimens mainly useful for biological monitoring and those suitable for 'collections for future reference', nor between those reflecting current exposure and body burden (see below). Before entries with ? are used, considerable further research work is necessary.

Tissues	As	Be	Cd	Cr	F	Pb	Hg	Mo	Mn	Ni	V	Zn	Se	Cu	Co	Pt/Pd	Sn	Methyl Hg	Other organo metallics (Pb, Sn)	Asbestos
Adipose tissue																				
Amniotic fluid																				
Aorta and major arteries						?														
Bile	?		?	?		?	?		?									?		
Blood	+	?	+	?	?	+	?	?	?	?	?	?	?	?	?	?	?	+		
Bone	0	?		0	+	+					?	?						?		
Bone marrow	?		?			?						?						?		
Brain	?					?	+		?	?		?						+	+	0
Cerebrospinal fluid																		?		0
Endocrine glands			?																	
Eye																				
Expired air	0	0	0	0	0	0	0	0	0	0	0	0	?	0	0	0	0	0		0
Faeces			+			+	?					?						?		?
Foetal tissue																		?		
Gall bladder																				

Pollutants Tissues	As	Be	Cd	Cr	F	Pb	Hg	Mo	Mn	Ni	V	Zn	Se	Cu	Co	Pt/Pd	Sn	Methyl Hg	Other organo metallics (Pb, Sn)	Asbestos
Gastric juice																				+
Hair and Nails	+		?	?	?	+	?	?	?	?	?	?	?	0			?	+		
Heart	?		?			?						?			?			?		
Intestine - G.I. tract																?	?	?		?
Kidney	?		+	?	?	+	+	?	?	?	?	?		?	?	?		?		
Liver	?		+	?	?	?	?	?	?	?	?	?	?	?	?	?	?	+		
Lung and adjacent tissues	?	?	?	?		?				?	?									?
Lung washings																				?
Lymph nodes																				?
Mammary glands																				
Milk			0			?						?						?		
Muscles			0									?						?		
Ovaries testis			?									?						?		
Pancreas	?		?			?						?						?		
Peripheral nerves	?																	?		

Tissues	As	Be	Cd	Cr	F	Pb	Hg	Mo	Mn	Ni	V	Zn	Se	Cu	Co	Pt/Pd	Sn	Methyl Hg	Other organo metallics (Pb, Sn)	Asbestos
Placenta			+		+	+	?					?						?		
Pleura and peritoneum																				?
Prostate			?									?								
Saliva							?													
Skin	?											?						?		
Sperm												?						?		
Spinal cord																		?		
Spleen	?		?			?						?						?		
Sputum	0																	0		?
Sweat						?	?													
Tears																				
Teeth	0	0	?		+	+												0		
Umbilical cord blood			?		+	+						?						+		
Urine	+	?	+	+	+	+	+	?	?	+	?	?	?	?	?			0		
Urinary bladder																				
Uterus & Vagina																				

Pollutants	Adipose tissue	Amniotic fluid	Aorta and major arteries	Bile	Blood	Bone	Bone marrow	Brain	Cerebrospinal fluid	Endocrine glands	Eye	Expired air	Faeces	Foetal tissue	Gall bladder
Silica															
DDT + organochlorine pesticides excluding phenoxyherbicides and pentachlorophenol	+			?	+	O		?				O	?	?	
Phenoxy herbicides					?	O						O			
Pentachlorophenol	?				?	O						O	?		
PCB - PBB - PCN	÷			?	?	O		?				O		?	
Tetrachloro-dioxin benzofurane and azobenzene	?			?	?	O		?				O		?	
Chlorinated solvents + plastic monomers	?			?	+	O		?				÷			
Fluorinated propellants	?			?	÷	O		?				÷	O		
Non substituted aliphatic + aromatic volatile hydrocarbons	?			?	+	O	?	?				+	O		
Polycyclic hydrocarbons	?			?	?	O						O			
Amino and nitro derivatives	?			?	?							O			
Nitroso derivatives					?										
Alcohols (including long chain)	?				+	O						÷			
Glycols				?	?	O									
Ethers					?	O						+			
Ketones				?	?	O						÷			
Aldehydes, Acids, Amides				?	?	O									
Phenol derivatives					?	O									
Organo phosphorus esters					+	O			?			O			
Phthalate esters	?				?	O									
Carbon monoxide	O	O	O	O	+	O	O	O	O	O	O	÷	O	O	O
Cyanide nitrile	O	O	O	?	?	O	O	O	O	O	O	O	O	O	O
Mycotoxins	?			?	?	O						O			
Antibiotics				?	?	?						O			
Hormonal substances	?			?	?							O			

Tissues	Silica	DDT - organochlorine pesticides excluding phenoxyherbicides and pentachlorophenol	phenoxy herbicides	Pentachlorophenol	PCB - PBB - PCN	Tetrachloro-dioxin benzofurane and azobenzene	Chlorinated solvents and plastic monomers	Fluorinated propellants	Non substituted aliphatic and aromatic volatile hydrocarbons	Polycyclic hydrocarbons	Amino and nitro derivatives	Nitroso derivatives	Alcohols (including long chain)	Glycols	Ethers	Ketones	Aldehydes, Acids, Amides	Phenol derivatives	Organo phosphorus esters	Phthalate esters	Carbon monoxide	Cyanide nitrile	Mycotoxin	Antibiotics	Hormonal substances
Gastric juice															0						0	0	0		
Hair and Nails									0	0	0		0	0	0	0					0	0			
Heart																					0	0			
Intestine - G.I. tract												?									0	0	?		
Kidney												?									0	0	?		
Liver		?	?	?	?	?	?	?	?	?		?						?		?	0	0	?	?	?
Lung and adjacent tissues	+						0			?											0	0			
Lung washings	?						0	0	0	?	0		0	0	0	0	0	0	0	0	0	0	0		0
Lymph nodes	?																				0	0			
Mammary glands																					0	0			
Milk		÷			+	?	?	?	?									?	?	?	0	0	?	÷	?
Muscles																					0	0		?	?
Ovaries testis																					0	0			?
Pancreas																					0	0			
Peripheral nerves							?		?												0	0			

Pollutants	Placenta	Pleura and peritoneum	Prostate	Saliva	Skin	Sperm	Spinal cord	Spleen	Sputum	Sweat	Tears	Teeth	Umbilical cord blood	Urine	Urinary bladder	Uterus and Vagina
Silica									+							
DDT and organochlorine pesticides excluding phenoxy herbicides and pentachlorophenol	?						?		0			0	+	?		
Phenoxy herbicides													?	+		
Pentachlorophenol													?	+		
PCB - PBB-- PCN	?				?		?		0		0	0	+			
Tetrachloro-dioxin benzofurane and azobenzene	?				?				0		0	0	?			
Chlorinated solvents and plastic monomers	?						?		0		0	0	?	+		
Fluorinated propellants									0		0	0	?			
Non substituted aliphatic and aromatic volatile hydrocarbons							?		0		0	0	?	+		
Polycyclic hydrocarbons	?								?			0	?	?		
Amino and nitro derivatives									0		0	0	?	?		
Nitroso derivatives														?		
Alcohols (including long chain)					0				0		0	0	?	+		
Glycols					0				0		0	0	?	?		
Ethers									0			0	?	?		
Ketones									0			0	?	?		
Aldehydes, Acids, Amides									0			0	?	?		
Phenol derivatives									0			0	?	?		
Organo phosphorus esters									0			0	?	+		
Phthalate esters	?								0			0	?	?		
Carbon monoxide	0	0	0	0	0	0	0	0	0	0	0	0	+	0	0	0
Cyanide nitrile	0	0	0	?	0	0	0	0	0	0	0	0	?	?	0	0
Mycotoxin									0			0	?	?		
Antibiotics				?					0			?	?	?		
Hormonal substances				?					0			?	?	?		?

34

The most important pollutants for which biological monitoring programmes could be implemented immediately lifted from Table III are listed here with the indicator specimens considered at the present time to be of greatest significance in a monitoring programme -

As	:	blood, urine, hair
Cd	:	blood, urine, faeces, kidney, liver, and sometimes placenta
Cr	:	urine
Pb	:	blood, urine, hair, faeces, kidney, liver, bone, and sometimes placenta and teeth
inorganic Hg	:	blood, urine, kidney, brain
methyl Hg	:	blood, brain, hair
organochlorine pesticides	:	adipose tissue, blood, milk
pentachlorophenol	:	urine
PCBs	:	adipose tissue, milk, blood
chlorinated solvents	:	blood, expired air, and sometimes urine
benzene	:	blood, expired air
CO	:	blood, expired air

The following additional comments regarding the above pollutants and their indicator specimens must be made. The presence of **arsenic** in blood or urine mainly reflects recent exposure, and since dietary arsenic may rapidly influence the arsenic concentration in blood and urine, the time of sampling should be standardized. The concentration of arsenic in hair integrates exposure during various periods of time, depending on the segments analysed.

The concentration of **cadmium** in the faeces reflects daily exposure. Its concentration in blood has probably two components : one in equilibrium with body burden, and the other influenced mainly by recent exposure. In the general population, the blood cadmium concentration does not appear to fluctuate very much, so that the time of sampling is not very critical. In the absence of excessive exposure (occupational circumstances), the concentration of cadmium in urine, kidney and liver, depends mainly on body burden.

The significance of the **lead** concentration in various indicator specimens seems well established. Its concentration in blood, urine, faeces and placenta is an indicator of recent exposure (in blood, urine and placenta, of exposure during the last weeks ; in faeces of daily exposure). In the absence of marked peak exposure (e.g. occupational conditions), the time of sampling does not appear to be critical. The lead concentration in teeth, hair, kidney, liver and bone reflects integrated exposures, but for varying length of time according to the tissue analysed (usually life-integrated exposure for kidney, liver and bone, and shorter exposure periods for hair and deciduous teeth).

The **inorganic mercury** level in blood and in urine is influenced by recent exposure. The time of sample collection does not appear to be very inportant. The body burden of **methylmercury** can be estimated by analysing blood, hair, kidney and/or brain.

The concentration of most **organochlorine pesticides** in the listed indicator specimens (adipose tissue, blood, milk) is usually an indicator of body burden. However, it has not yet been established whether the concentrations of PCBs in these tissues do actually reflect body burden or current exposure.

Chlorinated solvents and benzene are non-cumulative pollutants, quickly eliminated unchanged (expired air) or after metabolic transformation (urine). Their concentration in blood, expired air and urine correlates with the intensity of the last few hours exposure. The same applies to the **carbon monoxide** : carboxyhaemoglobin concentration in blood and/or CO level in expired air.

The following compounds are also considered as potentially inportant pollutants but the feasibility of, and interest in, biological monitoring of the general population should be further evaluated before initiating a large-scale monitoring programme :

- asbestos
- nickel
- phenoxy herbicides
- tetrachloro derivatives of dibenzo-p-dioxin, dibenzofurane and azobenzene
- plastic monomers, such as vinylchloride, styrene, acrylonitrile, chloroprene
- polycyclic hydrocarbons
- aromatic amino derivatives
- nitroso derivatives
- organophosphorus esters and carbamates
- mycotoxins
- antibiotics

Present knowledge concerning the stability of elements, minerals and some organo-halogenated compounds in biological tissues is consistent with the initiation of some pilot-scale 'collections for future reference', in order to establish base-line levels in the future.   A set of human tissues obtained at autopsy constitute the most appropriate indicator specimens for this purpose ; however, the applicability of available storage methods should be demonstrated before large programmes are implemented.   In some instances, tissues and fluids collected for biological monitoring may in addition be stored.

6. T E C H N I C A L   C O N S I D E R A T I O N S (FOR SPECIFIC CATEGORIES OF POLLUTANTS)

6.1. SPECIMEN COLLECTION, PREPARATION AND STORAGE

6.1.1. Feasibility of collection and storage of samples

Sampling in areas remote from laboratories requires special precautions.   **In vivo** samples that have been subjected to prolonged transportation under adverse conditions may be useless and collection should therefore be restricted to those samples that can be adequately preserved in the field.

Both **post mortem** and **in vivo** samples are valuable for both biological monitoring and biological specimen banking programmes.   Although legal restraints or local customs may complicate collection of **post mortem** samples, once authorized they are relatively easy to collect (with the exception of most body fluids).   Routine autopsies may not be representative of the general population, and careful statistical control and interpretation are required.   Good population representation can be achieved with **in vivo** samples, although these are, in general, limited to blood, urine, faeces, hair, nails and saliva.

Proper storage of samples for trace metal analysis is relatively easy, however storage for other analyses is much more difficult because of potential degradation, transformation, volatilization, etc.

6.1.2. Tissue excising and collection of body fluids

The purpose of the study will dictate to a large extent the size of the sample required and the precautions necessary to avoid contamination.

In establishing a 'collection for future reference' the specimen should be as large as possible consistent with the preservation technique to be employed.

With respect to contamination a primary consideration is what substances are to be determined ; for certain elements contamination risks are relatively less serious (e.g. cadmium), whereas in other cases (e.g. chromium and nickel) the ordinary procedures for sample collection may create considerable contamination problems. Precautions must also be taken to avoid contamination from the environment.

It is evident that the influence of contamination introduced by cutting will depend on the size of the tissue sample. For small samples, large errors may be introduced, whereas in some programmes using whole organs there appear to be no errors when ordinary stainless steel instruments are used. The recommended procedures for obtaining samples free from contamination include the use of quartz or borosilicate glass instruments, or those made of titanium, beryllium, beryllium oxide ceramic or carborundum. Titanium knives have beeen used and no contamination has resulted except for titanium. Such knives may be easier to use than the other types of instruments. Contamination by copper, manganese, chromium, nickel, iron, cobalt, silver, tin, antimony and tantalum has been demonstrated when using stainless steel instruments.

For **in vivo** blood collection, needles made from nickel or platinum can be used instead of the ordinary stainless steel instruments. The use of plastic catheter may also avoid contamination by metals. When sampling blood in venipuncture, a small initial portion should be discarded. Careful selection of an appropriate anticoagulant must be made if whole blood analysis is required.

External contamination is frequently a problem when working with hair and nails. However, this can be overcome by using special cleaning procedures and by making comparisons with the composition of hair taken from different parts of the body.

For organic compounds, instruments and other materials made of organic compounds, which come into contact with the samples, must be avoided (with the possible exception of plastic gloves in order to avoid contamination by skin oils) ; although when analysing for pthalates, plastic gloves should be used with caution.

For organochlorine pesticides, data are available showing the remarkably uniform distribution of these compounds in the adipose tissue from different sites of the body. Therefore an acceptable sample may be removed, in the case of surgical intervention, at almost any site of the body.

6.1.3. Additional supportive samples

Biological specimens from non-human organisms and other environmental samples (water, food, air) may often be useful, and in some instances particularly appropriate, for the evaluation of human exposure to certain pollutants. Careful consideration should be devoted to the collection of such samples, so that together with human biological samples they will provide the basis for the development of adequate models for the establishment of exposure/dose relationships.

6.1.4. Homogenization

Studies requiring data on the distribution of a substance within a tissue would, of course, involve the preservation of the intact tissue or whole organ. Homogenization of the tissue may be employed in instances where a substance is heterogeneously distributed or where replicate analyses are to be carried out by different investigators. However, great care must be exercised with the homogenization procedures to avoid contamination and to ensure that any portion taken is representative of the whole.

6.1.5. Containment of specimens

One of the greatest sources of error in analytical work is sample contamination, a source of which may be the specimen container. To reduce the possibility of contamination, the following characteristics should be observed :

- minimum interaction between specimen and container
- minimum interaction between specimen and external environment
- container capable of withstanding possible temperature changes.

The choice of container and cap material is dictated by the sample to be stored and the substance to be determined. In general, high pressure polyethylene, borosilicate glass, teflon and quartz should be considered. Such containers should be carefully cleaned by washing with acid and with doubly distilled deionised water prior to use. The cleaned container should be protected from environmental contamination (e.g. dust) before and during sample insertion. To reduce oxidation of the sample, the container may be filled with an inert gas. An empty sample container should be forwarded to the laboratory with the specimens for analysis of background contamination.

6.1.6. Storage methods

Possible approaches to long-term tissue preservation include :

6.1.6.1. Lyophilization (freeze drying)

Lyophilized tissue can be maintained with a high degree of integrity for long periods at room temperature. It may be necessary to store some samples in an inert atmosphere. The procedure can be recommended generally for inorganic but not organic analysis. Precautions must be taken to avoid contamination and losses.

6.1.6.2. Rapid freezing of tissue

To prevent losses of labile organic compounds and to preserve the potential for microscopic pathology without addition of chemical preservatives, rapid freezing of tissue samples at temperatures of $-40°$ C to $-70°$ C is required. Initial and maintenance costs may be factors to be considered. If good histological detail is to be preserved, only very small samples (milligramme amounts) can be used. There is also evidence that many organic contaminants are not stable indefinitely, even when stored at low temperatures, although experience with temperatures lower than $-40°$ C is very limited. For trace metal determinations (except mercury) hair and nails do not require freezing for storage.

6.1.6.3. Chemical preservation

Traditionally, formaldehyde has been used to stabilize and preserve human tissue chemically. This method has proved excellent for the purpose for which it was originally designed, i.e. for histological examination. At the present time however this method is not recommended for preservation prior to chemical analysis.

6.1.6.4. Radiation sterilization

It may be used for short-term storage, but should not be used for samples intended for 'collections for future reference'. In any case, it is applicable only for elemental analysis because of potential ionization damage to compounds, both organic and inorganic.

6.1.6.5. Ashing

This is a potential method for trace metal pollutants not subject to volatilization at the temperature used, but it is not applicable for organic chemicals and may present problems even for the analysis of certain elements.

6.1.6.6. Special considerations on storage of organochloringe pesticides

When sampling for organochlorine pesticides in adipose tissue, the samples are generally put in small non-plastic containers and analysed as soon as possible. They may be frozen and stored for short periods, up to one week. Data are scarce regarding the behaviour of the various organochlorine pesticide compounds under such storage conditions, but there is evidence to suggest that even under deep-freeze conditions (- 20° C), transformation of DDT into DDE takes place. The fate of these compounds in specimens for 'collections for future reference' is not known. The biological importance of the different metabolites of organochlorine pesticides and polychlorinated biphenyls is great enough to warrant the initiation of studies for better storage methods. The storage of blood samples for organochlorine pesticide analysis for future reference also needs study. Freeze-drying is another possibility but losses of volatile compounds such as hexachlorocyclohexane could be considerable, and volatilization of other compounds cannot be ruled out.

6.2.   ANALYTICAL ASPECTS

6.2.1.   Analytical procedures for elements

The precautions required for the analysis of elements start with sampling procedures, sample containment, and storage before analysis. All these steps, which have been discussed above, need to be followed if meaningful analytical results are to be obtained. Trace element analysis in itself can be effected by employing various instrumental methods and by using a wide range of instruments, all of which have their specific advantages and disadvantages. Many of the methods require sample pre-treatment, such as digestion and extraction procedures, which may create a risk of contamination or loss of elements if proper precautions are not taken.

Methods are currently available for the analysis of most of the elements of the periodic table in many biological tissues. These methods have been reviewed in the working papers for this workshop and only a few comments will be made. The choice of methods for the analysis of elements depends on a number of factors relating to the study in question. Some of these are : the number of elements to be determined in each sample, quantity of sample available, number of samples to be analysed, expected concentration range, precision and accuracy required, and economic limits.

For multi-element analyses in a single sample, spark source mass spectroscopy, neutron or photon-activation, emission spectroscopy, or X-ray fluorescence may be used. Some methods are non-destructive and allow subsequent analsyses on the same sample.

Other methods make it possible to determine minute quantities of trace elements in very small samples, and can be used to scan over a sample to facilitate the detection of concentration gradients in the sample (e.g. the electron probe microanalysis of subcellular particles in thin epon-embedded specimens). By analysis of several portions of the same sample, concentration gradients for many elements can be determined with sufficient precision and accuracy by some less expensive and more readily available techniques such as conventional and micro-colorimetric methods, and atomic absorption spectrophotometry.

6.2.2. Analytical procedures for organometallic compounds

Total metal analysis is often used as a screening method prior to the determination of organometallic compounds.   When it is decided that these determinations are warranted, special care must be exercised since these compounds may be incompletely extracted from the matrix and less stable organometallics may be destroyed.   At the present time, the most commonly performed analyses for organometallic compounds are those for methylmercury.   Interest in other organometallics is, however, increasing.

6.2.3. Analytical procedures for minerals

Because both physical and chemical information is necessary to identify minerals, there are no generally accepted routine methods for the accurate quantitative determination of minerals in biological or environmental samples.   Nevertheless, using a transmission electron microscope fitted with selected area diffraction and microanalysis capabilities, mineral contamination can be monitored in a reasonably quantitative way, even in cases of low pollutant concentration. When dealing with low concentrations, dust contamination must be avoided during the sample preparation stage ; ideally, a laboratory equipped with efficient air filters should be used.   The electron microscopy method has been extensively used for the biological monitoring of asbestos. Inter-laboratory comparisons and further research are needed especially for non-asbestos particles. Another problem in this field is the determination of organic compounds adsorbed on mineral particles.

6.2.4. Analytical procedures for organochlorine pesticides

The basic steps in the analysis of organochlorine pesticides in biological samples have been widely studied.   Progress in standardization and unification of methodologies, however, has been slow even for national programmes, and individual workers prefer their own modifications of similar procedures.   A possible direction for further development is the elaboration of procedures utilizing smaller fat samples, as has already been done for other human tissues.

The parameter of chromatographic mobility (retention time) is poor evidence for identification purposes.   This serious drawback of methodology based entirely on chromatographic techniques is well recognized and alternate methods and confirmatory tests are now obligatory ; a wide variety of interfering substances go through the whole procedure and can cause misinterpretations of the chromatogramme.

Combined gas liquid chromatograhy-mass spectrometry equipment has proved invaluable for the identification of pesticide residues and polychlorinated biphenyls.   This equipment is, however, very expensive and it will most appropriately be used in a reference laboratory for particular cases which fail to be resolved by other means.   A wide battery of techniques for identity confirmation are available including : microcoulometric detection systems, capillary columns for superior resolution, thin layer chromatography, synthesis (often done 'on column') of derivative compounds, and infra-red spectroscopy.

Often, very thorough clean-up is an absolute condition for the application of these techniques.

6.2.5. Analytical procedures for polyhalogenated biphenyls

The PCBs go through all steps of the analysis of organochlorine pesticides and interfere in the final identification by gas liquid chromatography with electron capture detectors.   It is now common practice to use various techniques to deal with this situation ; the most widely used is speration of the PCBs from the cleaned extract using column chromatography.   The PCB fraction is then injected into a gas chromatograph.   Because of the wide variability in PCB compositions, the interpretation of the chromatogramme and quantitation of individual PCBs is very difficult.

Various approaches have been employed, such as the use of the DDE response as a reference, perchlorination of the mixture to obtain a single peak, and using synthetic mixtures of PCBs.   There is no generally accepted method, but, when possible, quantitation by comparison of the peaks with those of a standard formulation most closely resembling the PCB pattern of the biological sample is widely used.   The above is also generally applicable to polybrominated biphenyls.

6.2.6. Other organics

The problems are so different for each group of chemicals that no generalizations can be made of analytical methodology.   However, in a number of cases the accuracy of the methods, particularly in the presence of biological materials, is not well established.   This is an area requiring further research.

6.2.7. Reporting of results

All information should be collected and all analytical results reported in a uniform and standardized manner.   Prepared forms for checking-off entries relating to the sample history and with minimum of writing are preferable.   The concentrations of pollutant residues should be expressed relative to both dry and wet sample weight, microgrammes per gramme organ weight (or for substances that deposit in fat, on a percent lipid basis), according to a standard format, together with information on the precision and accuracy of the analytical method used. All information necessary to define what is meant by 'wet' weight, and all factors needed to convert from wet weight to dry weight or to ash weight, should be included.

6.3.   STANDARDS AND QUALITY CONTROL

Assessment of environmental pollutants in biological media usually involves analytical procedures for very minute quantities and may often involve large analytical errors.   Because of the very low concentrations of pollutants to be analysed, laboratories should maintain strict control of the environment in which the analyses are performed.   This includes controlled ingress and egress of people in the laboratory and maintenance of scrupulous cleanliness to minimize contamination.

A thorough and reliable system of establishing and maintaining a high quality of analytical performance is essential.   In reporting data, the procedures used to ensure the quality of the results, along with estimates of accuracy and precision, should be included as far as possible ; preferably data for all the replicates should be included.   The procedures used to ensure quality control should be reported with the results.   The approaches which must be considered to ensure the quality of the analytical results are discussed below.

6.3.1. Intralaboratory controls

They involve scrupulous maintenance of cleanliness in the laboratory, purity of reagents and reliability of standard solutions, strict adherence to methods, and a systematic check on the performance of individual analysts.   Standard materials carefully prepared in the local laboratory , and similar in matrix and composition to the samples to be analysed, should be used at frequent intervals.

6.3.2. Interlaboratory checks

They must involve all participating laboratories in a programme.   These are best supervised by a central organization which takes overall responsibility for the analytical performance of the monitoring programme by :

-- determining the precision of the analytical methodology,
-- checking the precision and accuracy of analytical results of the individual laboratories,
-- keeping a constant watch over methodology and detecting deficiencies in the methods,
-- organizing interlaboratory comparison programmes to gauge and correct the performance of the laboratories,
-- distributing reference materials* such as those available from the International Atomic Energy Agency (IAEA), certified reference materials** from the U.S. Bureau of Standards (NBS), to evaluate accuracy ; it must be recognized, however, that in many instances certified reference materials have yet to be developed.

6.3.3. Use of independent analytical procedures

An additional means of establishing and confirming accuracy is the application of two (or more) independent methods to the same sample. When the same analytical result is obtained by two methods utilizing different instrumental principles, this gives a reasonable assurance of accuracy in the analysis.

Routine laboratories performing large series of analyses with one instrumental technique should send aliquots of some of their samples to a reference laboratory using several methods to assure the accuracy of their results.

6.3.4. Laboratory training

Even the best analytical method is inadequate in the hands of an untrained, unskilled, or disinterested operator. For this reason, participation in well-planned and carefully prepared training courses in the various analytical techniques and methods is essential before an operator moves into a laboratory position. Biological monitoring programmes and 'collection for future reference' programmes should give high priority to the provision of appropriate training. Training programmes should be complemented by periodic checks, examinations and seminars in order to maintain and update knowledge, methodology and analytical skills.

---

* Reference materials are materials which have been shown to be homogeneous ; composition data given are usually obtained from intercomparison programmes.

** Certified reference materials may be defined as those materials for which the composition data given are certified by a national or international standardizing body.

7. ORGANIZATIONAL ASPECTS OF "BIOLOGICAL MONITORING" AND "BIOLOGICAL SPECIMEN BANKING" PROGRAMMES

This chapter covers the various types of programmes that can be initiated, the concepts to be taken into account in designing a programme, the practical organisational aspects, the ethical and legal aspects to be considered, the advantages of collaborative programmes at international level, and an approach for cost estimates.

7.1. PROGRAMME DESIGN AND IMPLEMENTATION

The design of individual programmes will depend upon the type of programme under consideration, as well as the specimen types that will be collected.

For the pollutants and indicator specimens listed in Section 5.3 biological monitoring and pilot scale 'collection for future reference' programmes may be initiated immediately. For the other pollutants identified in the same section for which information is lacking on body distribution as well as biological effects, further research is necessary, but in some instances, pilot scale programmes may be considered.

7.1.1. Types of programmes

Both for biological monitoring programmes and for 'collections for future reference', the design and operation will depend significantly on the objectives and on the pollutants to be considered. In section 5.3., for the various pollutants a number of indicator specimens have been suggested with an indication of their significance with respect to exposure and body burdens. The objectives will determine the choice of the index specimens which will govern the sampling conditions.

7.1.1.1. Biological monitoring programmes
These programmes may be designed for at least three purposes :
- to assess general population exposure to one or several pollutants, thus obtaining base-line levels. These programmes will have to select the indicator specimen most representative for several pollutants, and reflecting, if possible, body burdens. Both **in vivo** and **post mortem** specimens may be considered. Sampling will usually cover a broad geographic area. The ratio of subjects selected with respect to the population may be small, but will have to follow strict statistical criteria ;
- to evaluate the situations where high exposures are indicated or suspected. These programmes will have to select the indicator specimen that is most representative of exposure to the pollutant of interest and is relatively accessible for sampling. Sampling will usually cover a confined geographic area, but the ratio of subjects selected with respect to the population will have to be higher than in programmes designed to obtain base-line levels. Stratification may not be necessary, but subjects should be selected essentially from the population group most suspected of being highly exposed. In the programme design, consideration must be given to the need for resampling in the same area, and for medical follow-up, if unusually high individual exposures are found ;

- to evaluate exposure in situations where toxic effects are present or suspected, for example following accidental exposures.   These programmes will have to select the indicator specimen most representative of exposure to that pollutant, with less consideration being given to its accessibility.   Sampling will usually cover a well-defined area and most of the individuals affected should be sampled.   In the design, special consideration will have to be given to the possible need for resampling the same individuals and for medical follow-up.

All three of the above-mentioned types of biological monitoring programmes will assist in the development and refinement of dose-response relationships.

7.1.1.2. Biological specimen banking

These programmes are usually aimed at determining pollutant levels retrospectively. They may be pollutant-oriented, in which case the indicator specimen to be selected should be most representative of the body burden, independent of difficulty of collection.   On the other hand, they may be oriented towards collecting tissues which are likely to contain the largest numbers of pollutants in order to discover possible future problem pollutants.   In any case, storage considerations as regards the index specimen are of prime importance. Geographical coverage will usually be very large and the number of stored samples limited.   The subject selection should be effected on very strict statistical criteria ; however, this is hampered by the fact that the indicator specimens selected will usually come from autopsy cases.

Programmes may be designed to cover both approaches, biological monitoring and collections for future reference, a fraction of the samples being analysed immediately, the reminder stored for future reference.

7.1.2. General guidelines for programme design

The Workshop stressed the need to consider the following general principles and guidelines in the design of all programmes dealing with the collection and analysis of human biological specimens :

-- studies should only be started when the overall purpose and objectives have been clearly identified, as these will determine the type of programme ;

-- expert statistical advice must be available from the outset to ensure that suitable statistical principles are incorporated in its design and that statistically valid methods are employed for the handling and interpretation of data ;

-- the donors and biological specimens selected should be representative of the target population and body burdens of interest ;

-- detailed pertinent information regarding the donor and environmental conditions should be collected and recorded for each sample ;

-- special attention should be given to specimen collection, as regards the use of trained staff, choice of container and transport conditions ;

-- storage conditions for the specimen will be determined by the pollutant being studied ;

-- suitable analytical methods should be chosen and careful attention paid to the availability of laboratory services ;

-- a protocol should exist for data analysis, evaluation and distribution and for further investigation or action if indicated.

If environmental monitoring and/or banking is in progress in a given location it may be desirable to integrate it with biological monitoring and/or 'collection for future reference' programmes in that same location. In a location where no effort has been made to monitor a pollutant of interest, biological monitoring should first be considered. If concentrations are low with respect to pre-established levels considered to constitute a health hazard, then environmental monitoring may be unnecessary. Conversely, in the cases of extensive high concentration levels of pollutants in the biological samples, it will be necessary to conduct environmental monitoring so as to establish the pollutant pathways in the ecosystem and the control measures which may be required.

A synoptic description of the various steps and requirements for the design and implementation of both biological monitoring and 'collection for future reference' programmes is given in Table IV.

7.1.3. Special Considerations

7.1.3.1. Statistical Requirements

One of the most important statistical problems is how many samples to collect to obtain useful results. The vast body of data on important pollutants (such as metals and halogenated hydrocarbons) shows that body burdens do not follow normal or Gaussian distributions and have in general a positive skew. This fact must be taken into account in the design of future sampling programmes and in the interpretation of the results.

When undertaking a programme for a specific pollutant or group of pollutants, the available data should be examined to estimate the ranges of expected levels and the variability for specific population groups. If this information is not available, then a sub-sampling of the population (50 to 100 samples if the population is homogeneous) should be carried out to give a first estimate of the pollutant distribution. The data on concentration ranges of pollutants, or the results from the sub-sampling should then be discussed with a statistician who should be given a definition of the programme aim, the parameters under consideration for the determination of the samples size, the population to be selected, and how the data will be treated. Account will also have to be taken of the analytical and contamination errors as well as the biological variability.

7.1.3.2. Selection of population groups and donors

Population groups and donors must be selected and sampled in a manner to represent accurately the study parameters stipulated in the study objectives. If stratification by age, socio-economic status, geography, health condition, degree of exposure or any other factors are sought, then appropriate statistical tests should be applied to determine the number of samples and levels of confidence for the varying groups, keeping in mind the considerations noted above regarding sample size.

The donors must be contacted in advance to encourage maximum cooperation and they have to be adequately informed as to the purpose of the study.

It is recognized that one of the most difficult aspects in collecting human biological specimens is the accessibility of the individual. The organisation of the sampling programmes should therefore be very carefully planned so as to maximize the information obtained. Further, it should be recognized that specimens contributed on a voluntary basis may introduce a bias since often, in a statistical sense, they may not accurately represent the target of interest.

7.1.3.3. Indicator specimen selection

The selection and manner of collection of specimens should take into account available information on the metabolic pathways of the pollutant(s) of interest ; such information is the most important determinant in the selection of appropriate samples as well as in the interpretation of results. Also, the distribution of a pollutant or its metabolite in a particular tissue or organ is an important parameter that must be considered in specimen selection and in the interpretation of results, because homogeneous distribution rarely occurs.

In planning the sampling programme, consideration should be given to the use of aliquots of biological specimens already being collected for other health related programmes.

TABLE IV
OUTLINE OF DESIGN AND IMPLEMENTATION REQUIREMENTS

Programmes stages	Requirements
Definition and planning of the programme, operation and management	- Full time staff - Consultants (in relevant disciplines) - Meetings and liaison with other programmes and collaboration at international level - Contacts with appropriate authorities
Sample selection	- Statistical advice - Consent for sampling
Sample collection	- Technical staff for sample collection - Administrative staff for questionnaire administration - Medical and/or scientific staff for supervision - Travel to sampling sites - Equipment for sample collection and quality control - Possibly special premises for sample collection
Sample transportation	- Special containers and rapid transportation prior to storage and analysis
Sample storage	-* Special premises and facilities -* Technical and administrative personnel necessary for the management of stored tissues -* In some instances, research facilities may be needed to evaluate and improve storage conditions

*) These items will be minor in the case of biological monitoring and predominant in the case of collections for future reference.

Sample analysis	- Analytical staff - Participation in quality control programme - Adequate analytical facilities - In some instances, research facilities may be needed to evaluate and improve analytical methods
Data treatment and analysis	- Technical and adminstrative assistance (to enter analytical results and information from questionnaires) - Statistical advice - Computing facilities
Data evaluation, distribution of information and follow-up activities	- Experienced staff including medical consultants where appropriate for data evaluation problems - Meetings for discussing results and for comparing with other programmes - Publication facilities - Feedback of results to sample donors and/or appropriate authorities - Meetings to discuss follow-up actions where necessary

7.1.3.4. Information on donor and indicator specimen

In any given programme all information should be collected and reported in a uniform and standardized manner. Prepared forms for checking-off entries with a minimum of writing are preferable. The design of the questionnaire must take into account the way the information will be handled later. All donors and specimens should be coded in relation to the programme to which they belong.

In general, information with respect to the following parameters should be systematically collected and recorded :

regarding the donor :

sex, age, ethnic origin, socio and economic level, health status, nutritional status, smoking habits, drinking habits, history of employment*, past and present residential environment*

*(include if possible the nature and concentration of the pollutants to which the donor has been exposed)

Other additional information on the donor may be required such as :

medication history, employment of the other family members, use of cosmetics and contraceptives.

regarding the biological specimen :

autopsy* or biopsy protocol (including equipment used), tissue collected, total tissue weight (wet), sample taken (if not the whole organ or tissue), sample preparation, method of storage, length of storage time, method of analysis, results of analyses.

*(including pathological diagnosis).

It should be stressed that in order to have comparable data from various programmes, and especially in the case of collaborative programmes, agreement must be reached as to how the above information will be obtained and reported. This is particularly true for defining and classifying health status, smoking habits, social and economic level, history of employment, past and present residential environment, and ethnic information.

It is essential that analytical results be reported in accordance with accepted standardized practice. (see section 6.2.7.)

7.1.3.5. Specimen transportation, storage and analysis

These items have been discussed in detail in chapter 6. The choice of laboratory services will be influenced by several factors including : the objectives and magnitude of the monitoring programme, complexity of methodology, availability of laboratory facilities and trained personnel, and cost considerations.

Analytical methodologies for trace residues of pollutants often require highly sophisticated and expensive equipment including automated procedures not readily available in smaller laboratories. In some programmes, it may be advantageous to establish regional laboratories, located adjacent to sampling areas. An additional regional approach may be instituted, whereby sampling and sample preparation will be carried out in field or satellite laboratories, then the samples shipped to a centralized laboratory for analysis and storage.

7.1.3.6. Data handling and storage

Factors to be considered in data storage and retrieval have to be based on user and specimen sample requirements, i.e. original data volume, data format, updating and amending of the data, data compressibility for storage, data processing and traceability and frequency of user access to data.

Where demographic data, as well as data on indicator specimens are entered into the data storage facility, the individual donor must be protected against indiscreminate use of the data. It is therefore essential to code data entered into a data bank. This code should be accessible only to health authorities to ensure confidentiality, and to provide for medical advice in the case of abnormal results.

7.1.3.7. Data presentation

Descriptive statistics should be calculated from the data to include reliable statistical measures of central tendency and of frequency of distribution. In cases where data are not normally distributed and cannot be made so by transformation, measures of central tendency and of dispersion should be calculated by appropriate non-parametric means. These descriptive statistics may include, but are not limited to, arithmetic mean, geometric mean, median, maximum and minimum, and dispersion (percentile, standard deviation, etc.). Some indication should be made as to the use and definition of 'trace' amounts.

7.1.3.8. Evaluation of results

The advice of statisticians is vital for the application of correct statistical techniques to ensure the best possible interpretation of the data. The results of statistical evaluations must be assessed in conjunction with biological implications. Extrapolation beyond the range of the original data should only be done with caution.

In a biological monitoring programme where repeated or follow-up sampling is undertaken on a population, it must be expected that a percentage of subjects will not report for a given sampling campaign. Thus careful records of the subjects reporting each time must be kept. Statistical evaluations and data interpretation must take this into consideration.

7.1.3.9. Further action necessitated by results

The results of monitoring are, in general, expected to show the general trends of human body burdens of environmental agents and to serve as a basis of long-term policy decisions for public health protection. In the cases where high values are found with respect to pre-established levels and following expert advice, further action may be required on either an individual or environmental basis. This may involve further sampling of the same or other donors, medical examinations, environmental monitoring and the determination of the sources of the pollutant with possible remedial action.

In the design of the programmes, the possibility for follow-up action, when required, should be built-in.

7.1.3.10. Management and operation

The management and operational plan for 'biological monitoring' and 'collection for future reference' programmes must include the development of practical guidelines and procedures for potential contributors and users as regards both input of and access to data and samples.

Field workers should be adequately trained and familiar with the programme before any monitoring activities are initiated. Where possible, a rehearsal should be conducted so that good and smooth coordination can be ensured among the collaborators.

As biological monitoring involves various organisations and expertise, negotiations and arrangements with the various parties are a prerequisite - in particular with local authorities and professional groups such as the medical associations - irrespective of their participation in the monitoring activities.

Feedback of results of monitoring to the participating donors and, where appropriate, to collaborative authorities is of prime importance to ensure further cooperation.

7.2.   COST ESTIMATES

The actual costs for planning and implementing programmes for the collection and analysis of human biological specimens will vary considerably according to the objectives and magnitude of the programmes, the country where they are carried out and the facilities available.

For 'biological monitoring' programmes, apart from initial capital expenditure, it is estimated that analytical costs will account for at least 50 % of the total operating budget, the remainder being allocated to scientific supervision, data handling and interpretation and shipment. Storage costs for biological monitoring programmes are negligible.

Personnel services generally constitute more than half of the total operating costs. In the U.S.A. personnel services (including overhead and indirect costs) range from about $30,000 to $50,000 per man-year. An example of the wide variability in cost is reflected in the estimates provided by the U.S. and Japan for the analysis of elements in tissues ; these ranged from $3 to $50 per element and per tissue depending on the type and number of analyses per tissue.

The costs of obtaining autopsy specimens will vary considerably as well. In the U.S. and WHO studies, institutions will often provide specimens at little or no charge in collaborative programmes. Generally the costs in the U.S.A. do not exceed $75 per autopsy set of twenty tissues per individual. For special programmes, like the Transuranic Autopsy Registry, a payment of $350 is made to the next of kin.

Shipment costs will vary depending upon the points of acquisition, storage, and analysis. As an example, a container holding sixteen autopsy sets and twenty-three Kg of dry ice for a total weight not exceeding 35 Kg costs approximately $30 to ship air-express, door to door, cross country in the U.S.A.

The above budget estimates refer only to 'biological monitoring' programmes and we have little information on the cost of 'collections for future reference' except for developmental aspects in the U.S.A. and the Federal Republic of Germany. In the U.S.A. a preliminary survey and evaluation study on specimen collections and sampling, storage and analysis techniques related to a National Environmental Specimen Bank (NESB) cost approximately $100,000. It is estimated that the development of detailed protocols for design, data storage, retrieval system, operation and management plan will cost an additional $300,000 to $400,000. It is anticipated that a major cost for 'collection for future reference' programmes in contrast to 'biological monitoring' programmes, will be for the storage of specimens.

It is thus clear that cost estimates in terms of money can be made only for a very specific programme, be it 'biological monitoring' or 'collection for future reference', in a given country. However, one can estimate the different steps necessary to implement any programme of this nature, and the type of requirements in terms of staff, technical equipment, space facilities, administrative assistance, etc. Table IV can be used as a framework for budget items to be considered in developing a programme.

International collaboration will undoubtedly be beneficial in providing a more cost effective and expeditious acquisition of high quality data for use in resolving problems of mutual interest. Increased cost-effectiveness will result, among other things, from :
- avoidance of duplication in resolving research problems of common interest ;
- centralized laboratory analytical services ;
- standardized reference material repository ;
- comparability of data for expediting decisions.

7.3.   ETHICAL AND LEGAL CONSIDERATIONS

There are differences among various countries and sometimes between states within the same country, with respect to the regulations, customs and restrictions that must be considered in planning and implementing programmes for the collection, storage, and analysis of human specimens. For example in some countries the regulations require a formal institutional committee review to ensure proper safeguards on the health of subjects, informed consent, and confidentiality of data. Each responsible investigator must be cognizant of and proceed according to the customs and legal restrictions applicable to his country and/or any collaborating nation. The investigator may find it desirable to seek legal advice before starting the programme.

Above all it should be recalled that the Nuremberg code of 1947 precludes any experiment on a human subject without his 'voluntary consent' and this principle has remained absolutely unchallenged. More recently the term 'informed consent' has become widely used. It is generally agreed that children, mental defectives, and the mentally deranged cannot give valid consent, although their parents or other legal guardians may, in certain circumstances, give consent on their behalf. Such consent for biological monitoring may be given, in particular, when there is a suspected exposure to environmental pollutants which may be detrimental to the health of the individual.

While the format of the 'informed consent' to be used may vary from country to country, with the circumstances and the types of indicator specimens to be collected, the following basic elements of information should be considered for inclusion in 'informed consent' forms :
- procedure to be followed for taking the biological specimen ;
- description of any attendant discomforts and risks which might reasonably be expected ;
- description of the purpose of the study and of the benefits reasonably to be expected for the individual and the community ;
- an assurance that the individual results will be kept confidential but that the individual (or/and his physician) will be informed, if he/she wishes, of the results with comments regarding their significance ;
- in the case of a study requiring repeated sampling, an instruction that the person is free to withdraw his consent and to discontinue participation at any time without prejudice to the subject.

'Informed consent' should be given as far as possible in writing.

In the case of collection of **post mortem** specimens, the concept of 'informed consent' should be replaced by 'permission of next-of-kin'. This 'permission' must be requested whenever appropriate and some information regarding the purpose of the study should be provided if requested.

Ethical and legal considerations generally will also differ depending on whether specimens are collected ante-mortem or post-mortem. Usually permission to acquire post-mortem specimens is more difficult to obtain than ante-mortem specimens because of legal reasons, as well as local customs or mores. The need for collaborating pathologists to perform autopsies in accordance with the laws of the country is emphasized. However, problems may arise in connection with the collection of material from cases of accidental death which in some countries are under the jurisdiction of the 'medical examiner' or a department or agency responsible for forensic cases. Often permission of next of kin is required.

In some countries there are no laws, or regulations regarding the confidentiality of information on results obtained on a group basis, although, autopsies often are not performed for religious and other reasons.

Even though ante-mortem specimens generally are provided on a voluntary basis they may nonetheless cause ethical issues and complex legal arrangements as part of the programme plan.

Whenever possible, when a biological specimen is to be obtained with invasive techniques, other non-invasive samples such as hair, nails and urine should be collected ; their collection is usually free of legal and ethical complications.

It is recognized that 'informed consent' may be more readily obtained if other analyses are offered to the individual as an incentive ; however, this approach should **only be used if the additional analyses can benefit the individual and be adequately followed up.** Any offer of additional analyses must be very carefully reviewed.

There appears to be little problem in the transportation of specimens, and although the issues are somewhat more complex when shipments are contemplated across frontiers, they can usually be resolved. Many types of ante-mortem and post-mortem specimens have been exchanged freely among many nations in cooperative studies.

7.4.   COLLABORATIVE PROGRAMMES

Since environmental pollutants occur quite independently of any geographical or political boundaries, collaborative programmes among states and nations are needed to characterize the environmental pathways and the distribution patterns of human exposures for many pollutants. Historically, coordinated national and international studies on human body burdens have been successfully carried out, since there was first concern about radioactive fallout almost 20 years ago. In more recent years there have been several international collaborative 'biological monitoring' programmes for other environmental chemicals.

Coordinated and collaborative programmes enable expertise and resources to be shared, and provide information on the demographic patterns of environmental pollutants with a degree of economy and effectiveness unobtainable by independent investigations. It is therefore concluded that efforts must be made to expand coordinated and collaborative programmes so as to enhance our knowledge on the environmental pathways of pollutants and their public health importance. However these programmes should be carefully planned and organized, and appropriate participating institutes selected.

The international coordination of laboratory analyses, distribution of 'reference samples' and the like, is also essential if results from different programmes are to be pooled together and thus provide a broader picture of the situation.

WORKING PAPERS

SUBMITTED FOR THE WORKSHOP

PESTICIDES AND OTHER PERSISTENT CHEMICALS: COLLECTION AND STORAGE OF BIOLOGICAL SPECIMENS FROM HUMAN POPULATIONS

Z. Bardodej

Department of Medical Chemistry, Medical Faculty of Hygiene, Prague

Summary

Chlorinated pesticides, polychlorinated biphenyls and mercury are very important contaminants of the living environment; the hazards of this contamination have been recognized on the basis of experiments on animals and of the medical investigation of workers exposed to these chemicals. The levels of persistent pesticides, PCBs, mercury and similar compounds in the environment have been determined as well as their residues in food and levels in human tissues, but more data are needed from different population groups for better evaluation of the hazard. Our knowledge on slowly developing changes in the body caused by chemicals is very limited; at present there is only unsatisfactory information on chemical carcinogenesis and mutagenesis in man. Studies on current exposure of human populations to man-made chemicals should be performed to a much greater extent, with standardized sampling, storage and analysis. Not only fat and blood but also other tissues may be valuable material for the evaluation of exposure, e.g. hair, nails and urine from living persons and liver, kidney and brain as post mortem samples. Specimens for future reference should be stored at -40° C.

The cost will not exceed U.S. $10.00 for one specimen sent across the border and U.S. $30.00 for an average analysis. In Czechoslovakia the level of some environmental contaminants is monitored and there are no principal obstacles for an investigation of human specimens provided the following provisions are respected: principles of medical ethics, and mail, anti-epidemic and customs regulations. The project must be approved by the Ministry of Health, which, no doubt, will adopt a positive attitude.

a.   Review of Past and Current Programmes

Biological monitoring of exposure to toxic substances was employed already before the second world war in industrial toxicology, where exposure tests serve for disclosing dangerous exposures to inorganic and organic compounds. To date about 50 limits (BTLV) have been recommended for noxious substances and metabolites in urine, about ten in blood and some in other biological material, e.g. in hair etc. Tests for pesticides are also now available, e.g. for cholinesterase activity and persistent pesticides in blood (WHO Reports 1975, Dale 1966, Jager 1970) as well as for nonpersistent and persistent pesticides in urine, insofar as these or their metabolites are excreted by urine (Davies et al 1976, Shafik and Bradway 1976, Linch 1974). Today nobody doubts the value of such investigations; often they are preferred to air analysis.

Exposure of the population to pesticides and other persistent compounds is much lower than of occupationally exposed persons and therefore damage to health would appear after a much longer time; determination of the dose-response relationship here is much more difficult. Nonetheless in this sphere, too, a great amount of data about the level of compounds in the environment and in biological material has accumulated in the course of years. Most attention has been focused on DDT and other chlorinated pesticides, chlorinated biphenyls and methylmercury. It is possible that health impairment will show itself only in the future thus adding importance to the data about now passing exposure. Apart from this some noxae are still unknown, for others suitable analytical methods are lacking, in other cases there is not enough information what to determine and where because data about biotransformation of foreign compounds are, particularly in low concentrations, incomplete. Data collection about present-day human exposure, as far as an analysis is possible, and storage of the material for future analysis and evaluation should be obligatory for workers in this field. It should be added that just as important as the time course of the level of body burden is also a possible development of changes which thus far cannot be evaluated for the simple reason that they are still unknown.

b.   Rationale for Interest or Concern

Persistent environmental pollutants include in particular chorinated pesticides, polyhalogenated aromatic hydrocarbons used for other purposes than against pests, various other organic compounds that are slowly degraded, e.g. TCDD, of phosphorous pesticides Trichloronat, and inorganic substances that have been employed as pesticides and which cannot be chemically destroyed, only diluted, e.g. mercury, etc.

Persistent chlorinated insecticides are chemically considerably stable compounds. Aldrin, Camphechlor or Toxaphene, Chlordane, DDT, Heptachlor, Lindane are chlorinated hydrocarbons, Dieldrin, Endrin, Isobenzan or Telodrin and Methoxychlor contain besides C, H and Cl in the molecule also 1-2 atoms of oxygen. They are solids under normal temperature, little soluble in water but well soluble in organic solvents and in fats and have a low vapour pressure (10^{-4} - 10^{-7} Torr). In the body they are fairly stable and are deposited in adipose tissues. The half-life of elimination from the body is long. Dechlorination, dehydrochlorination, oxidation, formation of alcohols, phenols, acids and conjugation occur during their biotransformation. Mercapturic acids may also be formed. The chief effect is neurotoxicity, possibly liver damage, and some have been suspected as carcinogens (DDT, Dieldrin, etc.).

Since the production and application of persistent pesticides are being reduced the environmental level is not expected to increase in the coming years. They get into the human organism to 90 % by food and only to a small extent by water and air. Their use in households may also be a source of contamination as well as occupational exposure during production and use.

Polychlorinated biphenyls (PCBs), polychlorinated terphenyls (PCTs) and bromobiphenyls are chemically related to chlorinated insecticides. PCBs are a numerous group of compounds differing in the number of chlorine atoms and their position. Of the possible 209 isomers several tens have been found in technical products; they are solid substances, their mixtures, however, are oily, viscous or sticky under normal temperature. The physical properties are influenced by the chlorine content. They are employed in the production of transformers and condensers, as hydraulic fluids, plasticizers, for heat tranfer, etc. They have a low vapour pressure, are hardly soluble in water but well soluble in fats and fat solvents, and are chemically stable. In the body they accumulate in adipose tissues. Biotransformation gives rise to chlorophenols and conjugates and perhaps also to mercapturic acids. PCBs are ubiquitous; they are carried into the organism chiefly by food, at occupational exposure also by other routes, especially by inhalation. PCBs produce chloracne, nervous symptoms and are also hepatotoxic. They induce formation of microsomal monooxygenases. Traces of chlorinated dibenzofuranes may be present as contaminants in PCBs and may be formed also by oxidation in the environment. Their toxicity approaches the toxicity of 2,3,7,8,-tetrachlorodibenzodioxine (DL_{50} in tens µg/kg).

2,3,7,8-Tetrachlorodibenzodioxine enters into the environment as the contaminant of pesticides e.g. 2,4,5-T and Trichloronat, and at accidents in industry, where it may be formed by condensation of two molecules of 2,4,6-trichlorophenolate. It produces chloracne, is hepatotoxic, carcinogenic and mutagenic. It is one of the most poisonous compounds and very stable. It is carried into the organism probably by food, at occupational exposure mainly by inhalation.

Organomercuric pesticides, used for seed dressing as fungicides, the production of chlorine and soda lye where Hg is used as cathode, and chemical plants where mercury compounds serve as catalysts have been important primary sources of environmental pollution with mercury. Alkyl, alkoxyalkyl and aryl-derivatives of which methylmercuric compounds are the most dangerous, are used in agriculture. They may be formed in the environment also from other mercury compounds by methylation. Methyl mercury gets most frequently into the organism by the consumption of fish, but there were also cases of community poisoning when grain, treated with methylmercuric pesticides, was misused for bread production, etc. Methylmercury poisoning develops very slowly; neurologic effects, blindness and often, after long suffering, death, have been observed. Methylmercury is eliminated slowly from the body; high levels have been found in hair.

There is an immense list of papers dealing with persistent pesticides, chlorinated biphenyls and metals as environmental contaminants. Many reviews and monographs have been published recently, e.g. by Brooks (1974), Edwards (1973), Friberg and Vostal (1972), Hutzinger et al (1974), IARC working group (1974), Jager (1970), Metcalf and McKelvey (1976), Ulmann (1973), an expert group (1971), from joint FAO/WHO meeting (1974), of a working group (1973) and of a workshop on epidemiological toxicology of pesticide exposure (1972). Investigation of chlorinated terphenyls and brominated biphenyls is in progress.

Some data on the toxicity of chlorinated pesticides, PCBs and mercury, of their half-life in man, daily intake, levels in diet and food, physical environment, human adipose tissues and blood, MACs in the air of workrooms and BTLVs in biological specimens from exposed workers are summarized in Tables I - VII.

c.   **Considerations for human sample selection, collection, containment, shipment and storage**

Various types of specimens are used for biological monitoring; material in which the compound is present in the highest concentration is preferred; the material must be accessible. In living persons blood, urine, possibly the hair and finger-nails, in dead persons also adipose tissues, liver, kidney, brain, etc. are analysed.

Specimens must be protected from contamination. For example, at mercury exposure contact of the specimen with mercury or its compounds used as antiseptics must be prevented. Substances leached out from plastic materials could interfere with the determination of some halogenated compounds.

For all types of specimens good quality glass containers (Pyrex) with a screw cap and an inlay made of a material which does not contain leachable or volatile substances can be recommended; these containers should be supplied to cooperating laboratories by a central source. Preservatives should be omitted. Specimens should be stored at a temperature of -40°C; for transport over a short distance dry ice, over a longer distance a refrigerator is required. Tissue specimens containing water may be freeze-dried.

d.   **Analytical Procedures**

For determining the compounds in question analytical methods have been developed which in a number of countries are standardized. One specimen should be analysed for more than one contaminant.

Chlorinated pesticides are determined by gas chromatography with ECD after extraction and cleaning up. Similar methods are used for the determination of chlorinated biphenyls.

Mercury is estimated by cold-vapour atomic absorption spectrophotometry, gas chromatography or neutron activation.

If analyses are not performed by a single laboratory then it is indispensable to use reference standards which are to be supplied by the leading institute. Prior to implementation of the program it appears necessary to check the work of the cooperating laboratories by means of reference samples. Just as important for the success of the program would be an interlaboratory check in the course of the work.

Methods for determination of pesticides, PCBs and mercury have been reviewed by Biros et al. (1971), in panel of hazardous trace substances (1972), by Fishbein (1970) and others. The best procedures have been accepted and recommended as standard methods by the Department of National Health and Welfare (1973), the Deutsche Forschungsgemeinschaft (1969), the Association of Official Analytical Chemists (1969), in Manual of analytical methods (1972), etc.

e.   **Program Design**

For a complex evaluation there should be available, if possible, besides analyses of the biological material also environmental levels of the compounds investigated, at least in the chief sources, from where they get into the body (food, water, air, etc.).

Donors of the biological material should live in different areas, be of different age, sex, social class and occupation. The groups should be sufficiently large to permit a statistical analysis.

The type of the sample for analysis depends on the type of the compound to be determined.

For the determination of chlorinated pesticides and biphenyls adipose tissues are suitable where the levels are, as a rule, by one or two orders higher than in the liver and by three orders higher than in blood. Some of these compounds may also be deposited in the hair, like mercury and arsenic. At present, urine is not being used for assessing exposure to persistent insecticides and halogenated biphenyls, with the exception of persons occupationally exposed to DDT. It is possible that hydrophilic conjugates of these compounds will be found in urine in the future.

The material to be examined and stored for future reference:
-    adipose tissues (halogenated pesticides and PCBs)
-    blood (halogenated pesticides, PCBs and methylmercury)
-    hair (methylmercury, halogenated compounds?)
-    finger-nails, liver, kidney, brain, urine (all substances?)

Identical forms should be used for the description of the donor containing the following data, which should be stored to a computer for processing:

Donor: Surname
           Name
           Number and labelling of the samples
           Date of birth
           Place of birth
           Sex
           Height and weight
           Education
           Domicile (in the last five years)
           Working place (in the last five years)
Exposure to chemicals: the extent, as far as is known
           Health status, illness, clinical diagnosis
           Autopsy diagnosis
           Remedies received
           Cosmetics used
           Chemical contraceptives used
Environment: Level of toxic compounds that are to be determined in the biological
           material, if possible   -   in the air
                                     -     in drinking water, in the donor's living place
                                     -     in foods in the area where he has been staying

f.   Organizational Aspects

Environmental pollution by persistent man-made compounds is being studied in most countries and the results are published.   The major part of these studies are performed by analytical methods based on the same principle and do not differ essentially from each other.   However, the levels determined are very low and might be affected in accuracy by various factors.   A recent investigation organized by the Health Protection Directorate, Commission of the European Communities in Luxembourg, provided evidence that the determination of common toxic substances, like lead and cadmium, is not devoid of complications; the present state was not found satisfactory (Lauwerys et al 1975).   In order to ensure reliability of results the specimens should be analysed by standardized methods and only by selected and controlled laboratories. Hence it is desirable that prior to initiating the program the laboratory personnel participating in the project should be first trained if it is found that preliminary results are not adequate as to precision, accuracy and reproducibility.   The use of identical reference standards of the compounds is absolutely necessary.

g.   Ethical and Legal Considerations

In this country and in most of the others with which the author is familiar there are no principal obstacles for an investigation of the living environment and for determining the extent of human contamination, provided the following provisions are respected:
-     principles of medical ethics
-     valid mail regulations, antiepidemic measures, required for transporting specimens of biological material and customs regulations for transportation across the border.   The whole project must be approved by the Ministry of Health which, no doubt, will adopt a positive attitude.

The above requirements apply for obtaining and transporting specimens from living persons as well as for post mortem specimens.

h.   Cost Estimates

The cost will vary if the material is only sampled and sent off, stored for a long time, or if it is analysed.   In Czechoslovakia medical performances are free of charge, thus an estimate is difficult; in such cases we shall have to take into account working hours required for the operation and its preparation; the cost for obtaining one specimen and its transportation would not exceed U.S. $10.00 (incl. chemicals, etc.).   The costs comprise: preparation 10%, collection and transport of specimens 20%, storage 5%, analysis of the specimen 60% and data processing 5%.   The estimate includes personnel, equipment and supervision.

TABLE I

Toxicity of Organochlorine Pesticides and some other Compounds* to Rats

Insecticide	Acute oral toxicity LD_{50} mg/kg
Aldrin	32 – 67
Camphechlor	40 – 150
Chlordane	457 – 590
DDT	113 – 250
Dieldrin	38 – 67
Endrin	30 – 220
Heptachlor	60 – 100
Hexachlorobenzene	10 000
Lindane	88 – 125
Methoxychlor	6 000
Telodrin	4,8 – 5,5
Chlorobiphenyls	1 300 – 11 300
2,3,7,8-Tetrachlorodibenzodioxine	0.010
Methylmercury	10

*   Compiled from Edwards (1973 a, p. 93), Panel on Hazardous Substances (1972) and Toxic Substances List (1974).

TABLE II

Half-life of Organochlorine Compounds and Methylmercury in Man*

Substance	Half-life
DDT	0.5 years
Dieldrin	0.73 years
Endrin	24 hours
Telodrin	2.77 years
Methylmercury	0.2 years

*   According to figures quoted by Metcalf and McKelvey (1976, p. 250), Jager (1970, pp 211-212), and Report from an expert group (1971, p. 107).

TABLE III

Organochlorine insecticides Found in Total Diet in the United States, 1965 - 1970*

Insecticide	Daily intake range mg
Aldrin	T – 0.002
Camphechlor	N.D. – 0.002
DDE	0.010 – 0.028
DDT	0.015 – 0.041
Dieldrin	0.004 – 0.007
Endrin	T – 0.001
Heptachlor	N.D. – T
Heptachlor epoxide	0.001 – 0.003
Hexachlorocyclohexane	0.001 – 0.003
Lindane	0.001 – 0.005
Methoxychlor	N.D. – 0.001
TDE	0.004 – 0.018

*   According to Edwards (1973 b, p. 341)
     N.D. : not detectable;   T : 0.0005

TABLE IV

PCBs in Food in the United States*

Food Article	PCBs average mg/kg
Fish	1.9
Cheese	0.2
Milk	2.3
Eggs	0.5
Composite diet	up to 0.4

*   As quoted by Hutzinger (1974, p. 217)

TABLE V

PCBs in the Physical Environment*

Sample	level	
Air	No data available	
particulate matter	50 μg/l	
rain	0.02 – 0.1 μg/l	
Freshwater	0.002 – 0.1 μg/l	Areas with little industrial activity
	0.02 – 2.1 μg/l	Industrialized areas
Seawater	0.005 – 0.020 μg/l	Coastal areas

*   As quoted by Hutzinger (1974, p. 216).

TABLE VI

Persistent Pesticides and PCBs in Human Adipose Tissues and in Blood
of General Population and of Occupationally Exposed in different Countries*
in μg/g

Compounds	General population		Occupationally exposed
	Adipose tissues	**Blood**	**Blood**
DDT total	2.2-26	0.013-0.06	0.11-1.36
DDT	0.3-16	0.005-0.025	0.21-0.57
Dieldrin	0.1-0.68	0.0005-0.003	0.25-0.07
Endrin	0.1		
Heptachlor epoxide	0.01-0.23	0.0008-0.0013	
Hexachlorocyclohexane	0.08-1.43	0.0004-0.010	
Lindane	T-1.7		
Telodrin			0.0067-0.01
Chlorobiphenyls	<1	0.005	0.036-1.9
Methylmercury		<0.01	0.180

*   Compiled from Edwards (1973b, pp.319, 320. 324 and 1973a p. 100), Karppanen and
       Kolho (1973), Report from an expert group (1971, pp. 220,221) and Friberg and Vostal
       (1971, pp. 220,221).
       T : traces

TABLE VII

MACs of Organochlorine Pesticides and Some Other Compounds in Workroom Air
and BTLVs in Biological Material of Exposed Workers

Substance	MAC USA	mg/m^3 USSR	BTLV*
Aldrin	0.25	0.01	
Camphechlor	0.5	0.2	
Chlordane	0.05	0.01	
DDT	1	0.1	0.5 µg/ml blood 3 mg DDA/l urine
Dieldrin	0.25	0.01	0.2 µg/ml blood
Endrin	0.1		0.05−0.1 µg/ml blood
Heptachlor	0.5	2	
Hexachlorobenzene		0.9	
Hexachlorocyclohexane			
(mixture of isomers)		0.1	
Lindane	0.5	0.05	
Methoxychlor	10		
Telodrin			0.15 µg/ml blood
Chlorobiphenyls		1.0	1 µg/ml blood (?)
(42 %chlorine)	1.0		
(54 %chlorine)	0.5		
Hexachloronaphtalene	0.2		
Tri-, tetra- and			
pentachloronaphtalenes		1.0	
Higher chlorinated naphtalenes		0.5	
Mercury	0.05	0.01	0.1 mg/l urine
Mercuric chloride		0.1	0.1 mg/l urine
Mercury - alkyl compounds	0.01		0.1 µg/ml blood 35 µg/g hair

* Compiled from Report of a WHO Study group (1975, p. 64), Report from an expert group (1971, pp. 339,344), Jager (1970, p. 209), Linch (1974, p. 128) and from TLVs adopted by ACGIH for 1975 and from Sanitarnyje normy projektirovanija promyšlennych predprijatij SN 245-71.

REFERENCES

BIROS, F.J. et al: Pesticides identification at the residue level. American Chemical Society, Washington, 1971.

BROOKS, G.T.: Chlorinated insecticides. Vol. I, II. CRC Press, Cleveland 1974.

DALE, W.E., CURLEY, A., CUETO, C.: Hexane extractable chlorinated insecticides in human blood. Life Sciences 5, 47 (1966).

DAVIES, J.E., SHAFIK, M.T., BARQUET, A., MORGADE, C., DANAUSKAS, J.K.: Worker re-entry Safety VII. A medical overview of re-entry periods and the use of urinary alkyl phosphates in human pesticide monitoring. Residue Rev. 62, 45−74 (1976).

DEPARTMENT OF NATIONAL HEALTH AND WELFARE, CANADA: Analytical Methods for pesticide residues in foods. 1973.

DEUTSCHE FORSCHUNGSGEMEINSCHAFT: Rückstandsanalytik von Pflanzenschutzmitteln. Mitteilung VI der Kommission für Pflanzenschutz-, Pflanzenbehandlungs- und Vorratsschutzmittel. Verlag Chemie GmbH, Weinheim 1969.

EDWARDS, G.A. (Ed.): Persistent pesticides in the environment. 2nd Ed. CRC Press, Cleveland 1973a.

EDWARDS, C.A. (Ed.): Environmental pollution by pesticides. Plenum Press London and New York 1973 b.

FISHBEIN, L.: Chromatographic and biological aspects of organomercurials. Chromatogr. Rev. 13, 83-162 (1970).

FRIBERG, L., VOSTAL, J. (Ed.): Mercury in the environment. CRC Press, Cleveland 1972.

HORWITZ, W. (Ed.): Official methods of analysis of the Association of Official Analytical Chemists. Association of Official Analytical Chemists, Washington 1975.

HUTZINGER, O., SAFE, S., ZITKO, V.: The chemistry of PCBs. CRC Press, Cleveland 1974.

IARC WORKING GROUP: Evaluation of carcinogenic risk of chemicals to man. Some organochlorine compounds. Vol. 5. Lyon 1974.

JAGER, R.W.: Aldrin, Dieldrin, Endrin, Telodrin. Elsevier Publishing Company, Amsterdam, London, New York 1970.

KARPPANEN, E., KOLHO, L.: The concentration of PCB in human blood and adipose tissues in three different research groups. PCB Conference II, National Swedish Environment Protection Board, Publications 4 E, 124-127 (1973).

LAUWERYS, R., BUCHET, J.P., ROELS, H., BERLIN, A., SMEETS, J.: Intercomparison Programme of lead, mercury and cadmium analysis in blood, urine and aqueous solutions. Clin. Chem. 21, 555-557 (1975).

LINCH, A.L.: Biological monitoring for industrial chemical exposure control. CRC Press, Cleveland 1974.

MANUAL OF ANALYTICAL METHODS. CB/PTSEL, NERC, EPA 1972.

METCALF, R.L., McKELVEY, J.J. Jr.: The future for insecticides. Needs and prospects. Y. Wiley and Sons, New York, London, Sydney, Toronto 1976.

PANEL ON HAZARDOUS TRACE SUBSTANCES. Environ. Research 5, 249-362 (1972).

REPORT FROM AN EXPERT GROUP: Methylmercury in fish. A toxicologic-epidemiologic evaluation of risks. Nordisk hygienisk tidskrift. Supplementum 4, Stockholm 1971.

REPORT OF A JOINT FAO-WHO MEETING: The use of mercury and alternative compounds as seed dressings. WHO, Geneva 1974.

REPORT OF A WHO SCIENTIFIC GROUP: Chemical and biochemical methodology for the assessment of hazards of pesticides for man. WHO, Geneva 1975.

REPORT OF A WHO STUDY GROUP: Early detection of health impairment in occupational exposure to health hazards. WHO, Geneva 1975.

SHAFIK, M.T., BRADWAY, D.E.: Worker re-entry safety. VIII. The determination of urinary metabolites — An index of human and animal exposure to nonpersistent pesticides. Residue Rev. 62, 59-77 (1976).

ULMANN. E. (Ed.): Lindan. Verlag. K. Schellinger, Freiburg im Br. 1973.

THE TOXIC SUBSTANCES LIST. U.S. Department of Health, Education and Welfare, Rockville 1974.

WORKSHOP ON EPIDEMIOLOGICAL TOXICOLOGY OF PESTICIDE EXPOSURE. Arch. environ. Health 25, 399 (1972).

SALIVA FOR BIOLOGICAL MONITORING

H. Ben-Aryeh and D. Gutman
Department of Oral and Maxillo-Facial Surgery, Laboratory of Oral Biology,
Rambam Medical Centre, Haifa, Israel

A. INTRODUCTION

Saliva is secreted by three pairs of major salivary glands: 25°/o by the parotids, 70°/o by the submaxillary and 4°/o by the sublinguals, the remaining 1°/o by the minor glands (1).

In a healthy population, the average rate of flow is 0.57 ml/min., the range: 0.1 - 1 ml/min. In the same individual, the rate of secretion is fairly reproducible, provided that the method of collection is standardized. During a 24 hour period 1000 to 1500 ml of saliva are secreted. A diurnal variation exists: during the day, the rate is 0.5 ml/min. and it decreases during the night to 0.05 ml/min. (2). The rate of secretion is lowered with age, in certain pathological states, after irradiation and as a side effect of several drugs. The rate of secretion increases during pregnancy, in diabetes or mercury poisoning (3).

Saliva consists of 99.5°/o water, organic components and inorganic salts. The salivary components measured in our laboratory are presented in Table I. This data was computed from a healthy random population (200) during a two-year period (Table I).

The composition of saliva is altered by stimulation (4). The contribution of individual glands varies and the rate of secretion of each chemical component changes. The concentration of sodium and chloride rises with increased secretion rate whereas the concentration of calcium magnesium, phosphate and protein is lowered. As a result, the stimulated saliva has a completely different composition from resting saliva. If a stimulated saliva is preferred, as in cases of lowered secretion, the mode of stimulation has to be standardized and appropriate controls used.

Salivary composition and rate of flow are of importance in oral health and may also be used as a diagnostic tool in systemic diseases (3).

B. THE USE OF SALIVA FOR BIOLOGICAL MONITORING

1. **Saliva as an indicator of systemic conditions**: Salivary composition reflects certain physiological and pathological systemic changes, salivary composition and rate of flow are regulated by the hormonal balance of the body. For example, sodium-potassium ratio reflects the rate of secretion of aldosterone and can be used in diagnosis of hypertension (5). In hyperthyroidism, the rate of salivary secretion is increased. In diabetes, the protein composition of saliva changes. Salivary phosphate concentration may be used as an indicator of ovulation (6).

2. **The effect of drugs on salivary glands**: Salivary glands serve as target organs not only for hormones but for certain drugs as well. For instance, digitalis inhibit the Na-K ATPase activity in the gland causing an increase in concentration of salivary electrolytes. Salivary calcium and potassium measurements are used for diagnosis of digitalis toxicity (7).

The rate of salivary secretion is also influenced; some drugs cause hypersalivation (see Table II) whereas others inhibit saliva secretion (8) (see Table III), or cause salivary gland enlargement (9) (Table IV).

3. **Monitoring of physiological components**: Direct measurement of various physiological compounds in saliva for monitoring was attempted. Saliva was suggested for follow-up of hemodialysis patients. Salivary urea and creatinine were found to be directly dependent on their concentration in blood (10).

Saliva was suggested as a medium for determination of human adrenocortical status (11).

4. **Monitoring of environmental pollutants**: Saliva was suggested for monitoring of certain organic and inorganic pollutants.

The inorganic components include Lead, Mercury, Silver, Copper, Zinc, Fluorine and Lithium. In some instances saliva proved preferable to blood or urine. Such is the case for the salivary lead determination by atomic absorption. The sodium interference is negligible owing to its lower concentration in saliva (12). However, there are divergent opinions on the use of saliva as a suitable medium for detection of lead poisoning (13).

Mercury was measured in saliva, blood and urine (14). An excellent correlation was found between blood and salivary levels.

The secretion of lithium was investigated in manic depressive patients. Lithium was found to be concentrated in saliva up to four times the plasma level. A good correlation with blood was found. No significant effect of salivary flow rate on concentration of lithium was detected (15).

Besides Lithium, Strontium and Iodine are also concentrated in the salivary glands.

Fluorine contents in mixed saliva of workers in a superphosphate plant was measured. A change in salivary fluorine concentration was apparent during a workday (16).

Estimation of Zinc concentration in parotid saliva in healthy individuals and in patients with idiopathic hypogeusia was performed (17).

Copper binding substances were found in saliva, gastric juices and in secretin (18).

The **organic components** measured in saliva include drugs, such as barbiturates, salicylic acid (19), antibiotics (20), amoxycillin (21), theophylline and morphine. For instance, the concentrations of theophylline in saliva and in blood were found to be in excellent linear relationship (22).

Heroin was analysed in saliva, blood and urine. Saliva was recommended for detection of high-dose abuse.

Tetrahydrocannabinol, the psychotoxic-principle of hashish was found to concentrate specifically in salivary glands, and can be monitored in saliva (24).

C.   METHODS

Collection of whole saliva for analysis can be performed by expectoration into a test-tube. Collection of saliva from the individual glands is done with the help of special devices, such as the parotid-cup or the Brock-Brotman Collector. Each method has its drawbacks.

An elegant method of saliva collection for monitoring of heroin was described. Saliva is collected by placing a Pen-Assay disc under the subject's tongue for 30 sec. The disc can be analysed directly by RIA. When dried, it can be easily stored for future analysis. This method could be adopted for other chemicals as well.

We use whole, unstimulated saliva. The method of saliva collection has to be standardized. The saliva should be collected at the same time of the day to eliminate diurnal variation. Duration of collection should be timed and the volume measured so that the rate of secretion can be estimated.

The collected saliva has to be centrifuged as soon as possible. The supernatant may be stored in tightly covered glass vials at 4°C for short term analysis or lyophilized for long term 'collection for future reference'.

D.   ANALYTICAL PROCEDURES

The analytical procedures are the same as for blood or urine: atomic-absorption spectrophotometry, flame-photometry, spectroscopy, gas chromatography or radio immunoassay. Some special adaptations for saliva were developed and could be further extended as the need arises.

E.   DISCUSSION

Saliva may be used for monitoring of all those substances that are secreted by the salivary glands. It provides a possible alternative method to repeated blood sampling. While monitoring by blood is invasive and requires medical personnel, collection of saliva is uninvasive and could be performed by the patient himself. Salivary monitoring is simpler than that of urine. Obtaining urine samples is often difficult. It involves observed urine collection, and handling and shipping of large volumes. The collection of saliva is simple, uninvasive and inexpensive.

In order to recommend saliva to biological monitoring, the existing data base has to be enlarged.

First, the normal salivary concentration of the specific chemical has to be determined in a healthy population. The intersubject and intrasubject variability has to be estimated. The relationship between the concentration of the chemical in the plasma and saliva has to be established. The mechanisms of excretion of each component should be investigated because individual chemicals are handled differently by the salivary glands.

To overcome the problem of variability in concentration with change of secretion rate there are two possibilities:

1. By internal control, using such chemicals whose concentration does not change with rate of flow, such as urea or creatinine.
2. By calculating the rate of secretion, defined as concentration multiplied by flow rate.

Extensive research is needed on the possibility of using 'saliva for biological monitoring'. This may be justified if we consider the advantages of this media: ease of collection, handling, storing and shipping.

SUMMARY

Saliva is recommended for biological monitoring of environmental pollutants, both organic and inorganic.

It can be collected by simple, uninvasive methods, easily stored and analysed.

However, before full recommendation of saliva for biological monitoring will be possible, extensive research is still required. Normal salivary concentrations of the specific chemicals have to be determined in a healthy population and the relationship between the concentration in plasma and saliva established.

TABLE I

Salivary Components

	Average	Range
Rate of flow	0.57	(0.1 - 1.0) ml/min.
pH	6.75	(5.6 - 7.6)
Electrolytes		
Potassium (K)	20	(14 - 38) mEq/L
Sodium (Na)	10	(2 - 15) mEq/L
Magnesium (Mg)	0.58	(0.2 - 1) mEq/L
Calcium (Ca)	5.8	(2 - 10) mg/100ml
Total Phosphate (p)	19	(8 - 30) mg/100ml
Protein		
Total	170	(100 - 400) mg/100ml
Albumin		(2 - 0.1) mg/100ml
Immunoglobulin (sIgA)	9	(2 - 18) mg/100ml

TABLE II

Chemicals that cause hypersalivation

Alkylphosphates (Parathion etc.)	Metaldehyde
Aminita muscaria	Muscarine
Ammonia	Neostigmine
Botulism	Nicotine
Bromine	Phenol
Cantharidin	Phosphorus
Castrix	Physostigmine
Coniine	Picrotoxin
Cresol	Pilocarpine
Curare	Quinine
Cytisine	Santonin
Daphne	Saponins
Emetine	Silver nitrate
Fluorides	Strychnine
HCL	Tabun
Iodism	Tetraethylpyrophosphate
Lead	Thallium
Manganese	Trichloroethylene
Mercury	Xylene

TABLE III

Chemicals that cause dryness of the mouth
Substances which inhibit the secretion of saliva

Aconite	Benadryl
Benzedrine	Hyosciamine
Antihistaminic agents	Lobeline
Atropine derivatives	Opiates
Barium	Scopolamine
Belladonna derivatives	Solanum
Chlorpromazine	Artane
Delphinine	Trifluperidol

TABLE IV

Chemicals that cause salivary gland enlargement

Oxyphenbutazone	Sulphisoxazole
Phenylbutazone	Vincristine
Pyrazolone derivatives	

REFERENCES

1. MASON D.K. and D.M. CHISHOLM. Salivary Glands in Health and Disease. W.B.Saunders Co. Ltd. ed. 1975, London.
2. GUTMAN D. and H. BEN-ARYEH; The influence of age on salivary content and rate of flow. Int. J. Oral Surg. 1974: 3:314-7.
3. MANDEL I.D. and S. WOTMAN. The Salivary Secretions in Health and Disease. A.H. Melcher and G.A. Zarb ed. Toronto, 1976 Munksgaard, Copenhagen, Oral Sciences Reviews 8: 25-47.
4. DAWES C. The Effects of Flow Rate and Duration of Stimulation on the Concentrations of Protein and the Main Electrolytes in Human Parotid Saliva. Archs. oral Biol. 14: 277-94, 1969.
5. LAULER D.P., R.B. HICKLER and G.W. THORN. The Salivary Sodium-Potassium Ratio. A Useful 'Screening' Test for Aldosteronism in Hypertensive Subjects. New. Engl. J. of Medicine 267(22): 1136-7, Nov. 29, 1962.
6. BEN-ARYEH H., S. FILMAR, D. GUTMAN et al. Salivary phosphate as an indicator of ovulation. Am. J. of Obstetrics and Gynecol. 125(6): 871-874, Jul. 15, 1976.
7. WOTMAN S., J.T. BIGGER, I.D. MANDEL et al. Salivary Electrolytes in the Detection of Digitalis Toxicity. New Engl. J. of Medicine 285(16): 871-6, Oct. 14, 1971.
8. MOESCHLIN Sven. Poisoning: Diagnosis and Treatment. Grune & Stratton ed. 1965, p. 665.
9. MEYLER L. and A. HERXHEIMER. Side effects of Drugs. Excerpta Medica Foundation, 1968.
10. DAHLBERG W.H., L.M. SREEBNY and B. KING. Studies of parotid saliva and blood in hemodialysis patients. J. Appl. Physiol. 1967, pp. 100-8.
11. SHANNON I.L. and J.R. PRIGMORE. Parotid fluid as a medium for the determination of human adrenocortical status. Oral Surg., Oral Med. and Oral Pathol. 13(7): 878-82, July 1960.

12. DI GREGORIO G.J., A.P. FERKO, R.G. SAMPLE, et al. Lead Determination in Human Parotid Saliva. J. Dent. Res. 52(5): 1152, Sept.-Oct., 1973.

13. FUNG H.-L., et al. Blood and salivary lead levels in children. Clin. Chim. Acta 61(3): 423, 1975.

14. JOSELOW M. and R. RUIZ. Absorption and excretion of mercury in man. Arch. Environ. Hlth. 17: 35, 1968.

15. LAZARUS J.H., G.S. FELL, J.W.K. ROBERTSON, et al. Secretion of lithium in human parotid saliva in manic depressive patients treated with lithium carbonate. Archs. oral Biol. 18: 329-35, 1973.

16. MEZGILBAEVA. A Fluorine content in mixed saliva of the workers of a superphosphate plant. Gos. Med. Inst. 43: 28-30, 1971.

17. HENKIN R.I., C.W. MUELLER and R.O. WOLF. Estimation of Zn concentration of parotid saliva by flameless atomic absorption spectrophotometry in normal subjects and in patients with idopathic hypogeusia. J. Lab. Clin. Med. 86(1): 175-80, 1975.

18. COLLAN J.L. Nature of complexes formed by Copper with alimentary secretions and their influence on Copper absorption in the rat. Clin.Sci.Mol.Med. 49(3): 237-45, 1975.

19. GRAHAM G. and M. ROWLAND. Application of salivary salicylate data to biopharmaceutical studies of salicylates. J. Pharm. Sci. 61: 1219, 1972.

20. SUKCHOTIRATANA M., A.H. LINTON and J.P. FLETCHER. Antibiotics and the Oral Streptococci. J. Appl. Bacteriol. 38(3): 277, 1975.

21. STEWART S.M. et al. Amoxycillin levels in sputum, serum and saliva. Thorax 29: 491-3, 1974.

22. SOYSOOKO R., E.F. ELLIS and G. LEVY. Relationship between theophylline concentration in plasma and saliva of man. Clin. Pharmacol. and Therap. 15(5): 454-60, 1973.

23. GORODETZKY Ch.W. and M.P. KULLBERG. Validity of screening methods for drugs of abuse in biological fluids. II. Heroin in plasma and saliva. Clin. Pharmacol. and Therap. 15(6): 579-87, 1974.

24. JUST W.W., G. WERNER, G. ERDMANN et al. Detection and identification of 8 and 9 Tetrahydrocannabinol in saliva of man and autoradiographic investigation of their distribution in the different organs of the monkey. Strahlentherapie, Sonderb. 78: 90-7, 1975.

TEETH FOR BIOLOGICAL MONITORING

H. Ben-Aryeh and D. Gutman
Department of Oral and Maxillo-Facial Surgery, Laboratory of Oral Biology,
Rambam Medical Centre, Haifa, Israel

A.   INTRODUCTION

The main components of teeth are enamel and dentine. Enamel contains 36% water and 0.6-0.7% organic matter: keratin and collagen. Dentine contains 10% water and 20% organic matter, mainly collagen. The inorganic material of teeth is similar to that of bone, except that it is denser and less soluble (1).

The chemical composition is:

	Ca	P	Mg	Co_3
Enamel: percent of ashweight	38	18	0.2	0
percent of material dried at 105°C	36	17	0.4	2.5
Dentine: percent of ashweight	38	18	0.9	3.3
percent of material dried at 105°C	37	13	---	----

The minor elements in teeth are (percent of material dried at 105°C):

	Enamel	Dentine
Cl	0.2 - 0.3	0.00 - 0.03
Fl	0.01 - 0.0034	0.024 - 0.076
Na	0.71 - 0.9	0.3
K	0.05 - 0.3	0.07 - 0.1
Fe	0.0008 - 0.04	0.007
Cu	0.00017 - 0.0009	—
Zn	0.021 - 0.026	0.021 - 0.026
Pb	—	0.005

In addition other elements such as Ag, Al, B, Ba, Cu, Ni, Si, Sr, Ti and V have been detected spectroscopically in teeth. They could be derived from fillings (2).

B.   TEETH FOR BIOLOGICAL MONITORING OF INORGANIC ELEMENTS

Many studies have been done on trace element concentrations in teeth, for example:
An extensive study was performed in the USA. The base line data for 21 trace elements in enamel was obtained: Cd and Zn were analysed by atomic absorption. Ag, Al, B, Ba, Be, Co, Cr, Cu, Fe, Mn, Mo, Ni, Pb, Si, Sn, Sr, Ti, V and Tr were analysed by optical emission spectroscopy (3).

A study on Zn, Pb, Cu and Cd in human teeth was reported from Japan (4); another study on trace elements in the enamel of teeth from New Zealand and the U.S.A. (5), and another from Norway (6).

Some studies on strontium in teeth were published (7, 8), so were others on silver (9), iodine (10) and mercury (11). Many studies on lead concentration in teeth as indicators of exposure to lead were made (12, 13, 14, 15).

C.   METHODS

The sources of teeth for monitoring could be deciduous teeth, extracted teeth or teeth taken out at autopsy.

Teeth have to be rinsed under running water, dried at room temperature, weighed and stored in polythene containers (14). The enamel has to be separated from the dentine (16).

D.   The analytical procedures are the same as for bone analysis: atomic absorption spectrophotometry, optical emission spectroscopy, X-ray emission spectrography or microprobe analysis.

Special methods were also developed, such as direct atomization from the solid state of Cd and Pb (17).

E.   DISCUSSION

Teeth may be used for biological monitoring of all those elements that are incorporated into the calcified tissues. Teeth are preferable to bone since:
1.   They are easy to obtain.
2.   Variations with age are small compared to those of bone.

The use of teeth for biological monitoring requires baseline data on the trace elements that may occur in enamel and dentine. The following parameters have to be taken into consideration:

Origin of the tooth, history of the patient, age and tooth type.
Methods of preparation and analysis have to be standardized.

SUMMARY

Teeth may be used for biological monitoring of all those elements that are incorporated into the calcified tissues. Teeth are preferable to bone as they are obtained by an uninvasive method and change less with age.

REFERENCES

1.   BLOOM W. and D.W. FAWCETT.   A textbook of Histology. W.B. Saunders Comp. ed. 1962.
2.   EASTO J.E. In: Biochemist Handbook. Long C. ed., London 1961, Spon, 721.
3.   LOSEE F.L., M.E. CURZON and M.E. LITTLE.   Trace Element Concentrations in Human Enamel. Archs. oral Biol. 19: 467-70, 1974.
4.   KANEKO Y. et al.   Zinc, Lead, Copper and Cadmium in Human teeth for different geographical areas in Japan. Bull. Tokyo, Den. Coll. 15(4): 233-43, 1974.
5.   CURZON M.E. et al.   Trace elements in the enamel of teeth from New Zealand and the U.S.A. New Z. Dent. J. 71 (324): 80-3, 1975.
6.   HONGSLO J.K.   Trace elements in teeth. Nor. Tannhaegeforen Tid. 85(8): 310, 1975.
7.   KUBOTA J. et al.   Determination of strontium in ground and whole teeth by X-ray emission spectrography. J. Dent. Res. 53(5): 1276-9, 1974.
8.   RYTOMAA I.   Str.-90 in deciduous teeth in Finland. Acta Odontol Scand. (Suppl.) 30(60): 1-29, 1972.
9.   MACINTYRE E.H. et al.   Identification of silver in a periapical lesion of a tooth. Am. J. Clin. Pathol. 60: 613, 1973.
10.   LIIV S.E. et al.   Determination of iodine level in the hard tissues of human teeth. Lab. Delo. 5: 295, 1973.
11.   KEVORKIAN J. et al. Mercury Content of Human Tissues. AJPH April, 1972.
12.   STEWART D.J.   Teeth as indicators of exposure of children to lead. Arch. Dis. Child. 49(11): 895-7, 1974.
13.   MALIK S.R. et al.   A study of Lead distribution in Human Teeth, using charged particle activation analysis. Caries Res. 8: 283-92, 1974.
14.   BURKITT A. et al.   Lead in teeth during the perinatal period. Postgrad. Med. J. 51 (601): 778-9, 1975.
15.   LOCHERETZ W.   Lead content of deciduous teeth of children in different environments. Arch. Environ. Health 30(12): 583, 1975.
16.   LOSEE F.L. et al.   Natural elements of the periodic table in human dental enamel. Caries Res. 8: 123, 1974.
17.   LANGMYHER F.J. et al.   A Ab. Spectrometric determination of cadmium and lead in dental material by atomization directly from the solid state. Anal. Chim. Acta 73(1): 81-85, 1974.

REVIEW OF SOME FACTORS RELEVANT TO THE ASSESSMENT OF EXPOSURE TO ASBESTOS DUSTS

J. Bignon* — P. Sebastien** — M. Bientz*

*Université de Paris - Val de Marne
Centre Hospitalier Intercommunal
40 Avenue de Verdun
94010 Créteil

**Laboratoire d'Etude
des Particules Inhalées
37 bd St Marcel
75013 Paris

SUMMARY

The different parameters (chemicals and physical) that are involved in the aetiology of asbestos related diseases are first reviewed. Indications are given on the possibilities of exposure and on the levels of air and water asbestos pollution. Taking into account the presence of fibres in the pulmonary and gastro-intestinal tracts, the cellular effects and the locus of pathogenicity are described.

The review of previous studies related to measurement of asbestos in human samples brought to light the failure in establishing body-burden/effects relationships because of the great differences in sampling programmes and analytical procedures. However, the previously reported findings could be a basis for the planning of a coordinated large-scale programme.

A general design of a biological monitoring programme is proposed for detection of people at risks. This programme is based upon the study of the relationships between pattern, indicator of retention during life and occurrence of diseases.

1. INTRODUCTION

The world production of asbestos in 1973 was about 5,200,000 tons. Chrysotile is the most common, accounting for approximately 95 per cent of the total. More than 3,000 applications of asbestos could be cited.

The first report on the adverse health effects of asbestos on man was drawn up by MURRAY in 1907. Only a few reports on pulmonary diseases due to asbestos dust appeared during the following two decades. After this, numerous investigations on the association of occupational exposure to asbestos and subsequent development of diseases were published. Since 1960, the presence of asbestos fibres in air, water and food grade materials has become a subject of health and environmental concern. In 1973, CEC and WHO decided to classify asbestos in the first category of pollutants whose effects are to be studied in priority.

The factors relevant to the assessment of public health risks of exposure to asbestos have been recently reviewed by ZIELHUIS in a CEC document. It is well documented that exposure to asbestos dust can lead to the development of lung fibrosis, bronchogenic carcinoma, pleural plaques, pleurisy, mesothelioma, gastro-intestinal tumours and perhaps other unexpected diseases. The most critical point today is the establishment of dose-response relationships. Adequate data to establish a threshold limit are not yet available. "The existence of a theoretical no-effect level may even be doubted; however, there may exist practical no-effect levels, below which any excess incidence cannot be adequately established" (ZIELHUIS, 1976).

As far as asbestos is concerned, because of the various possibilities of exposure, it is difficult to define retrospectively sharp conditions of exposure. So, the exposure-effects relationships are not very reliable and greater reliance should be put upon biological monitoring. Asbestos metrology in human samples could provide information about the most important questions arising for the assessment of dose-effects relationships and for the subsequent definition of prevention practices:

1.   What is the biological significance of physical and chemical properties of fibres (length, diameter, associated pollutants....) regarding the induction of diseases (particulary tumours)?

2.   Is there any relationship between one or several body-burden parameters at autopsy and the cause of death, sex, age and possibilities of exposure? The problem is that the latency period of asbestos induced diseases can be very long (30 to 40 years). As the accumulation of fibres in man occurs in a dynamic way (related to inhalation and clearance mechanisms), only the residue-burden can be investigated at autopsy. Research is needed to establish eventual relationships between autopsy residue-burden and burden at the time of disease onset.

3.   What is the most suitable external indicator of body-burden during life? Such a contamination indicator, if it exists and if available for monitoring, could be very helpful for the detection or the survey of exposed people. If relationships could be established with related diseases or with any biological test, this kind of survey should be specifically relevant to biological monitoring.

4.   Can the accumulation of fibres in humans be quantitatively evaluated from data on pollution levels and conditions of exposure? Some models for deposition of fibres in the human respiratory system have been proposed. The verification of such models by a comparative measurement study of conditions of exposure and body-burden could lead to define more appropriate standards or quality guides, giving them a biological significance.

This lack of precise knowledge in dose-effects relationships for asbestos may affect the general design of programs for the "biological monitoring" and the "collection of specimens for future reference". Perhaps it will be interesting in a first step to concentrate efforts upon the assessment of dose-effects relationships by means of measurement in human samples.

2.   RATIONALE FOR INTEREST OR CONCERN

Asbestos is a generic term for a variety of hydrated silicate minerals which have one common attribute, namely, the ability to be separated into relatively soft, silky fibres. They are derived from two large groups of rock-forming minerals, the serpentines and the amphiboles. Chrysotile is the only species of the serpentine group; the amphibole group   five major types of asbestiform minerals: amosite, crocidolite, anthophyllite, tremolite and actinolite.

As asbestos are naturally occurring minerals, their chemical and physical properties are dependent on their geological origin. Nevertheless, it seems interesting to provide data from analytic studies of the five UICC* standard reference samples of asbestos. These samples have been prepared for use in medical research. They are considered to be representative of most commercially available asbestos materials; many laboratories have used them for relating the different types of asbestos fibres to their biological effects.

2.1.   Chemical and physical properties

2.1.1. Crystal structure
The basis of the chrysotile structure is an infinite silica sheet $(Si_2O_5)n$. Attached to one side of this sheet is a brucite layer $Mg(OH)_2$ (SPEIL and LEINEWEBER, 1969). The mismatch in the dimensions of the silica and brucite sheets introduces a strain in the structure. The relief of this strain is accomplished by a curvature of the crystal lattice. By means of high resolution electron microscopy, YADA (YADA, 1971) has shown that ultimate chrysotile fibrils have a hollow cylindrical form. The outer and inner diameters of such fibrils are in the range 22 - 27 nm and 7 - 8 nm, respectively, dependent on the geographical origin of the sample.   Chrysotile fibres are in fact formed by the association of numerous such ultimate fibrils disposed concentrically in a direction parallel to the fibre axis.

The basic crystal from of the amphibole minerals is less complicated than that of serpentines. The basic structural unit is a double silica chain (Si_4O_{11}). The chains are paired "back-to-back" with a layer of hydrated cations to satisfy the negative charges of the silica chains. The various minerals in the amphibole group are characterized by the cations which occur in the structure: magnesium, iron, calcium and sodium. In practice, the idealized formulas are never achieved as the amphiboles structure allows great flexibility in ionic replacement.

2.1.2. Chemical composition
The compositional analysis of the UICC samples have been first published by TIMBRELL in 1970 (TIMBRELL, 1970 a) (see Table I). In all cases, analysis has shown that the chemical composition differs very little from the idealized one. The most common impurities in chrysotile are iron and aluminium. But the attention was especially drawn to the amount of trace metals in UICC samples:

Ni 0,1 °/o in chrysotile and anthophyllite
Cr 0,1 °/o in chrysotile A and anthophyllite
Mn 1,5 °/o in amosite

In view of these analysis results, the carcinogenetic effects of asbestos dust has been related to the presence of such trace metals. In fact, it was difficult to believe that such metals were completely incorporated into the crystal structure of asbestos minerals (GERMAIN, 1974). GERMAIN has studied the associated non-asbestos minerals of the UICC samples. Examination of Table I shows that these accessory minerals can contribute to the observed values of minor constituent concentrations. The composition of material separated magnetically from chrysotile was examined using radioactive tracer methods (MORGAN et al., 1973). Information regarding the place of trace metals in the chrysotile structure was obtained using comparative leaching

----

* Union Internationale contre le Cancer

procedure. The conclusion was that all metals considered can replace magnesium in the brucite layer of chrysotile; however, with the possible exception of scandium, they are also present in accessory minerals associated with the fibres. It seems to be a final conclusion; however, the question must remain under close scrutinizing to assess in a quantitative way what amount of trace metals are really related to the asbestos fibre structure.

The association of benzo(a)pyrene and other organic impurities with asbestos minerals has also been described (HARINGTON, 1965). The amount of benzo(a)pyrene in chrysotile seems to be very low compared to the amount in amphibole fibres (especially crycidolite: up to 24pg of benzo(a)pyrene for 100 g of crocidolite from North West Cape in South Africa). The amount of benzo(a)pyrene is greater for commercially available asbestos than for virgin samples collected in the field; this suggests that some of the benzo(a)pyrene is introduced during the processing or shipping of the fibre.

2.1.3. Fibres shape and size

Studies in recent years have indicated that physical factors are deeply involved in the aetiology of diseases associated with exposure to asbestos dust (STANTON, 1973; TIMBRELL, 1965).

As asbestos fibres can be easily separated and broken mechanically the size distributions are very dependent on the nature of the emission source and of the environmental conditions. For this reason, our concern will be restricted to general considerations on physical parameters of fibres sampled in different circumstances of pollution and of fibres in human samples.

The individual amphibole fibre is generally straight. The ultimate fibril of chrysotile can be straight or curly; short fibrils are often straight. Chrysotile fibres tend to consist of fluffy bundles of fibrils which are often curvilinear with splayed ends.

A fibre can be defined by measuring its true diameter and length. Measurement made with an aerosol spectrometer (TIMBRELL, 1965) showed that the falling speed of asbestos fibres was only dependent on the true diameter and that an approximate value for the aerodynamic diameter was obtained by multiplying the true diameter of the fibre by 3. However, as asbestos fibres can be curly (especially chrysotile), a complete mathematical description of their shape is difficult. For this reason, TIMBRELL (TIMBRELL, 1970b) has defined the coil dimensions: length and diameter of an imaginary cylinder enclosing the fibre. Both true and coil dimensions are important for the deposition, clearance and biological effects of asbestos fibres in humans.

In working environments, airborne fibres as long as $200\mu m$ can be found. Such fibres can penetrate deeply in the lung if their diameter is small enough; however, most of the fibres recovered in autopsic lungs are less than 5 μm in length and their diameter rarely exceeds 0,5 μm. In case of water and beverage pollution, fibres are generally shorter (2 μm mean length).

2.1.4. Surface characteristics

The surface characteristics of the asbestiform minerals are very important in relation to their interaction with whatever environment they may be exposed to. The external surface of chrysotile fibres consists of magnesium hydroxide. The pH of a suspension of chrysotile in distilled water is 10.3, comparable to a value of 10.37 for magnesium hydroxide suspension under the same conditions (PUNDSACK, 1955). This can be attributed to the removal of hydroxyl groups from the chrysotile surface. When suspending chrysotile in acidic solutions the dissociation of the surface is more pronounced because of the interaction of surface hydroxyl groups with hydrogen ions and the surface charge is strongly positive. Below pH 3, the magnesium ions are removed and the silica surface exposed.

Chemically, the surface of the amphiboles is similar to that of silica. It is polar in nature, but not as highly polar as chrysotile.

The surface area of chrysotile is generally high, dependent on the degree of fibre bundle openness (up to 50 m^2g^{-1} for fiberized material). It has been shown that leaching of magnesium from chrysotile results in an increase of the surface area (450 m^2g^{-1} for 95°/o leached chrysotile) (JOHAN et al., 1973). The surface area of amphibole asbestos is considerably lower than that of chrysotile (15 m^2g^{-1} for fully fiberized material).

The adsorption of various materials on the surface of chrysotile has been studied from both the liquid and vapor states: nitrogen, argon, carbon monoxide, acetylene, n-butane, trimethyl amine, ammonia, water vapor, ethanol, benzene, hexane, human serum albumin. The adsorption data show that the polar surface of chrysotile has a greater affinity for polar molecules than for nonpolar ones. Amphiboles do not exhibit such behavior and by contrast, dispersion by shaking or by ultrasonic treatment produces little change in uptake (MORGAN, 1974).

2.1.5. Chemical instability of asbestos

Asbestos has often been called the "indestructible mineral". In reality, this is far from the case and the solubility of chrysotile and amphiboles has been studied in various mixtures.

The most interesting features are the effects of acid or salt solutions, of water and of certain anionic wetting agents. Dissolution of fibres in vivo has also been assessed. Thus, recently the leaching of magnesium from chrysotile fibres in human lung has been demonstrated using electron microprobe analysis (JAURAND et al , 1976).

2.2. Human exposure to asbestos dusts

2.2.1. Emission sources and possibilities of exposure

The numerous uses of asbestos must be known by the physician concerned with biological monitoring. He must also be aware that asbestos material is in fact the association of microscopic fibrils (the weight of an ultimate fibril of chrysotile is of the order of 10^{-15}g), any operation on asbestos or asbestos containing products contributes to a mechanical desintegration of asbestos. Released fibres become readily airborne because of their low falling speed.

Generally, the different possibilities of exposure are classified according to the different occupations known as potentially at risk and according to the various para-occupational or environmental situations able to give rise to an asbestos pollution (ZIELHUIS, 1976; BECKLAKE, 1976):

- Direct occupational exposure, including asbestos mining, milling, handling, spraying, products manufacturing.
- Indirect occupational exposure, including bystanders (workers in the vicinity of asbestos contaminated work situations) and workers who use the newly manufactured products if they are sawn, disrupted or cut in any way.
- Para-occupational domestic exposure to members of a household.
- Neighbourhood exposure: vicinity of asbestos mines, factories, etc.
- Natural exposure in countries with asbestos related geology.
- True environmental exposure through ambient air, food, water, beverages etc.

The definition of this category is not very clear and probably a subject will be called "true environmentally exposed" if, after careful inquiries, none of the previously listed possibilities of exposure can be discovered. In fact, unexpected exposure can occur and the search for exposure in the background of patients with mesothelioma has brought to light various forms of such unexpected exposures. As an example, it has been recently found that the presence of an insulating asbestos layer in buildings can lead to the establishment of a serious indoor air pollution by asbestos (SAWYER, 1974; NICHOLSON et al , 1975; SEBASTIEN et al , 1976 a).

The aforecited kinds of potential exposure to asbestos could theoretically provide accurate information on the amount of fibres inhaled per year by a group of exposed people, and, when knowing the duration of the exposition, it could be possible to work out the body-burden.

In fact, different points prevent such indirect evaluation:

a)   The distinction between the various conditions of exposure is more qualitative than quantitative, not taking into account the exposure levels in the ambient environment; so far, there are few quantitative data available on the occurrence of asbestos in the environment.

b)   Another point is the difficulty to define groups of people with the same quantitative body-burden of asbestos. Indeed, even if people are exposed to the same risk, accumulation of asbestos in the human body is related to numerous individual factors (penetration, clearance, healthy or diseased people, personal susceptibility). For the general population, these parameters although poorly known must have a wide range of variations from case to case.

Elsewhere there is so far no direct information on the number of people actually exposed in each category. These reasons enhance the need for biological monitoring in order to assess the integrated past-exposure for humans.

2.2.2. Levels of environmental pollution
2.2.2.1.Asbestos air pollution

The release of asbestos fibres to the atmosphere occurs mainly during industrial processes. It will be interesting to distinguish the level of emission at the source (directly related to the occupations at risk) between the impact of such sources on the general environment (more related to the true public health hazard).

The different factors relevant to the occupational exposure to airborne asbestos have been recently reviewed (ACGIH-AIHA, 1975). Many techniques have been used for assessing airborne asbestos in the workroom air. Concerning sampling, almost every type of instrument has been used: konimeter, impinger, thermal precipitators, membrane filters, open filters, electrostatic precipitators, respirable dust sampler and light scatter instruments. The analytical procedures reported are: optical microscopy (fibre counting), optical microscopy using phase contrast illumination (fibre counting), electron microscopy, optical sizing of airborne particles, ash determination, magnesium determination, infrared spectroscopy, X-ray diffraction, trace constituents determination, orientation in a magnetic field. These procedures can express levels of pollution in different ways: numerical concentration of fibres (dependent on the analytical instrumentation used, light or electron microscope), weight concentration of asbestos dust, weight concentration of total dust and proportion of asbestos.

These studies have shown that:

-    many fibres are smaller than the resolution limit of light microscopy,
-    long chrysotile fibres are frequently curly, the others are mainly straight,
-    amphibole fibres frequently occur as single fibres,
-    the diameters of individual fibres in the air seldom exceed 5 μm,
-    the fibres lengths range from 0,2 μm to 1000 μm,
-    large clumps of fibres have been observed frequently,
-    the pollution level is very dependent on the nature of the operation on asbestos materials and on the existence or not of a protection system(air ventilation, hoods, etc....)

(HARWOOD, 1971). As an example, more than 100 optically visible fibres per cc of air have been found during asbestos spray processing (REITZE et al, 1972).

The standard regulations in force in different countries have been reviewed by ZIELHUIS in his CEC document. The most common regulation is 2 or 5 fibres/cc of air determined by the membrane filter method and the fibre count under the light microscope. Such standards have been proposed only in recent years (1960). In the past, workers were probably exposed to greater concentrations because the prevention against dust exposure was less thorough than it is now. The asbestos industry discussed the feasibility of using such regulations or projected lower ones (Federal register, 1975).

The impact of asbestos use on the atmospheric pollution of the general environment could occur in two general ways. First, it is obvious that fibres can escape from places where great quantities of asbestos are processed (asbestos factories, shipyards, etc......). Even in cases of controlled sources (ventilation system and dust removal) the numerical concentration of escaped fibres can be high because of the difficulty in controlling fine dust emissions (HARWOOD et al , 1975). This type of sources ensures a continuous emission in time. They are generally localized in space and the possibility of exposure can be discovered by means of residential inquiries. However, the presence of small factories is often ignored by the public and can be incidentally discovered during a large-scale program on air pollution monitoring (SEBASTIEN and BIGNON, 1976b). The second way of contamination is related to the extensive use of asbestos containing products: asbestos spray processing (SELIKOFF et al , 1972; SKIDMORE and JONES, 1975), use of insulating and other asbestos containing compounds (ROHL et al, 1975) weathering of insulating asbestos layers in buildings (LUMLEY et al , 1971; SEBASTIEN et al., 1976a), asbestos cement products installation, floor tile installation (MURPHY et al , 1971) brake maintenance (ROHL et al , 1976), brake lining decomposition (ALSTE et al , 1976), use of asbestos contaminated talc powders (ROHL and LANGER, 1974) and occasional use of specific asbestos containing products (ZIELHUIS et al , 1975).

The level of air pollution has been monitored in many circumstances (see Table II). The results have been expressed in two ways: numerical concentration of optically visible fibres as defined by the industrial hygiene method, and gravimetric concentration as provided by means of the quantitative morphometric study with the transmission electron microscope (SEBASTIEN and BIGNON, 1976c). Only a few attempts have been made to relate the results provided by both methods (ROHL et al , 1976). The experience of this laboratory shows that, because of the small size of fibres encountered in air pollution, the light microscope is useless for air pollution monitoring in non-industrial circumstances. The conclusions of the CEC working group on metrology for asbestos are in agreement with it (WORKING GROUP ON ASBESTOS METROLOGY, 1976). Table II shows a background of asbestos air pollution and higher levels in local circumstances. The fact that pollution levels were found in the same range inside buildings insulated with asbestos and in the vicinity of asbestos plants where mesothelioma cases were reported, should be a subject of health concern.

2.2.2.2. Water and beverages contamination

The presence of asbestos in beverages is to be related to their filtration through asbestos containing filters (PONTEFRACT and CUNNINGHAM, 1973; SEBASTIEN et al , 1976d). In cases of filtered beverages, the concentrations are in the range 10^6-10^7 TEM size fibres per liter.

In case of water, natural contamination can occur depending on the local geology. The use of cement pipes for drinking-water supplies has also been described as a source of water pollution (CASTELMAN and BLUM, 1975) but the deposits from hard or soft water on pipe surface can protect emission (WEBSTER, 1974). Examination of Table III shows that the most important concentrations have been found in case of surface water contamination occurring during industrial processes (NICHOLSON, 1974; SEBASTIEN et al , 1976e).

2.3. Cellular effects and locus of pathogenicity in humans

Asbestos fibres are able to induce two kinds of diseases in humans: fibrosis, mostly of lung and pleura, and tumour of various organs.

From human and experimental data, different cell types appear as susceptible targets to asbestos fibres: interstitial cells, such as fibroblasts, in relation to fibrosis and various epithelial cells and perhaps more specifically mesothelial cells susceptible to transformation and carcinogenesis. Asbestos fibres before inducing an adverse effect at the level of these target cells have an initial biological effect on macrophages. This interaction of fibres with the macrophage metabolism has been studied, either in vitro or in vivo. In vitro, asbestos fibres are responsible for hemolysis (HARINGTON et al , 1971) and for the release of cytoplasmic enzymes (LDH) from macrophages (PARAZZI et al , 1968; BECK et al , 1972). These effects have been interpreted as due to a chemical interaction of asbestos fibre with cell plasma membrane (ALLISON, 1971). The release of lysosomal enzymes occurs (DAVIES et al , 1974) as with very cytotoxic dust such as quartz, in spite of a better viability of the cells and this effect seems mostly related to phagocytosis of asbestos fibres (BIGNON et JAURAND, 1976). Thus, the initial cytogenic effects of asbestos at the level of macrophages look more like a metabolic stimulatory effect than like a cytotoxic effect. However, it is possible that the substances released during phagocytosis of asbestos by macrophages play an important intermediate role for the induction of fibrogenesis (NOURSE et al, 1975) or perhaps cancerogenesis. In vivo, the relationship between asbestos fibres and macrophages has been studied in the lung of different species. After their penetration into the alveoli, short fibers (less than 5 µm) are phagocytosed by alveolar macrophages and sequestrated within phagocytic vesicles. In contrast, long fibres are attacked by more than one macrophage, but cannot be sequestrated within the cells because of their size. A very low proportion of fibres (2°/o or less) mostly long fibres, is transformed into coated fibres, by deposi - tion of mucopolysaccharids and iron around the fibres (DAVIS , 1970; GOVERNA and RO-SANDA, 1972; NOURSE et al, 1975). The thickness of this coating varies from very thin to 5 µm (SUZUKI and CHURG, 1969; POOLEY, 1972b). Coated fibres when non identified are called ferruginous bodies (FB), (UTIDJAN et al, 1968). Coated asbestos fibres are called asbestos bodies (AB). It is very easy to recognize FB under the light microscope and FB have been described or counted in many measurement studies on human samples. Fibre size seems to be an important factor for the genesis of FB; the ferroprotidic coating is preferentially formed around large fibres (greater than 5 µm in length) which cannot be completely engulfed by one macrophage. Concerning asbestos, AB seem to form preferentially around amphibole type fibres. There is so far no demonstrated information regarding the fibrogenic effect to asbestos. The original hypothesis of a stimulating effect of the fibroblastic activity due to a physical irritation by fibres is not absolutely demonstrated; other factors relevant to the solubility of fibre or to the susceptibility of the host (immunological factors) might be important.

The carcinogenetic effects of asbestos dust is now demonstrated by human data as well as experimental data. All commercial forms of asbestos are carcinogenic in animals, producing lung carcinoma and pleural or peritoneal mesothelioma, whatever route used for introducing the fibres (GROSS et al, 1967; REEVES et al, 1971; WAGNER et al, 1973/1974; POTT et al, 1976). Concerning carcinogenesis, there are now many biological data relevant to the mechanisms of pathogenecity of asbestos fibres. However, these mechanisms are still poorly elucidated and some data appear controversial. Till recently, it was strongly believed that the carcinogenetic effect of asbestos fibres was due to chemical contaminants. Powerful carcinogens, such as 3.4 benzo(a)pyrene could come from natural oils and waxes (HARINGTON, 1962) and from contaminant oils during milling of the fibre (HARINGTON and ROE et al, 1966) or storage in plastic bags (COMMINS and GIBBS, 1969). SHABAD et al., (1974) have shown that chrysotile is able to absorb benzo(a)pyrene in vitro. This sorptive property should be increased in lung tissue where the specific surface area of chrysotile fibres must increase due to leaching of magnesium from the crystal(JAURAND et al., 1976). However, in animal, fibres from which the oils had been removed, gave the same results as natural fibres (WAGNER and BERRY, 1969; WAGNER et al, 1973).

A carcinogenic effect of trace metals is deduced from the presence of traces of cobalt, nickel, chrome, iron and so on, associated with different asbestos samples (HARINGTON, 1965, 1973; HARINGTON and ROE, 1965). However, the role of metals has not yet been demonstrated.

Recently, experimental data have stressed upon the fact that the carcinogenic effect of asbestos was mostly due to physical irritation. The shape, the length and above all the diameter of the fibre seemed important factors (STANTON and WRENCH, 1972; STANTON, 1973; POTT et al , 1976). Moreover, other fibrous minerals, such as fibreglass, were also able to induce cancer if their diameter was identical to asbestos fibres diameter. At present, it seems that fibres less than 0,5 µm in diameter are most active in producing tumours. The length is another parameter and the biologically active fibres seem to be longer than 3 or 5 µm (POTT et al , 1976).

Dose effect relationship of biological response to asbestos

- The fibrogenic effect in the lung seems related to the dose of asbestos dust retained in the lung and also to the size of the fibres; the longer the fibres the more fibrogenic. However, there are also host factors, related to the immunological surveillance system.

- Regarding the carcinogenic effect, there is evidence of a dose response relationship in humans from the epidemiologic studies of mesothelioma cases (NEWHOUSE and BERRY, 1976) and of bronchogenic carcinoma (ENTERLINE, 1976; ZIELHUIS, 1976). Until now, as far as cancer is concerned, there is no answer to the question of a safe level of asbestos fibre in the environment. However, it seems that mesothelioma can occur even with brief periods and low levels of exposure, in animals (WAGNER et al, 1973) as well as in humans (BECKLAKE, 1976; ZIELHUIS, 1976; JONES et al, 1976) implying a lack of a dose relationship to exposure.

3.   REVIEW OF MEASUREMENT STUDIES IN HUMAN SAMPLES

Several studies have been carried out on asbestos metrology in human samples. However, there appears to be no direct information on the existence of programmes of collection for future references. A critical review of published data shows that the establishment of such a programme is urgently needed: because of the great variability in samples studied and analytical procedures used, the data published until now provide information only on limited fields of interest. Another general remark is that it seems very difficult to integrate and coordinate all published data in order to answer many questions arising for the assessment of biological effects of asbestos exposure by means of measurement studies in human samples. Nevertheless, this chapter will review the most important data presently available and discuss in which manner the published studies have contributed to the knowledge of different topics relevant to the biological monitoring.

3.1.   What could be the definition of body-burden for asbestos?

The actual amount of pollutant in humans at any time is called retention. The retention of particles in humans occurs in a dynamic way and reaches an equilibrium level depending on the relative rate constants of deposition and clearance processes. Models of lung retention based on the ICRP Task Group report have been described (BRAIN and VALBERG, 1974; TAULBEE and YU, 1975). The general scheme of particles deposition sites and clearance processes is shown in fig. 1 (TASK GROUP ON LUNG DYNAMICS, 1966). So far, the penetration and retention of fibres through the gastro-intestinal tract have not been intensively investigated. Anyway, whatever route is used for penetration, the retention of fibres in the human body must be related to many other factors, most of them poorly known. As asbestos measurement in organs requires a destructive process, the retention of asbestos fibres cannot be controlled continuously and for each case studied, a measurement of asbestos in organs provides information on asbestos retention at a very definite time: time of death for autopsic material or time of surgical intervention for biopsic samples. However, few attempts have been made for asbestos retention monitoring by means of a process involving no sampling (COHEN, 1973) or by means of relating body-burden to the amount of asbestos in sputum (BIGNON et al, 1974a), gastric juice (BIGNON et al, 1975) and pulmonary washing-fluid (NOLIBE et al, 1975). These studies of asbestos content in different samples have provided information regarding the different factors relevant to the establishment of body-burden: deposition, penetration, clearance, retention, distribution and translocation of fibres in the human body.

3.1.1. Deposition

Distinction will be made between the two pathways for human exposure to asbestos: the pulmonary tract (PT) and the gastro-intestinal tract (GIT).

TIMBRELL has reviewed the mechanisms by which particles deposit in the respiratory system and has addressed specifically the problem of fibre deposition (TIMBRELL, 1965). He identified settling, inertial impaction and Brownian diffusion as deposition mechanisms which operate for both compact particles and fibres. In addition, he listed a fourth mechanism, direct interception, which is of little significance for compact particles but which may be of marked importance for fibres. In this view, a model for deposition of fibres in the human respiratory system has been described (HARRIS and FRASER, 1976). The effectiveness of these deposition mechanisms depends on the anatomy of the respiratory tract, the effective aerodynamic diameter of the particles (size, shape, density) and the pattern of breathing.

According to the first three listed mechanisms of deposition, it is likely that airborne asbestos fibres can readily deposit after touching a surface either in the trachea, bronchi and bronchioles or the alveolated peripheral airways. Measurements in lung parenchyma have shown that the great majority of fibres did not exceed 0.5 μm in diameter. These findings are in good agreement with the theoretical deposition pattern prevision of the ICRP report and with TIMBRELL's theory saying that the aerodynamic diameter of asbestos fibres is equal to the true diameter x 3. However, the size parameters measured in autopsic samples cannot be directly related to the original size of the inhaled fibres because of the possibilities for asbestos fibres, specially for chrysotile, to split longitudinally under the mechanical action of the air flow and fluid movement in the airways or the chemical action of enzymes or other potent biological reagents present in lung fluid and in alveolar macrophages (OTOUMA and TAKE, 1975; BIGNON et al, 1976a).

Another confirmation of TIMBRELL's theory concerns the fourth mechanism of deposition of fibres by direct interception. POOLEY (1972a) has shown that chrysotile fibres can be located at airways bifurcations in human lungs. Similar findings were made by MORGAN et al (1975) in experimental studies on rats using activated asbestos. Thus it appears that the frequency and angles of branching are important parameters for the regional deposition of asbestos fibres inside the lung. Nevertheless, these theoretical points of view on fibrous particles deposition do not explain why the concentration of asbestos fibres has been found higher in peripheral areas of the human lung (SEBASTIEN et al, 1975).

Asbestos fibres can also deposit in the gastro-intestinal tract (GIT) either directly (because of the presence of asbestos in water, beverages and food) or indirectly (fibres coming from the respiratory airways and being swallowed). There appears to be no direct information on the mechanisms of fibre deposition in the human GIT. Most studies have been carried out on animals in order to answer the following question: do ingested fibres penetrate tissue and cause cancer? (GROSS et al, 1974a).

It is obvious that more quantitative information on the deposition of asbestos fibres in humans cannot be obtained because of clearance and translocation mechanisms occurring simultaneously during lifetime. What we measured in the human body is the result of all these mechanisms.

3.1.2. Clearance

Fibres that are deposited on the mucus blanket covering the surface of trachea and bronchi are moved towards the pharynx by cilia. Clearance of inhaled particles by these mechanisms is believed to be more than 98 % effective for most deposited particles (GROSS and de TREVILLE, 1972). The fibres deposited at the surface of the alveoli are taken by alveolar macrophages and more or less cleared towards the ciliated airways. For chrysotile, this type of clearance might be important since WAGNER and SKIDMORE (1965), WAGNER et al (1974) found that a large percentage of chrysotile asbestos entering the lungs of rats may be removed from the lung within 58 days. The cleared fibres are swallowed as demonstrated by the study of EVANS et al (1973) using inhaled neutron activated asbestos. Up to 75 % of this asbestos was found in the faeces within 30 days.

Measurements related to clearance in humans have been carried out in several kinds of samples: sputum (SLUIS–CREMER, 1965; STUMPHIUS, 1971; BIGNON et al, 1974a), gastric juice (BIGNON et al , 1975) and feces (CUNNINGHAM et al , 1976). Generally, the findings of asbestos in such samples were related to past exposure, to pulmonary burden or to pathological features. The feasibility of using such samples as indicators of body-burden will be discussed later.

The most clearance-related paper in humans was by BIGNON (BIGNON et al , 1974b). It was shown that asbestos can be found in sputum more than 30 years after the end of the exposure, even in case of continuous low level exposure or in case of short moderate exposure. The proportion of coated/total fibres (visible with the light microscope) in sputum increases with the length of time elapsed since the last exposure and reached a constant value of about 0.75 for elapsed period longer than 15 years. This striking fact has not been explained for the moment (see fig. 2).

3.1.3. Penetration, distribution and translocation of asbestos fibres in the human body.

Measurements in tissues using the transmission electron microscope (TEM) have revealed the presence of numerous fibres and fibrils far more than was ever imagined when the fibre population was evaluated by light microscopy alone. These findings, occurring even in case of moderate exposure and long elapsed time from last exposure, suggest a very high penetration and retention rate for TEM size fibre. In humans, asbestos fibres have been found in lung parenchyma, bronchial tissue, lymph nodes (GROSS et al, 1973), parietal pleura (SEBASTIEN et al, 1976f), pleural fluid (POOLEY, 1976), peritoneum (HOURIHANE, 1965), liver (FONDIMARE and DESBORDES, 1974), stomach (HENDERSON et al, 1975), bowel walls (POOLEY, 1974), colon (ROSEN et al, 1974).

Within the lung, there appears to be a tendency for fibres to accumulate in the peripheral regions (SEBASTIEN et al, 1975). The regional distribution of asbestos fibres in lung parenchyma might be influenced by pathological features (fibrosis, tumours) or individual breathing patterns (smokers). In this laboratory, fibre concentrations were always less important in the tumour areas than in non-involved areas of the lung. Additionally, in the same area of lung parenchyma, higher local concentrations could be found, especially when TEM size fibres were considered; in the same lung, differences of two orders of magnitude in fibre concentrations could be encountered from an area to another. So far, we do not know if fibres which have penetrated the lung tissue will remain almost indefinitely where they are or move towards other places. Some clearance does occur via interstitial space and lymph channels to hilar and mediastinal lymph nodes and perhaps also to bronchial lumens and blood-stream according to the general model of lung clearance (TASK GROUP ON LUNG DYNAMICS, 1966). Measurements have been made in lymph nodes (GROSS et al, 1973) but no correlation was found between fibre concentration in lymph nodes and in the lung. In view of these findings, an hypothesis of the lymphatic transport of inspired dust to the parietal pleura has been formulated (TASKINEN et al, 1973). However, the mechanism by which fibres can be transported from lung to pleural cavity is still a subject of controversy.

In the same manner, less is known about the penetration of ingested fibres through the wall of the gastro-intestinal tract (GROSS et al , 1974a). The relevance to human diseases, such as peritoneal mesothelioma, remains to be determined.

3.2. Asbestos exposure and body-burden

The difficulty in relating the actual retention of asbestos in any specific human tissue sample to exposure resides principally in the fact that the individual conditions of exposure are not known exactly. So, the asbestos exposure can only be described in terms of the general categories previously listed. Only a few attempts have been made for measuring the asbestos retention of diversely exposed people (GROSS et al , 1974b; SEBASTIEN et al , 1975). Generally measurements have been made in one category of exposed people only (asbestos workers, urban dwellers) or in pathological cases and matched controls. As in such conditions a statistical bias is introduced, it is probable that a wide range of exposures has not been investigated so far.

84

If we agree with the fact that mesothelioma can occur after various conditions of asbestos exposure, from occupational to environmental levels, measurements of asbestos fibres in meso-thelioma cases could indirectly lead to the investigation of a wide range of exposures. An example of such a study is the paper by POOLEY (POOLEY, 1973a).

Another general remark is the need for expressing the measurement results in a quantitative way. Expressing results in terms of prevalence (positive or negative case) provides only crude data concerning the proportion of positive cases in a group of people and with poor accuracy because it has been shown that the prevalence tends to increase with the intensity of the search for fibres and depends also on the amount of tissue examined. As an example, numerous papers have been concerned with the prevalence of ferruginous bodies in lungs of city dwellers and prevalence data were published in many countries (BECKLAKE, 1976). UTIDJIAN et al, (1968) and BIGNON et al, (1970) have demonstrated that, using a suitable preparation technique of the sample, ferruginous bodies were found in lungs of every city dweller ; these findings clearly brought to light the need for quantitative studies in the field of asbestos biological monitoring.

When trying to quantitate the amount of asbestos in lungs of diversely exposed people, it appears that the observed differences between several groups depend upon the instrumental analysis used: it seems easier to differentiate each group by means of a light microscopic study than by means of a TEM study (cf fig. 3). These findings are in agreement with the hypothesis of a higher retention rate for submicroscopic fibres: because of the small size of fibres encountered in case of true environmental exposure it may happen that the total amount of such fibres in true environmental aerosols be of the same order of magnitude as the proportion of submicroscopic fibres in industrial aerosols. This could explain the generally narrow range concentration of optically visible fibres and the widespread range concentration of TEM size fibres in controls. This and the fact that possibilities of asbestos exposure are numerous and can be undiscovered by inquiries enhance the difficulty in defining body-burden base-line values.

Information on body-burden base-line values have been mainly obtained by looking for ferruginous bodies with the aid of the light microscope in the lungs of city dwellers from necrospy series (BECKLAKE, 1976). Unfortunately the great majority of results have been expressed in terms of prevalence (positive or negative cases). The largest survey by this method has been published by SELIKOFF (SELIKOFF and HAMMOND, 1970) who reported data concerning 1,975 autopsy cases from the New-York City population. A large-scale measurement programme for multi-centre survey of asbestos bodies was initiated by POOLEY in 1966 (POOLEY et al, 1970) to determine if the incidence of asbestos in the lungs of the general population had changed over the last decades and to study geographical differences for the prevalence of ferruginous bodies in several countries. It was shown that the occurrence of ferruginous bodies in the lungs of Finnish cases was exceptionally high. Secular trends in pulmonary asbestos bodies indicate that the proportion of positive cases appears to be rising by about 1°/o per year in persons over the age of 30 living in the London area (OLDHAM, 1973).

Are such findings useful in establishing relationships between the levels of asbestos fibre pollution in the environment and asbestos body burden? Ferruginous bodies could only be used as an index of the degree of atmospheric pollution by asbestos in a given community if the following criteria are met: ferruginous bodies are to be specific for asbestos; a quantitative relationship must exist between ferruginous bodies and asbestos fibres; and the ferruginous bodies found in a given lung might originate only from the asbestos fibres inhaled with the environmental air and not coming from other source and location (occupational) (DAVIS and GROSS, 1973). Although ferruginous bodies can be formed around other fibres than asbestos, investigations using the electron microscope have demonstrated that asbestos fibres were actually present in the lungs of city dwellers (LANGER et al, 1971). However there appears to be no relationship between ferruginous bodies and asbestos fibres concentrations (DAVIS and GROSS, 1973). But the most important criticism is the failure in defining comparable conditions of exposure for a group of people.

These considerations may affect the general purpose of a biological monitoring programme. The usefulness of such a programme is the possibility of assessing the actual retention of asbestos fibres in individual cases. In fact the statistical data obtained by monitoring a large group of people can be only related to general considerations such as the consumption of asbestos, by example.

Another important point is the establishment of standards or quality guides for asbestos pollution and its consequences on body-burden. Up to now, no data is available in this field. The development of continuous monitoring on sharply defined small groups of exposed people would be very useful to improve theoretical models and allow the definition of biological significant standards.

3.3. Body-burden and effects

3.3.1. Lung fibrosis (asbestosis)

This field has not been investigated on a large-scale coordinated programme. Some authors have tried to relate the grade of fibrosis to one parameter of lung-burden on cohorts of people generally professionally exposed. The results appear to-day unsatisfactory because the investigated parameters and the analytical procedures were different.

We know that some asbestos fibres in the lung can be converted into asbestos bodies by the deposition of globules of protein and iron, producing an easily recognized and quite characteristic structure. Occasional references to asbestos bodies, assessed by light microscopy, are found in the literature from 1900 onwards. In the period 1930 - 1940, a great deal of work seems to have been done on a very small number of lungs. The parameters investigated were the quantitative numerical concentration of optically visible fibres and the amount of mineral dust expressed in weight concentration. In 1961, BEATTIE and KNOX published data on mineral content and particle size distribution in the lungs of 50 asbestos textile workers; a very interesting feature was the study of the accumulation rate of mineral material in the lung. A comparable paper was by NAGELSCHMIDT in 1965 who studied dust content and composition in 20 lungs with asbestosis. These authors failed to demonstrate any clear correlation between the severity of the fibrosis and the content of asbestos dust as determined in samples of lung tissue by ashing and acid extraction, and with chemical estimation of silica. The paper by ASHCROFT and HEPPLESTON in 1973 presented fibre counts from 35 asbestosic lungs showing a full spectrum of pathological features: in mild and moderate asbestosis there was a progressive increase in concentration of asbestos fibres with increasing severity of fibrosis, whereas in severe asbestosis no correlation existed between fibre concentration and the form or the extent of the pathological fibrous reaction; it was suggested that the severe fibrosis resulted from the supervention of a non-specific inflammatory process. The results of SEBASTIEN et al (1975) concerning a limited number of autopsic cases with asbestosis are in good agreement with ASHCROFT and HAPPLESTON' findings. At present, lung fibrosis has been observed in relation with heavy occupational exposure and the concentrations of asbestos fibres in the lung tissue were high. However, recently in a case of apparently idiopathic lung fibrosis, a significant number of TEM size asbestos fibrils has been reported (MILLER et al., 1975).

3.3.2. Lung cancer

The increase of lung cancer risk for occupationally exposed people has been demonstrated by epidemiological investigations. Paradoxally, most of the measurement studies have been carried out in cases with low asbestos exposure, comparing the prevalence of ferruginous bodies in the lungs of cancer patients and matched controls series. The relationships between the lung-burden in asbestos bodies and bronchogenic carcinoma in a population not specifically exposed to asbestos has been found significant (WARNOCK and CHURG, 1975) or not significant (MEURMANN et al , 1970; DONIACH et al , 1975). Unfortunately, so far no data is available concerning the amount of TEM size fibres in these cases.

Many reasons can be involved for the actual failure to answer the following question: what level of burden in humans can produce asbestos related lung cancer?

- Lung cancer is now very frequent in man and its incidence is increasing in woman. This is mostly related to cigarette smoking, which is the major factor. However asbestos, even in cases with low exposure, can act as a multiplicative factor (SELIKOFF et al , 1968).
- Many other carcinogenetic agents are present in the environment, and synergetic effects can occur. It is not easy to isolate the specific role of asbestos in the production of tumours.
- The heterogeneous distribution of fibres in the lung (POOLEY, 1972a; SEBASTIEN et al , 1975) could be responsible for areas with very high concentration, able to induce carcinoma. But is carcinoma of the lung more easily induced by high local concentration than by moderate diffuse concentration of a carcinogen? Studies on the carcinogenetic effects of radioactive particles have led to the conclusion that the non-uniform distribution of plutonium particles in the lung is less hazardous than if the plutonium was uniformly distributed (BAIR et al , 1974).

It appears that studying thoroughly the lung lung-burden characteristics (fibre concentration, regional deposition, size distribution, mineralogical type, shape, associated pollutants) in a wide range of concentrations could be very helpful in assessment of dose-effect relationships for asbestos related cancer.

3.3.3. Pleural and peritoneal mesothelioma and other pleural disease

Epidemiological findings suggested that mesothelioma could occur after various degrees of asbestos exposure (ZIELHUIS,1976). Fibre counts in lung parenchyma are in agreement with that (See fig. 3) (ASHCROFT, 1973; FONDIMARE et al., 1973; POOLEY, 1973a). Thus it seems that the occurrence of mesothelioma is not directly related to the fibre count in lung parenchyma. This puzzling fact leads to the question: in which manner can asbestos fibres induce mesothelioma?   Perhaps fibre count in lung parenchyma is not the significant parameter for relating body burden to the occurrence of mesothelioma. Only a few quantitative data are available concerning the asbestos contents in pleura and peritoneum of diversely exposed people. The TEM study of SEBASTIEN et al , (1975) on a limited number of cases showed that in any one case there was no correlation between the concentration of asbestos bodies in the lung and the parietal pleural plaques. Moreover there were small variations of the FB concentration in pleural plaques. Moreover there were small variations of the FB concentration in pleural plaques in diversely exposed patients, as opposed to the variations of the number of fibres in lung parenchyma.

The presence of fibres in the pleural or peritoneal cavity involved transport mechanisms which can be dependent on fibre size, shape and perhaps solubility (reaction in the lymph nodes). Research is needed in this field to study the mechanism of transport and to specify which types of fibres are of biological significance for mesothelioma and which is the most suitable sample for biological monitoring. The same remarks should be made for the genesis of other pleural diseases (pleural plaques and pleural effusions).

The CEC have taken the initiative to assess the number of mesothelioma cases in the community by means of mesothelioma registers. A programme has been defined by a group of pathologists (MESOTHELIOMA PANEL, 1976). Taking lung samples for measurement is considered in this programme.

3.3.4. Other tumours

In the paper by DONIACH (DONIACH, 1975) a statistically significant relationship has been found between the presence of FB in the lung and the occurrence of breast cancer. No more data are available in this field for the present.

A few TEM size fibres were found in stomach tumours (HENDERSON et al , 1975; BIGNON and SEBASTIEN, 1976a) but no ferruginous bodies were found in the bowels of patients with primary carcinoma of the colon (ROSEN et al, 1974). Another surprising fact for asbestos related malignancies is that epidemiological findings indicated an increase of gastro-intestinal tumours for exposed people and that fibres could not be readily found in the bowel wall (POOLEY, 1974), although the gastro-intestinal tract is an important pathway for particles clearance.

3.4. External indicators of body-burden

Different types of samples can be used for estimation of body-burden in human during life-time. The usefulness of these samples to appreciate the asbestos body-burden, depends on the feasibility for sample recovery and the manner in which the amount of asbestos found in the sample is related to body-burden.

The feasibility for collection depends on the possibility to be used in a large scale, even in not diseased people. The only samples which can be used for monitoring asbestos body-burden in community are feces (CUNNINGHAM et al, 1976), blood and sputum when available (BIGNON et al, 1974a). In Table IV, the feasibility for collection is graded for − to ++++, according to the possibility to obtain data in the community related to public health.

3.4.1. Sputum

It has been demonstrated in this laboratory and by others that the amount of FB in the sputum was significantly related to the asbestos exposure (BIGNON et al, 1974; SLUIS-CREMER, 1965) and to the amount of FB in lung parenchyma further measured at the autopsy time (BIGNON et al, 1975) (Fig. 4). This test is very simple and can be used as a retrospective proof of asbestos exposure, even a long time after the exposure. Another advantage is that the coating around the fibres is the evidence that the fibres have stayed in the lung.

This test is good even in the case of light exposure if the TEM is used. As an example, in this laboratory have been studied the sputum from people working inside buildings insulated with sprayed asbestos containing material. The TEM examination has shown the presence of TEM size asbestos fibres, mostly of chrysotile type, in 23 out of 78 cases. But when dealing with uncoated fibres in sputum, the problem is to ascertain the lung provenance of such fibres. Nevertheless, if the presence of uncoated fibres in sputum in people presently exposed to asbestos cannot be related to lung retention, it indicates a specific exposure at the time of sample recovery. The analysis of sputum specimens sampled at different periods of time, during exposure and at a distance of exposure, might provide information about cleared fibres from the deep lung. But, in a large-scale epidemiological survey, the major inconvenience of sputum analysis is that it lacks in many people (normal non-smokers and women) who do not expectorate.

3.4.2. Bronchial secretions

Pure bronchial secretions can only be obtained by means of bronchoscopy. Although the fibre optic bronchoscope makes bronchoscopy much easier to do, this kind of sampling can only be used in diseased people. This technique is very reliable, providing more inorganic material than sputum. Moreover, there is less contamination from inorganic particles deposited in upper airways.

3.4.3. Lung washing fluid

Lung biopsy, even needle or fibre optic bronchoscopic biopsy, cannot be performed as an usual monitoring tool. This is the reason why we are now investigating the possibility of alveolar lavage to quantitate the lung content of asbestos fibres. Indeed, it has been shown in the baboon that pulmonary washing was an efficient procedure for the recovery of particles from the deep lung (NOLIBE et al, 1975). At present, the number of cases with asbestos exposure studied by this method is too limited to provide definite conclusions. The recovery by this technique of particles deposited at the alveolar surface should provide very interesting information on the actual deposit of fibres. Regarding the cases to be selected for this type of analysis, we have the same limitation as for bronchial secretions, because we need to do a fibre optic bronchoscopy to perform the alveolar lavage.

3.4.4. Gastric juice

One should have presumed that, as for the diagnosis of tuberculosis gastric catheterization should be a simple technique in order to estimate the amount of asbestos fibres cleared from the lung or ingested. Actually, this kind of investigation has been poorly accepted by diseased people (BIGNON et al, 1975) and cannot be reasonably planned for monitoring normal non sputing people. Moreover, such samples, to provide reliable data, need to be recovered early in the morning and many other non-defined factors can contribute to the variability of the results (BIGNON et al , 1975).

3.4.5. Feces

In order to have an easy access to human samples, value   has recently been set on the measurement of asbestos fibres in feces (CUNNINGHAM et al , 1976). The first results seem to be very promising and this technique, needing a small amount of feces, could be the most useful and the less troublesome one for providing quantitative data for a large survey of various populations exposed to asbestos intake from air, food, beverages and water. The published results show that the asbestos fibres in feces are numerous (up to 10^8 per g of wet feces) even in non-exposed people. So this method appears as a very sensitive one allowing detection of low intake of asbestos fibres.

3.4.6. Blood

There appears to be no direct information on the presence of asbestos fibres in human blood. However, such fibres have been found in rats after intragastric injection of asbestos (CUNNINGHAM and PONTEFRACT, 1973). Research is needed in this field; the fibres in blood could be related to the fibre penetration.

3.4.7. Pleural fluid

The search for asbestos fibres is also possible in pleural fluid and has been found positive in our laboratory in 2 cases of asbestos-related pleural effusion. This technique might be a helpful means for the diagnosis of idiopathic pleuresies.

3.4.8. Biopsy material

This technique is only available in patients, where needle pleural biopsy, peritoneal biopsy and lung biopsies can be carried out. The information provided by lung needle biopsy seems too small in comparison with the risk of complications. Surgical lung biopsy or even alveolar lavage brings more detailed information.

4.   CONSIDERATION FOR HUMAN SAMPLING

4.1.   Technical recommendations

In Table IV are listed informations concerning the different types of samples, their usefulness and their feasibility for collecting and analysis. It is obvious that biopsic samples cannot be used for determination of retention rate in humans for complete study of fibres distribution in the body; their interest is only related to the diagnosis of asbestos-related diseases. One inconvenience is that, generally, biopsic samples are too small for providing significant quantitative results.

Another remark is that the examination of tumours and organs invaded by the tumour has been found to provide unreliable quantitative data because of the important pathological changes within the tissues.

There is no special precaution for collecting and storage except guarding against any exogenous contamination (talc). All samples should be fixed in 10°/o formalin, previously filtered through 0.2 µm pore size filter. In case of liquids, the added quantity of formalin must be recorded. A convenient way for assessing asbestos concentration in lung parenchyma is to express results per cm^3 of lung parenchyma. To respect physiological conditions, the autopsic lung must be fixed by inflation with 10°/o formalin infused through the trachea or the bronchi. Such fixed samples could wait several years before analysis. Indeed, the chemial solubility of asbestos in formalin has not been demonstrated (JAURAND et al , 1976), it is likely that in such conditions fibres will preserve their morphological features and crystal structure. Polyethylene containers are very convenient for shipment and storage.

An important parameter for measurement in biological samples is the amount of material available for the mineralogists:

- For sputum, it has been found that study of three consecutive sputa ensures a good recovery of fibres (BIGNON et al., 1974).
- In case of liquids (gastric juice, pleural fluid, lung washing fluid) a few millilitres are sufficient for TEM analysis.
- For surgical biopsy and autopsy samples the largest amount of material is desirable because it will enable the study of the regional distribution of fibres in organs. In case of small-size biopsy samples the localization of the sampling site must be recorded. Especially for the autopsic lungs, a complete sagittal slide must be available.

4.2. Ethical and legal considerations

In each country, there are regulations concerning the autopsy procedure in public hospitals. In France, according to a 1947 - 1948 law, autopsy can be carried out in all general hospitals 24 hours after the death certificate. However, in University Hospitals, an early autopsy is permitted on condition that death be certified by two physicians from the concerned hospital confirming death by codified tests (arteritomy). Viscera sampling is allowed only if it does not alter the external integrity of the body. There are many various conditions where autopsy is not allowed in general hospitals: after an objection previously raised by the subject himself or from the relatives, for religious or racial matters and for legal purpose. In that field, it is noteworthy that in France, autopsy can only be carried out by a coroner on the body of people compensated for an occupational disease. This practice will cause major problems for the working out of a European program on the determination of dose-effect relationship in mesothelioma cases. For the purpose of epidemiological study, there is an urgent need for a standardisation of the regulation in the EEC.

Collecting biological specimens on living people is totally different: now biomedical research is under serious challenge if it causes some predictable or unexpected injury to the investigated subject. For the biological monitoring of asbestos, samples such as sputum, feces or blood will present no ethical or legal problem. Sampling the gastric juice implies the cooperation of the patient and, moreover needs technical improvement to become reliable (BIGNON et al, 1974).

Biopsy (lung, pleura), even when surgical, is justified to confirm the diagnosis of malignancies. When an asbestos-related disease is suspected, a biopsy can be performed on a consenting patient in order to confirm an occupational disease subject to compensation.

Alveolar washing is a new procedure, producing no injury. However, as it is performed during fibreoptic bronchoscopy, it needs to be carried out on volunteer patients, informed of the interest of this investigation for diagnosis as well as for scientific purposes.

5. ANALYTICAL PROCEDURES

5.1. Instrumental analysis

The most meaningful data concerning the nature and identification of microparticles may be obtained from the analysis of single individual particles. This and the fact that in tissue samples, mixed particulate populations are encountered limit the usefulness of bulk analysis methods like X-ray diffraction techniques, infra-red spectrometric analysis or differential thermal analysis. So, presently, only light and electron microscopy can be used for assessing asbestos fibres in tissue. Both microscopic techniques are needed to assess all the fibres within the samples for the following reasons:

- large fibres are not numerous enough to be significantly counted by electron microscopy, because only a small aliquot of the sample (10^{-15} of the lung) can be analyzed by this technique.

-   small fibres, which outnumber the large ones, are not optically visible and need electron microscopy.

On the basis of morphological features and electron diffraction patterns, it is very easy in TEM to recognize chrysotile and amphibole type fibres from other particles. To distinguish the different varieties of amphibole and identify non-asbestos particles, micro-analysis equipment is necessary. It must be pointed out that identification of every single microparticle by electron microprobe technique is still a very controversial research field. Ideally, both electron diffraction and microanalysis should be performed on the same particle, but this method is very time-consuming and electron diffraction pattern cannot be obtained from thick particles.

5.2.   Preparation methods

The preparation method is the most critical point in quantitative determination of particulate matter in biological specimens, because the recovery of material is very dependent on the technique involved. For example, the percentage of non-occupationally exposed cases with ferruginous bodies in their lungs ranged, in the literature, from 9 to 100 $^{\circ}$/o. 100 $^{\circ}$/o has been obtained using chemical digestion of lung samples and direct filtration on Millipore membrane.

If a large-scale measurement program is introduced, the measurement working group has to define a single convenient preparation method for analysis of biological specimens. First, if a sufficient amount of tissue is available, the study of bulk samples seems to be more promising for quantitative evaluation of asbestos burden than study of thin sections. The second point is that microfiltration of a liquid mixture containing particulate matter provides a good recovery of these particles; then the filter can be directly examined under the light microscope and small filter pieces can be transferred on to electron microscope grids. Transferring particles from the filter on the grid seems more efficient than allowing a drop of the mixture to dry on the grid. These two observations (bulk samples and recovery of particles by filtering the mixture) could be considered as basic points for choosing a convenient preparation method.

The major point is to concentrate the particles removed from the tissue:

a)   Digestive procedure with sodium hypochlorite presents the advantage of being performed at room temperature on both fresh and fixed tissue. The experience of this laboratory shows that this technique ensures good results except for calcified pleural plaques. The number of operations is limited and after the tissue has been destroyed, the mixture is directly filtered. It has been demonstrated that using this technique, the Mg content of the chrysotile fibres was not leached. But the use of sodium hypochlorite can lead to a chemical contamination by Cl, unsuitable when microprobe analysis is performed (JAURAND et al, 1976). Another inconvenience of sodium hypochlorite digestion is that this solvent does not destroy all organic particles and in the case of city dwellers a great amount of such particles is generally encountered.

b)   Ashing procedure is also used to destroy tissue and organic particles. This technique seems to avoid structural and chemical changes of most mineral dusts. Ashing large quantities of tissues has been found unsuitable for TEM examination, because of the large quantity of ash remaining in the sample. The suitable size of sample for ashing is to be discussed.

5.3.   Results

Before debating on a convenient method for counting and sizing identified particles, it seems important to define what has to be measured.

As far as asbestos fibres are concerned, the following parameters should be measured:

-   Numerical concentration of optically visible coated and uncoated fibres, identified by their optical properties.
-   Numerical and gravimetric concentration of electron microscope size asbestos fibres identified by their morphological features, their electron diffraction pattern or their microanalysis spectrum. One should discuss whether a distinction be made between each mine-

ralogic type of asbestos fibres or only between chrysotile and amphibole types.
- Size distribution (length and diameter) of asbestos fibres in light and electron microscopy

Quantitative data should be expressed both per cm^3 of fixed tissue and per gram of dried tissue.

If other particles are to be considered, considerable difficulties arise because each type of particles must be positively identified. This important problem is to be discussed and cannot be developed extensively here. At the present time, a lot of quantitative data concerning asbestos fibres contaminations are missing; the point is to know if information concerning non-asbestos particles is also needed. Perhaps, it might be interesting to define first in which conditions asbestos can be considered a major pollutant and which concentrations are of interest.

Concerning the count of asbestos fibres under light and electron microscopes, statistical methods must be developed in order to improve quantitative evaluations. A very promising technique now in progress in this laboratory is to add a known quantity of latex spheres to the mixture and to count simultaneously latex spheres and asbestos fibres. The counts should be recorded on a calculator and statistically computed.

A second way of improving quantitative evaluations should be the separation of asbestos from other materials in order to obtain more concentrated mixtures. No routine technique is presently available in this field.

5.4.   Interlaboratory check and organizational aspects

First experience with the CEC working group on metrology for asbestos indicates that an intercomparison programme within several laboratories (3 or 4) is the only way to enhance reliability of the results. The check could be performed on a limited number of samples only. Each step of the analytical procedure should be tested separately by the different laboratories. Another remark is that, as such measurements require specialized people and improved equipment, the work should be concentrated on a limited number of laboratories depending obviously   on the importance of the country (no more than 2 or 3 for a European country).

It should be realized that the studies mentioned require the input of highly specialized manpower and equipment; they will not give an adequate answer within a short period of time. It will be necessary to combine the efforts of specialized institutes on an international scale. Only a high degree of cooperation and   coordination could provide reliable and perhaps definite results in this field. The actual failure in biological monitoring for asbestos may be related to the dispersed efforts of laboratories without a highly coordinated programme.

6.   PROGRAMME DESIGN

Such a programme should be defined by a cohort working group of hygienists, pathologists, epidemiologists and mineralogists. Only general guidelines will be developed here.

It seems that the fundamental interest of biological monitoring, compared to epidemiological investigations, is that results may be of immediate importance and utility for individual cases. As the use of asbestos will not be forbidden in the near future and because exposure occurs in an individual way, the feasibility of detecting people at risk is of great importance. In this view great value   should be set upon indicators of body-burden during life-time. A general design of the programme should be proposed in this sense:

a)   Study of the relationships between body-burden pattern and occurrence of disease.

Review of past studies in this field indicates that a condition of success to obtain quantitative information on dose-effects relationships is that examination should be performed on a wide range of exposed people, and that many parameters should be assessed (regional distribution and concentration, physical information on fibres, associated pollutants, etc......). These measurements should be principally performed on autopsic cases fully examined by pathologists. Cases with truly authenticated mesothelioma represent an ideal material for the assessment of the dose-effects relationships.

b)   The search for a suitable indicator of body-burden during life-time.

Measurement in easily collected samples (sputum, feces, gastric juice, washing fluid, blood) in which the amount of pollutant is related to exposure and clearance mechanisms may provide information on the actual retention of fibres in humans. It is also possible that the presence of fibres in a definite organ enhances the release of a specific compound by a biochemical process unknown for the moment. Research is needed in this field.

It seems very difficult to give statistical indications for such a programme because the influence of personal factors in asbestos related diseases is not known for the moment. The validity of measurement results should be continuously controlled by statisticians. Concerning the cost, an indication can be given for a complete autopsic examination: in the range of 10.000 FF.

TABLE I.: Data on properties of UICC standard reference asbestos samples: compositional analysis, associated minerals. (Timbrell, 1975; Germain, 1974).

	Rhodesian Chrysotile. A.	Canadian Chrysotile. B.	Amosite	Crocidolite	Anthophyllite
Major Constituents (%)					
Aluminium	0.40	0.27	0.34	0.47	0.72
Iron	0.88; 1.7	1.14; 2.6	15.1; 28	15.1; 27	4.4; 1.98
Magnesium	31	32	11.0	3.6	24
Oxigen					
Sodium	—	0.08	—	4.4	—
Sodium as Na_2O	0.04	0.02	0.11	5.8	0.08
Silicon as SiO_2	39,1	38.06	50.3	49.1	58.2
Free SiO_2	0.01	0.13	3.0	2.06	0.23
Minor Constituents (ppm)					
Cobalt	55	45	7 - 11	2; 9	24; 50
Chromium	1,390	490	35	16; 22	870; 571
Manganese	430	510	15,000; 13,900	870; 864	988; 1,200
Nickel	1,250	990	34	13	424; 1,360
Antimony	4	—	2	2	—
Scandium	6	5	5	0,5	5
Associated Minerals. (listed by decreasing occurrence)	Magnetite Pyrrhotine Pentlandite Millerite Chromite Awaruite	Magnetite Chromite Pentlandite Linneite Awaruite	Pyrite Magnetite Pyrrhotine Hematite	Magnetite Pyrite Iron oxydes	Pyrrhotine Pentlandite Chromite Magnetite Smythite

TABLE II.: APPROXIMATE RANGES OF ASBESTOS CONCENTRATIONS IN DIFFERENT CIRCUMSTANCES

TYPE OF SAMPLE AND LABORATORY	LIGHT MICROSCOPE (fibres/ml)	ELECTRON MICROSCOPE (nanograms/m^3)
AMBIENT AIR Urban Sites, EPA 200 Samples in 50 US Cities, Environmental Sciences Laboratory Major City centre locations in U.K., Asbestosis Research Council Rural locations in U.K., Asbestosis Research Council Industrial town centres in U.K. Asbestosis Research Council 300 Samples in Paris, Laboratoire d'Etude des Particules Inhalées		0.5 - 15 0.1 - 100 0.1 - 10 1 0.1 - 1 0.1 - 10
NEAR ASBESTOS SPRAY OPERATIONS Health and Safety Executive, London Environmental Sciences Laboratory, New York	0.6 - 0.008	10 - 1000
IN THE VICINITY OF ASBESTOS PLANT Health and Safety Executive, London Asbestosis Research Council Environmental Sciences Laboratory, New York Laboratoire d'Etude des Particules Inhalées, Paris	0.02 - 0.1	1 - 100 10 - 5000 10 - 3000
HOMES OF ASBESTOS WORKMEN Environmental Sciences Laboratory, New York		100 - 5000
INSIDE BUILDINGS FIREPROOFED WITH ASBESTOS Health and Safety Executive, London Environmental Sciences Laboratory, New York Laboratoire d'Etude des Particules Inhalées, Paris	0.01 - 0.1	1 - 800 1 - 800

TABLE III.: ASBESTOS WATER POLLUTION

SAMPLING PROGRAM	X-RAYS (μg/litre)	LIGHT MICROSCOPY (fibres/litre)	ELECTRON MICROSCOPY (10^6 fibres/litre or μg/litre)
RANDOM SAMPLING 38 samples in USA — drinking water State of Vermont, USA — drinking water Netherlands		10^3 - 10^4 10^4 ϵ-10	 0.1
SURFACE WATER CONTAMINATION Great lakes basin	200		1 - 170
ASBESTOS CEMENT PIPE Glendale, Arizona, USA Netherlands		 ϵ-10	0.01 μg/l 0.1
NATURAL CONTAMINATION Malvern, Pennsylvania, USA			0.04 μg/l

TABLE IV.

TYPE OF SAMPLE	USEFULNESS	FEASIBILITY FOR COLLECTION	FEASIBILITY FOR ANALYSIS
RELATED TO CLEARANCE PROCESS			
— Sputum	+++	+++	+++
— Bronchial aspirate	+++	+	+++
— Gastric juice	++	++	+++
— Feces	+++	++++	—
RELATED TO ACTUAL RETENTION			
a) During life time			
— Bronchial biopsy	—	+	++
— Surgical lung biopsy	+	— —	+++
— Lung washing fluid	+++	+	+++
— Surgical pleura biopsy	++	— —	+
— Pleural needle biopsy	++	—	+
— Pleural fluid	+++	—	+++
— Gastric biopsy	—	+	+
— Peritoneal biopsy	+++	+	+++
— Tumour (any location)	—	— —	+
— Blood	++	++++	— —
b) At time of death			
— Lung (a complete sagittal slide)	++++	+++	+++
— Parietal pleura	++	+++	++
— Lymph nodes	++++	++	+++
— Pleural plaques	++	++	—
— Liver	+	+++	—
— Bowel wall	++	+++	—
— Peritoneum	++	+++	++
— Tumour (any location)	+	+++	+

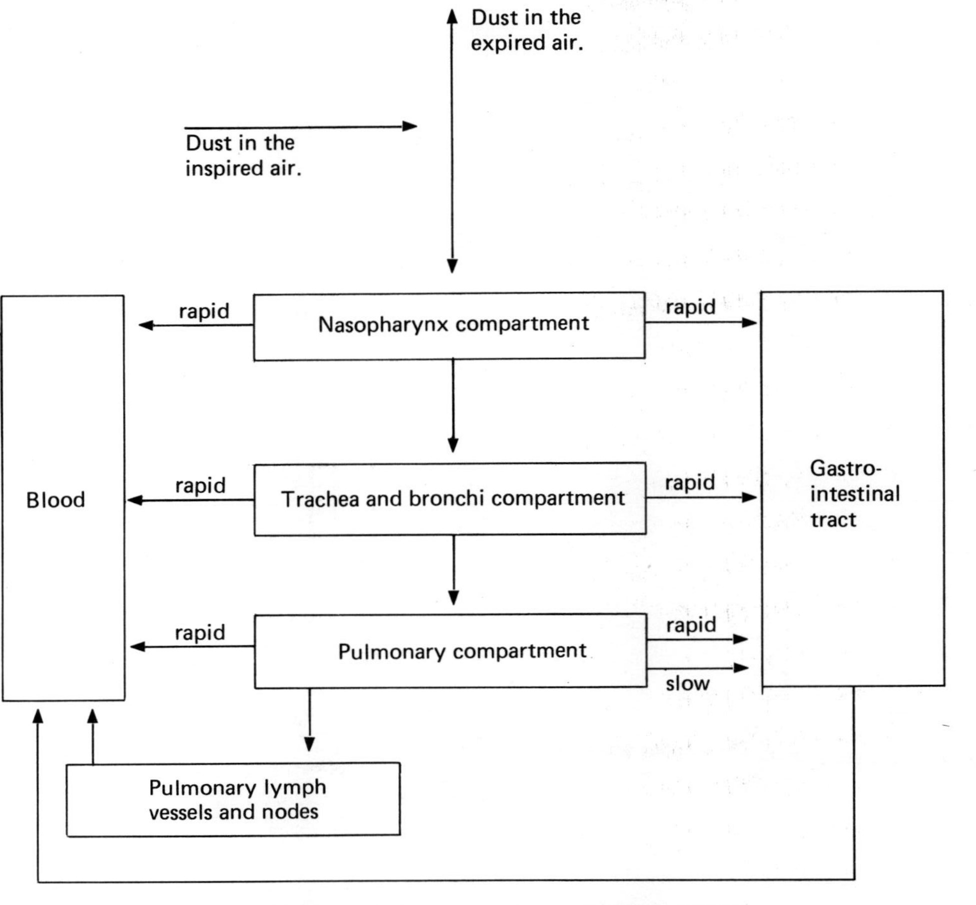

Figure 1. Particle deposition sites and clearance processes based on ICRP lung model, (TASK GROUP ON LUNG DYNAMICS, 1966).

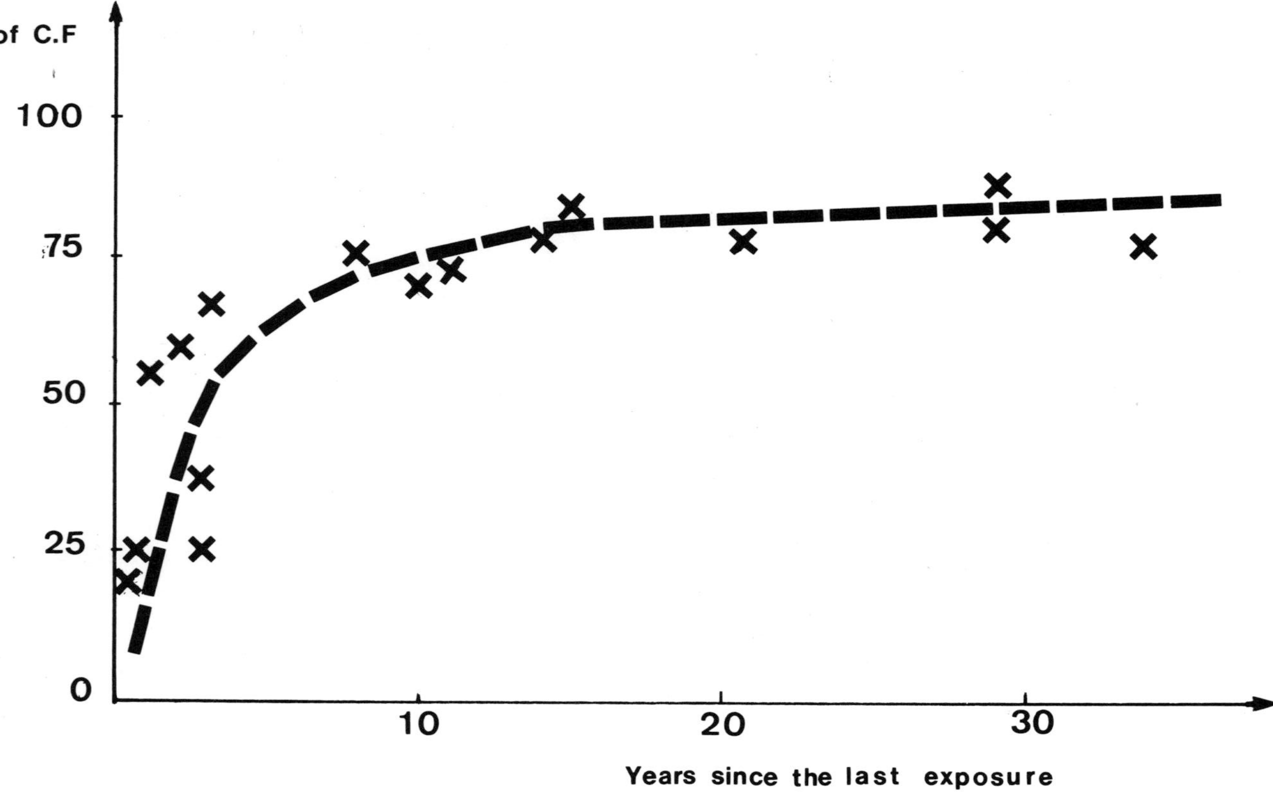

Figure 2. Fibres from lung parenchyma of diversely exposed people. Increase of the proportion of coated fibres (CF) with increase of the time elapsed since the last exposure (light microscope count).

Figure 3. Ranges of fibre concentrations in lung tissue. As technical procedures were different for each author, the results have been expressed in multiplicative factors of the lowest value (LwV) encountered in controls.

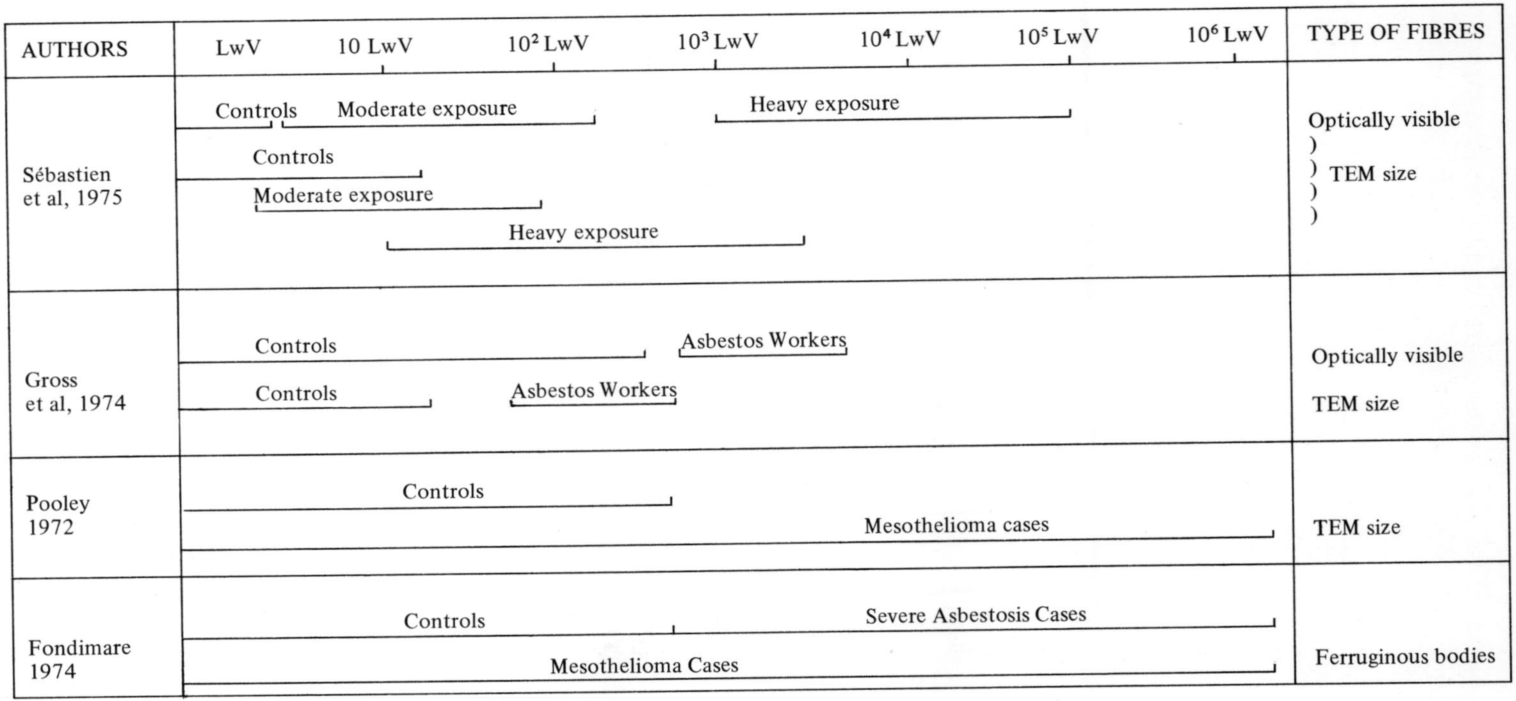

AUTHORS	LwV — 10 LwV — 10^2 LwV — 10^3 LwV — 10^4 LwV — 10^5 LwV — 10^6 LwV	TYPE OF FIBRES
Sébastien et al, 1975	Controls — Moderate exposure — Heavy exposure / Controls / Moderate exposure / Heavy exposure	Optically visible))) TEM size))
Gross et al, 1974	Controls — Asbestos Workers / Controls — Asbestos Workers	Optically visible / TEM size
Pooley 1972	Controls / Mesothelioma cases	TEM size
Fondimare 1974	Controls — Severe Asbestosis Cases / Mesothelioma Cases	Ferruginous bodies

Figure 4. Quantitative correlation between the maximal number of ferruginous bodies (FB) in sputum and the type of occupational exposure. For every patient with FB in sputum, this number is plotted in on the logarithmic scale.
(from Environmental Health Perspectives Vol. 9, pp. 155-160, 1974)

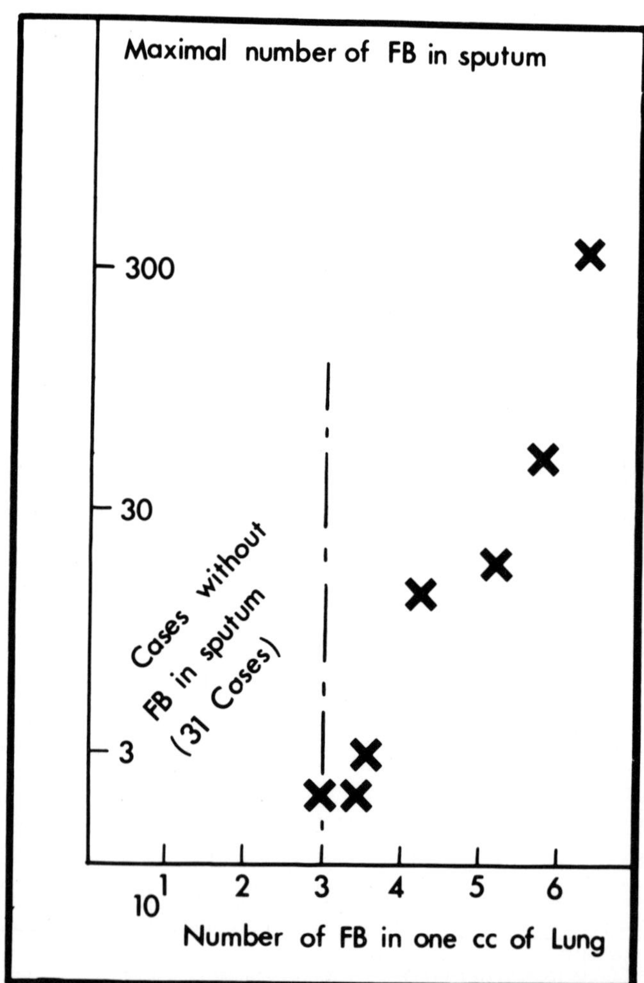

REFERENCES

1 – ACGIH–AIHA. Joint Aerosol Hazards Evaluation Committee (1975). Background documentation on evaluation of occupational exposure to airborne asbestos. Am. Ind. Hyg. Assoc. J., 36, 91-103.

2 – ALLISON, A.C. (1971). Lysosomes and the toxicity of particulate pollutants. Arch. Intern. Med., 128, 131-139.

3 – ALSTE, J., WATSON, D. and BAGG, J. (1976). Airborne asbestos in the vicinity of a free way. Atmospheric Environment, 10, 583-589.

4 – ASHCROFT, T. and HEPPLESTON, A.G. (1973). The optical and electron microscopic determination of pulmonary asbestos fibre concentration and its relation to the human pathologic reaction. J. clin. Path., 26, 224-234.

5 – ASHCROFT, T. (1973). Epidemiological and quantitative relationships between mesothelioma and asbestos on Tyneside. J. clin. Path., 26, 832-840.

6 – BAIR, W.J., RICHMOND, C.R. and WACHHOLZ, B.W. (1974). A radio-biological assessment of the spatial distribution of radiation dose from inhaled plutonium. United States Atomic Energy Commission, Document WASH-1320.

7 – BEATTIE, J. and KNOX, J.F. (1961). Studies on mineral content and particle size distribution in the lungs of asbestos textile workers. In Inhaled Particles and Vapours, edited by C.N. Davies, pp. 419-433. Pergamon Press, Oxford.

8 – BECK, E.G., HOLT, P.F. and MANOJLOVIC, N. (1972). Comparison of effects on macrophage cultures of glass fibre, glass powder, and chrysotile asbestos. Brit. J. Industr., Med., 29, 280-286.

9 – BECKLAKE, M.R. (1976). Asbestos-related diseases of the lung and other organs: their epidemiology and implications for clinical practice. Am. Rev. Respir. Dis., 114, 187-227.

10 – BIGNON, J., GONI, J., BONNAUD, G., JAURAND, M.C., DUFOUR, G. and PINCHON, M.C. (1970). Incidence of pulmonary ferruginous bodies in France. Environ. Res., 3, 430-442.

11 – BIGNON, J., SEBASTIEN, P., JAURAND, M.C. and HEM, B. (1974a). Microfiltration method for quantitative study of fibrous particles in biological specimens. Environ. Health Persp., 9, 155-160.

12 – BIGNON, J., SEBASTIEN, P., MONCHAUX, G. et BONNAUD, G. (1974 b). L'épuration à long terme des particules fibreuses chez l'homme. Colloques de l'I.N.S.E.R.M., 29, 205-218.

13 – BIGNON, J., HEM, B., BONNAUD, G., SEBASTIEN, P. et MONCHAUX, G. (1975). Evaluation en microscopie optique du degré de l'empoussiérage pulmonaire asbestosique par microfiltration de l'expectoration et du suc gastrique. In Recent Advances in the Assessment of the Health Effects of Environmental Pollution, Proceedings of an International Symposium, Paris, 24-28 June 1974, pp. 1189-1197. Published by CEC, Luxembourg.

14 – BIGNON, J., JAURAND, M.C., JAUBERT, F. et CHAHINIAN, P. (1976 a). Les protéines seriques de la surface de l'alvéole. Rev. Fr. Mal. Resp., 4, Suppl. 3., 49-66.

15 – BIGNON, J., SEBASTIEN, P. and MONCHAUX, G. (1976 b). Mesure de l'amiante dans une série de biopsies gastriques (unpublished Data).

16 – BIGNON, J. and JAURAND, M.C. (1976). Contrat CCE.

17 – BRAIN, J.D. and VALBERG, P.A. (1974). Models of lung retention based on ICRP Task Group Report. Arch. Environ. Health, 28, 1-11.

18 – CASTLEMAN, B. and BLUM, D. (1975). Asbestos-ciment pipe should not be used for drinking water supplies. A Mary PIRG Report, 2nd. Edition, October, 1975. University of Maryland, College Park, MD. 20742.

19 – COHEN, D. (1973). Ferromagnetic contamination in the lungs and other organs of the human body. Science, 180, 745-748.

20 – COMMINS, B.T. and GIBBS, G.W. (1969). Contaminating organic material in asbestos. Brit. J. Cancer, 23, 358-362.

21 – CUNNINGHAM, H.M. and PONTREFACT, R.D. (1973). Asbestos fibres in beverages, drinking water, and tissues: their passage through the intestinal wall and movement through the body. J. AOAC, J6, 976-981.

22 – CUNNINGHAM, H.M., PONTREFACT, R.D. and O'BRIEN, R.C. (1976). Quantitative relationship of fecal asbestos to asbestos exposure. Journal of toxicology and Environmental Health, 1, 377-379.

23 – DAVIES, P., ALLISON, A.C., ACKERMAN, J., BUTTERFIELD, A. and WILLIAMS, S. (1974). Asbestos induces selective release of lysosomal enzymes from mononuclear phagocytes. Nature, 251, 423-425.

24 – DAVIS, J.M.G. (1970). Further observations on the ultrastructure and chemistry of the formation of asbestos bodies. Experimental and molecular pathology. 13, 346-358.

25 – DAVIS, J.M.G. and GROSS, P. (1973). Are ferruginous bodies an indication of atmospheric pollution by asbestos? Biological Effects of Asbestos. Proceedings of a working conference at IARC Lyon, October, 2-6, 1972. Edited by Bogovski, P., Gilson, J.C., Timbrell, V. and Wagner, J.C., pp. 238-242. IARC Scientific Publications No. 8.

26 – DONIACH, I., SWETTENHAM, K.V. and HATHORN, M.K.S. (1975). Prevalence of asbestos bodies in a necropsy series in East London: association with disease, occupation, and domiciliary address. Brit. J. industr. Med., 32, 16-30.

27 – ENTERLINE, P.E. (1976). Estimating health risks in studies of the health effects of asbestos. Am. Rev. Resp. Dis., 113, 175-180.

28 – FEDERAL REGISTER (1975). Occupational exposure to asbestos. Notice of Proposed Rulemaking. Federal Register, 40, No. 197.

29 – FONDIMARE, A., DESBORDES, J., PERROTEY, J., TAYOT, J. et ERNOULT, J.L. (1973). Etude semi-quantitative de l'empoussiérage par l'amiante dans quatorze observations de mesothelioma pleuraux. Arch. Anat. Path., 22, 55-60.

30 – FONDIMARE, A. and DESBORDES, J. (1974). Asbestos Bodies and fibres in lung tissues. Environ. Health Persp., 9, 147-148.

31 – GERMAIN, D. (1974). Minéraux accessoires des Asbestes-Standards de l'Union Internationale contre le Cancer. Thèse, Faculté des Sciences, Université libre de Bruxelles.

32 – GOVERNA, M. and ROSANDA, C. (1972). A histochemical study of the asbestos body coating. Brit. J. Industr. Med. 29, 154-159.

33 – GROSS, P., de TREVILLE, R.T.P., TOLKER, F.D., KASCHAK, M. and BABYAK, M.A. (1967). Experimental asbestosis. The development of lung cancer in rats with pulmonary deposits of chrysotile asbestos dust. Arch., Environ., Hlth. 15, 343-355.

34 – GROSS, P. and de TREVILLE, R.T.P. (1972). The lung as an embattled domain against inanimate pollutants. Am. Rev., Respir., Dis., 106, 684-691.

35 – GROSS, P., DAVIS, J.M.G., HARLEY, R.A. and de TREVILLE, R.T.P. (1973). Lymphatic transport of fibrous dust from the lungs. J. Occup. Med., 15, 186-189,

36 – GROSS, P., HARLEY, R.A., DAVIS, J.M.G. and CRALLEY, L.J. (1974 b). Mineral fibre content of human lung. Am. Ind. Hyg. Assoc. J., 35, 148-151.

37 – GROSS, P., HARLEY, R.A., SWINBURNE, L.M., DAVIS, J.M.G. and GREENE, W.B. (1974 a). Ingested mineral fibres. Arch. Environ. Health, 29, 341-347.

38 – HARINGTON, J.S. (1962). Occurrence of oils containing 3:4 benzopyrene and related substances in asbestos. Nature (Lond), 1962, 193, 43-

39 – HARINGTON, J.S. (1965). Chemical studies of asbestos. Ann. N.Y. Acad. Sci., 132, 31-47.

40 – HARINGTON, J.S. (1973). Chemical factors (including trace elements) as etiological mechanisms. Biological effects of asbestos. IARC. Scientific publications No. 8. pp. 304-311.

41 – HARINGTON, J.S., MILLER, K. and MACNAB, G. (1971). Hemolysis by asbestos. Environ. Res., 4, 95-117.

42 – HARINGTON, J.S. and ROE, F.T.C. (1965). Studies of carcinogenesis of asbestos fibres and their natural oils. Ann. N.Y., Acad., Sci., 132, 439-450.

43 – HARRIS, R.L. and FRASER, D.A. (1976). A model for deposition of fibres in the human respiratory system. A. Ind. Hyg. Assoc., J. 3, 73-89.

44 – HARWOOD, C.F. (1971). Asbestos air pollution control. Illinois Institute for Environmental Quality, document No. PB-205 238. Edited by National Technical Information Service, Pringfield 22151.

45 – HARWOOD, C.F., OESTREICH, D.K., SIEBERT, P. and STOCKHAM, J.D. (1975). Asbestos emissions from baghouse controlled sources. Am. Ind. Hyg. Assoc. J., 36, 395-603.

46 – HENDERSON, W.J., EVANS, D.M.D., DAVIES, J.D. and GRIFFITHS, K. (1975). Analysis of particles in stomach tumours from Japanese males. Environ. Res., 9, 240-249.

47 – HOURIHANE, D.O.B. (1965). A biopsy series of mesotheliomata, and attempts to identify asbestos within some of the tumors. Ann. N.Y. Acad. Sci., 132, 647-673.

48 – JAURAND, M.C., GONI, J., JEANROT, P., SEBASTIEN, P. et BIGNON, J. (1976). Solubilité du chrysotile in vitro et dans le poumon humain. Rev. fran. Mal. Resp., 4, supp. 2, 111-120.

49 – JOHAN, Z., GONI, J., SARCIA, C., BONNAUD, G. et BIGNON, J. (1973). Influence de certains acides organiques sur la stabilité du réseau du chrysotile. Dans Advances in Organic Geochemistry, pp. 883-903. Editions Technip. Paris.

50 – JONES, J.S.P., POOLEY, F.D. and SMITH, P.G. (1976). Factory populations exposed to crocidolite asbestos, a community survey (in press).

51 – LANGER, A.M., SELIKOFF, I.J. and SASTRE, A. (1971). Chrysotile asbestos in the lungs of persons in New-York City. Arch. Environ. Health. 22, 348-360.

52 – LUMLEY, H.P.S., HARRIES, P.G. and O'KELLY, F.J. (1971). Buildings insulated with sprayed asbestos: a potential hazard. Ann. occup. Hyg., 14, 255-257.

53 – MESOTHELIOMA PANEL (1976). Dose/effect relationships (criteria) for asbestos. Hôpital Laënnec Meeting, 23-24 March, 1976. CEC Document No. V/F/1351/76 e.

54 – MEURMANN, L.O., HORMIA, M., ISOMÄKI, M. and SUTINEN, S. (1970). Asbestos bodies in the lungs of a series of Finnish lung cancer patients. In Pneumoconiosis, Proceedings of the International Conference, Johannesburg 1969. Edited by H.A. Shapiro, pp. 404-407. Oxford University Press, Cape Town.

55 – MILLER, A., LANGER, A.M., TEIRSTEIN, A.S. and SELIKOFF,I.J.(1975). "Nonspecific" interstitial pulmonary fibrosis. Association with asbestos fibres detected by electron microscopy. N. England. J. Med., 292, 91-93.

56 – MORGAN, A., LALLY, A.E. and HOLMES, A. (1973). Some observations on the distribution of trace metals in chrysotile asbestos. Ann. occup. Hyg., 16, 231-240.

57 – MORGAN, A. (1974). Absorption of human serum albumin by asbestiform minerals and its application to the measurement of surface areas of dispersed samples of chrysotile. Environ. Res., 7, 330-341.

58 – MORGAN, A., EVANS, J.C., EVANS, R.J., HOUNAM, R.F., HOLMES, A. and DOYLE, S.G. (1975). Studies on the deposition of inhaled fibrous material in the respiratory tract of the rat and its subsequent clearance using radioactive tracer techniques II.Deposition of the UICC standard reference samples of asbestos. Environ. Res., 10, 196-207.

59 – MURPHY, R.L., LEVINE, B.W., AL BAZZAZ, F.J., LYNCH, J.J. and BURGESS, W.A. (1971). Floor tile installation as a source of asbestos exposure. Am.Rev., Respir., Dis., 104, 576-580.

60 – MURRAY, H.M. (1907). Report on Departmental Committee on Compensation for industrial Disease, c.d. 3495.

61 – NAGELSCHMIDT, G. (1965). Some observations of the dust content and composition in lungs with asbestosis made during work on coal miners pneumoconiosis. Ann, N.Y. Acad., Sci., 132, 64-76.

62 – NEWHOUSE, M.L. and BERRY, G. (1976). Predictions of mortality from mesothelial tumours in asbestos factory workers. Brit. J. Industr., Med., 33, 147-151.

63 – NICHOLSON, W.J. (1974). Analysis of amphibole asbestiform fibres in municipal water supplies. Environ. Health Persp., 9, 165-172.

64 – NICHOLSON, W.J., ROHL, A.N. and WEISMAN, I. (1975). Asbestos contamination of the air in public buildings. Contract EPA No. 68-02-1346.

65 – NOLIBE, D., METIVIER, H., MASSE, R. and LAFUMA, J. (1975). Therapeutic effects of pulmonary lavage, in vivo, after inhalation of insoluble radioactive particles. Fourth International Symposium on Inhaled Particles and Vapours of the BOHS, Edinburgh, 22nd to 26th September 1975. (in press).

66 – NOURSE, L.D., NOURSE, P.N.,, BOTES, H. and SCHWARTZ, H.M. (1975). The effects of macrophages isolated from the lungs of guinea pigs dusted with silica on collagen biosynthesis by guinea pig fibroblasts in cell culture. Environ., Res., 9, 115-127.

67 — OLDHAM, P.D. (1973). Asbestos in lung tissue. In Biological Effects of Asbestos. Proceedings of a working conference at IARC, Lyon, October, 2-6, 1972. Edited by Bogovski, P., Gilson, J.G., Timbrell, V. and Wagner, J.C., pp. 231-235. IARC Scientific Publication No. 8.

68 — ORCEL, L., MARTIN, R. et GIORGI, H. (1970). Législation de la mort, prélèvements sur le cadavre. Vie. Med., 40, 5463-5494.

69 — OTOUMA, T. and TAKE, S. (1975). Effect of anionic surface active agent on chrysotile. In Proceedings of the Third International Conference on the Physics and Chemistry of Asbestos Minerals, paper, 5-21, Quebec, Canada, August 17th to 21st 1975.

70 — PARAZZI, E., PERNIS, B., SECCHI, G.C. and VIGLIANI, E.C. (1968). Studies on "in vitro" cytotoxicity of asbestos dusts. Med. Lav., 59, 561-576.

71 — PONTEFRACT, R.D. and CUNNINGHAM, H.J. (1973). Penetration of asbestos through the digestive tracts of rats. Nature, 243, 352-353.

72 — POOLEY, F.D., OLDHAM, P.D., UM, C.H. and WAGNER, J.C. (1970). The detection of asbestos in tissues. In Pneumoconiosis, Proceedings of the International Conference, Johannesburg, 1969. Edited by H.A. Shapiro, pp. 108-116. Oxford University Press, Cape Town.

73 — POOLEY, F.D. (1972 b). Asbestos bodies, their formation, composition and character. Environ. Res., 5, 363-379.

74 — POOLEY, F.D. (1972 a). Electron microscope characteristics of inhaled chrysotile asbestos fibre. Brit. J. Industr., Med., 29, 146-153.

75 — POOLEY, F.D. (1973 a). Mesothelioma in relation to exposure. In Biological Effects of Asbestos, Proceedings of a working Conference held at the IARC, Lyon, France, 2-6 October 1972, pp. 222-225. IARC Scientific Publications No. 8.

76 — POOLEY, F.D. (1973 b). Methods for assessing asbestos fibres and asbestos bodies in tissue by electron microscopy. In Biological Effects of Asbestos, Proceedings of a Working Conference held at the IARC, Lyon, France, 2-6 October 1972, pp. 50-53. IARC Scientific Publications No. 8.

77 — POOLEY, F.D. (1974). Locating fibres in the bowel wall. Environ., Health Persp., 9, 235.

78 — POOLEY, F.D. (1976). Personal communication.

79 — POTT, F., DOLGNER, R., FRIEDRICHS, K.H. and HUTH, F. (1976). Experiences sur animaux concernant l'effet oncogene de poussières fibreuses. Interprétation des résultats en relation avec la cancérogénèse chez l'homme. (to be published).

80 — PUNDSACK, F.L. (1955). The properties of asbestos. I. The colloidal and surface chemistry of chrysotile. J. Phys., Chem., 59, 892-895.

81 — REEVES, A.L., PURO, H.E., SMITH, R.G. and VORWALD, A.J.: Experimental asbestos carcinogenesis. Environ., Res., 1971, 4, 496-511.

82 — REITZE, W.B., NICHOLSON, W.J., HOLADAY, D.A. and SELIKOFF, I.J. (1972). Application of sprayed inorganic fibre containing asbestos: occupational health hazards. Am. Ind., Hyg., Assoc., J., 33, 178-191.

83 — ROE, F.J.C., WALTERS, M.A. and HARINGTON, J.S. (1966). Tumour initiation by natural and contaminating asbestos oils. Int. J. Cancer, 1. 491-495.

84 – ROHL, A.N. and LANGER, A.M. (1974). Identification and quantitation of asbestos in talc. Environ. Health Persp., 9, 95-109.

85 – ROHL, A.N., LANGER, A.M., SELIKOFF, I.J. and NICHOLSON, W.J. (1975). Exposure to asbestos in the use of consumer spackling, patching and taping compounds. Science, 189, 551-553.

86 – ROHL, A.N., LANGER, A.M., WOLFF, M.S. and WEISMAN, I. (1976). Asbestos exposure during brake lining maintenance and repair. Environ. Res., 12, 110-128.

87 – ROSEN, P., SAVINO, A. and MELANED, M. (1974). Ferruginous (asbestos) bodies and primary carcinoma of the colon. A.J.C.P., 61, 135-138.

88 – SAWYER, R.N. (1974). Yale art and architecture building asbestos contamination: pas., present, and future. (Private communication).

89 – SEBASTIEN, P., FONDIMARE, A., BIGNON, J., MONCHAUX, G., DESBORDES, J. and BONNAUD, G. (1975). Topographic distribution of asbestos fibres in human lung in relation with occupational and non-occupational exposure. Fourth International Symposium on Inhaled Particles and Vapours of the BOHS, Edinburgh, 22nd to 26th September 1975. (in press).

90 – SEBASTIEN, P., BIGNON, J., GAUDICHET, A., DUFOUR, G. et BONNAUD, G. (1976 Les pollutions atmosphériques urbaines par l'asbeste. Rev. franç. Mal. Resp., 4, Supp. 2, 51-62.

91 – SEBASTIEN, P. et BIGNON, J. (1976 b). Contribution à l'étude de la pollution particulaire de l'air ambiant de la Ville de Paris par les microfibrilles d'amiante. Contrat Ministère de la Qualité de la Vie No. 206.

92 – SEBASTIEN, P. and BIGNON, J. (1976 c). Measurement in asbestos air pollution. CEC document No. V/F)1115/76.

93 – SEBASTIEN, P., BIGNON, J. and BONNAUD, G. (1976 d). Asbestos fibres in wines. (Unpublished Data).

94 – SEBASTIEN, P., GONI, J., DUFOUR, G. and BIGNON, J. (1976 e). Water contamination by asbestos during industrial processes. (Unpublished Data).

95 – SEBASTIEN, P., BIGNON, J. and MONCHAUX, G. (1976 f). Asbestos fibres in parietal pleural and in pleural fluid. (Unpublished Data).

96 – SEBASTIEN, P., BIGNON, J., BADER, J.P., MONCHAUX, G. et BONNAUD, G. (1976 g). Etude de l'amiante dans une série de biopsies gastriques. (Unpublished Data).

97 – SELIKOFF, I.J. and HAMMOND, E.C. (1970). Asbestos bodies in the New-York City population in two periods of time. In pneumoconiosis. Proceedings of the International Conference, Johannesburg, 1969. Edited by H.A. Shapiro, pp. 99-107. Oxford University Press, Cape Town.

98 – SELIKOFF, I.J., HAMMOND, E.C. and CHURG, J. (1968). Asbestos exposure, smoking and neoplasia. J. Am. med. Ass. 204, 106-112.

99 – SELIKOFF, I.J., NICHOLSON, W.J. and LANGER, A.M. (1972). Asbestos air pollution. Arch. Environ. Health, 25, 1-13.

100– SHABAB, L.M., PYLEV, L.N., KRIVOSHEEVA, L.V., KULAGINA, T.F. and NEMENKO, B.A. (1974). Experimental studies on asbestos carcinogenicity J. Nat. Cancer Inst., 52, 1175-1187.

101— SKIDMORE, J.W. and JONES, J.S.P. (1975). Monitoring an asbestos spray process. Ann. occup. Hyg., 18, 151-156.

102— SLUIS-CREMER, G.K. (1965). Asbestosis in South Africa - Certain geographical and environmental considerations. Ann. N.Y., Acad. Sci., 132, 215-234.

103— SPEIL, S. and LEINEWEBER, J.P. (1969). Asbestos minerals in modern technology. Environ. Res., 2, 166-208.

104— STANTON, M.F. (1973). Some etiological considerations of fibre carcinogenesis. In Biological Effects of Asbestos, Proceedings of a Working Conference held at the IARC, Lyon, France, 2-6 October 1972, pp. 289-294. IARC Scientific Publications No. 8.

105— STANTON, M.F. and WRENCH, C. (1972). Mechanisms of mesothelioma induction asbestosis and fibrous glass. J. Nat. Cancer. Inst., 48, 797-821.

106— STUMPHIUS, J. (1971). Epidemiology of mesothelioma on Walcheren Island. Brit. J. Industr., Med., 28, 59-66.

107— SUZUKI, Y. and CHURG, M.D. (1969). Structure and development of the asbestos body. Amer. J. Pathol., 55, 79-107.

108— TASK GROUP ON LUNG DYNAMICS (1966). Deposition and retention models for internal dosimetry of the human respiratory tract. Health Phys., 12, 173-207.

109— TASKINEN, E., AHLMANN, K. and WILKERIE, M. (1973). A current hypothesis of the lymphatic transport of inspired dust to the parietal pleura. Chest, 64, 193-196.

110— TAULBEE, D.B. and YU, C.P. (1975). A theory of aerosol deposition in the human respiratory tract. J. Appl. Physiol., 38, 77-85.

111— TIMBRELL, V. (1965). The inhalation of fibrous dusts. Ann. N.Y. Acad. Sci., 132, 255-273.

112— TIMBRELL, V. (1970 a). Characteristics of the international union against cancer standard reference samples of asbestos. In Pneumoconiosis, Proceedings of the International Conference, Johannesburg 1969, edited by H.A. Shapiro, pp. 28-36. Oxford University Press. Cape Town.

113— TIMBRELL, V. (1970 b). The inhalation of fibres. In Pneumoconiosis, Proceedings of the International Conference, Johannesburg 1969, edited by H.A. Shapiro, pp. 3-9. Oxford University Press. Cape Town.

114— TIMBRELL, V. (1972). Inhalation and biological effects of asbestos. In Assessment of Airborne Particles, edited by T.T. Mercer, P.E., Morrow and W. Stöber, pp. 429-445. C.C. Thomas Publisher, Springfield, Illinois.

115— UTIDJIAN, H.M.D., GROSS, P. and de TREVILLE, R.T.P. (1968). Ferruginous bodies in human lungs. Arch. Environ. Health, 17, 327-333.

116— WAGNER, J.C. and BERRY, G. (1969). Mesotheliomas in rats following inoculation with asbestos. Brit. J. Cancer, 23, 567-581.

117— WAGNER, J.C., BERRY, G. and TIMBRELL, V. (1973). Mesotheliomata in rats after inoculation with asbestos and other materials. Brit. J. Cancer. 28, 173-185.

118— WAGNER, J.C., BERRY, G., SKIDMORE, J.W. and TIMBRELL, V. (1974). The effect of the inhalation of asbestos in rats. Brit. J. Cancer. 29, 252-269.

119— WARNOCK, M.L. and CHURG, A.M. (1975). Association of asbestos and bronchogenic carcinoma in a population with low asbestos exposure. Cancer, 35, 1236-1242.

120— WEBSTER, I. (1974). The ingestion of asbestos fibres. Environ. Health Persp., 9, 199-202.

121— WORKING GROUP ON ASBESTOS METROLOGY (1976). Dose/effect relationships (criteria) for asbestos. Second Meeting of National Experts, Luxembourg, 28-29 April, 1976. Progress Report. CEC Document No. V/F/1353/76 e.

122— YADA, K. (1971). Study of microstructure of chrysotile asbestos by high resolution electron microscopy. Acta Cryst., A27, 659-664.

123— ZIELHUIS, R.L., VERSTEEG, J.P.J. and PLANTEIJDT, H.T. (1975). Pleura mesothelioma and exposure to asbestos. Int. Arch. occup. Environ. Hlth., 36, 1-18.

124— ZIELHUIS, R.L. (1976). Public health risk of exposure to asbestos. ECE, Directorate Social Affairs, contract dd. 18-6. 1975.

MERCURY, BIOLOGICAL SPECIMEN COLLECTIONS

T.W. Clarkson and M.R. Greenwood
Department of Radiation Biology and Biophysics
University of Rochester
School of Medicine
Rochester, New York

Considerable care is needed in the collection, transport and storage of biological specimens for mercury. Eventually, these specimens will be used for analytical determinations of mercury so as to assess human exposure and body burdens. Errors involved in the early stages of collection, transport and storage will accumulate into the final error in determining mercury in the specimen and in correlating mercury in the specimen with exposure and body burden. A diagrammatical representation of the summation of errors is given in Table 1.

The choice of the biological specimen is determined by many factors. The overriding factor is that the specimen will represent a suitable indicator medium for human exposure (for full discussion on definition of indicator media, see TGMA 1973 and Subcommittee on Toxic Metals, 1976). However, the choice of sample may also be influenced by the type of analytical procedures that are currently available. For example, the use of hair samples in recapitulating past exposure of mercury has become available only after substantial increase in sensitivity of analytical methods for mercury. The analytical procedure may also determine the quantity of sample that should be collected and therefore influence other factors such as the means of transport and storage of the specimen. General increase in sensitivity of methods for both total mercury, inorganic mercury, and methylmercury have resulted in collecting samples of smaller weight or volume which enter in a simplified transportation and storage.

Mercury exists in a variety of physical and chemical forms. However, the most important forms of mercury with regard to human exposure are metallic mercury and methylmercury. This review, therefore will deal predominantly with these two forms of mercury.

METALLIC MERCURY VAPOR

(a) Rationale for Choice of Indicator Media

The metabolic model for inhaled mercury vapor in man and animals is complex (for full discussion see TGMA, 1973, Subcommittee on Toxic Metals 1976). In general, the clearance half-times of inhaled mercury vapor differ in various body compartments so that when the person is in a non-steady state condition it is difficult, if not impossible, to choose an indicator medium that truly reflects mercury concentrations in the critical organ, in this case the central nervous system. Under steady state conditions, one would expect that the brain concentrations would eventually assume a constant ratio to the observed concentration in the indicator medium. Although, as yet, we do not have any direct evidence for this in man, studies in occupationally exposed workers who have been exposed for six months or more, indicate a constant ratio between urinary concentrations and time weighted average air concentrations on a group basis. Similar constant relationships have been observed for whole blood levels of total mercury and time weighted average air concentrations (Smith et al. 1970). Observations on volunteers inhaling tracer doses of radioactive vapor indicate that the half-time of clearance from the body is about 60 days and that half-times in various regions of the body are not in excess of this figure. (Hursch et al. 1976). Thus one would expect occupationally exposed individuals would tend to reach a state of balance after six months. In this sense, therefore, samples of urine and blood in people in steady state conditions on a group basis, would indicate exposure and probably reflect, in an indirect way, the accumulated body burden in these people.

The problem arises, however, that part of the mercury measured in either urine or blood, might represent recent exposure and in part long-term exposure. Studies on volunteers inhaling tracer doses of radioactive vapor and other individuals who had received high exposure, indicate that at least two exponential factors are involved in clearance from blood.

110

The tracer data indicated a clearance half-time from blood of about three days and data on people receiving high exposures indicate a second half-time of about thirty days. When these observations are extrapolated to conditions of steady state exposure, it would indicate that approximately half the mercury in blood represents recent exposure and half a longer term exposure. The recent exposure would reflect mercury intake of the last one or two weeks whereas the thirty day component would be influenced by mercury exposure over the last five months. Data on urinary excretion in occupationally exposed workers would also indicate that at least two clearance components are present and that, although they are not precisely described as in the case of blood, the urinary concentrations also would in part reflect recent exposure and in part a longer term exposure.

Hair specimens are probably not suitable for estimates of body burdens of inhaled vapor in man. One of the chief problems is that of direct absorption of the vapor on the hair sample. Doherty and co-workers (unpublished observations) observed that samples of human hair left in a mercury contaminated atmosphere, absorbed large amounts of mercury. Although washing removed a substantial amount of the absorbed mercury, it was not clear whether the washing procedure removed only the absorbed mercury but also mercury incorporated into the hair from the blood stream. Until these problems are resolved, it is unlikely that hair samples will be useful in assessing exposure to mercury vapor.

Studies on animals indicate that measurement of mercury in faeces would offer no special advantage over measurement in urine. Apart from the difficulties in collection, transport, and storage as well as in analytical determinations in faeces, faecal samples would be influenced by dietary intake of mercury due to the appearance of unabsorbed mercury in the faeces.

Little information is available on the appearance of mercury in human milk following exposure to mercury vapor. In view of the fact that women of childbearing age are often employed in industries handling metallic mercury, this would seem to be a serious deficit in our knowledge of the metabolism of mercury at this time.

In summary, therefore, it would appear that our knowledge of the metabolism of the inhaled vapor in man and animals suggests that no really satisfactory indicator media are yet available for this form of mercury. Indirect evidence suggests that in conditions of steady state exposure, probably on a group basis, measurement of mercury in urine and blood could provide the best means of assessing body burdens in man.

(b) Collection, Transport, and Storage

Blood samples, approximately 10 ml, should be collected by venipuncture using heparinized vacutainers. The samples should be gently agitated after collection to ensure dissolution of the heparin to avoid clotting of the sample. If vacutainers are not available, the usual hypodermic syringe and needle can be used, collecting the blood in glass containers with heparin as anti-coagulant. Mercury vapor exposure generally results in the red cell concentration being approximately a factor of two higher than concentration of mercury in plasma so that it may be desirable to determine the plasma to red cell ratio. In this event, it is preferable to separate plasma from red cells prior to storage, if facilities allow. In this case, a larger volume of blood should be collected approximately 20 ml, the haematocrit determined and then a portion of this blood separated by centrifugation and the plasma removed and stored separately. The determination of mercury in a sample of whole blood and in a sample of plasma will allow calculation of the red cell concentration if the haematocrit is known.

After collection, the blood sample should be stored in the refrigerator but not frozen. Transport should be in insulated containers usually using polystyrene as the insulator. For long distances, transport should be by air and many commercial airlines now have available small package delivery systems which allow transport of the material virtually from all points on the globe within a 24 hour period.

Storage of blood samples for periods beyond several weeks is difficult because of the problem of haemolysis. Considerable care should also be taken to avoid bacterial infection as this can result in the volatilization of mercury (Magos et al. 1966). Long-term storage of blood may be achieved by freeze drying the specimen. However, inadequate information is available on the question of loss of mercury by volatilization during the freeze drying procedure. After freeze drying, difficulties are often found in redissolving the solid sample and in relating the amount of mercury to the original blood volume. Expressing the result per gramme of haemoglobin may be useful but it is a procedure that has not been common in studies of occupational exposures due to mercury vapor.

Ideally, urine collection should be over a 24 hour period with the separate collections well mixed and a representative sample taken for analysis. Under most practical conditions the collection of a complete 24 hour sample is usually impossible and the collector can never be sure that he has obtained a complete sample. The alternative is to collect an early morning urine sample with the view that creatinine determinations could be used to correct variations in the concentration in the urine. However, the value of the creatinine collection has not yet been established as far as exposure to mercury vapor is concerned (see Smith et al. 1970). The urine sample should be collected away from contaminated areas and care should also be observed that the contaminated clothing of the individual does not release microdroplets of mercury into the collection vessel. It should be noted that under many conditions of occupational exposure to metallic mercury, droplets of the metal can be carried home and collection of the urine sample at home by no means guarantees lack of contamination.

Glass vessels may be used for collection of the urine sample after they have been carefully acid washed. Plastic vessels are more convenient for transport and storage but care should be observed with regard to the fact that certain types of plastic allow passage of mercury out of the biological sample (Greenwood and Clarkson, 1970). After collection, the sample should be frozen as quickly as possible and transported and stored in the frozen state. If this is not possible, acid should be added to the sample immediately after collection (for discussion see Magos and Cernick, 1969). If urine samples are allowed to stand for several days without the addition of acid and without freezing, a change in the form of mercury occurs which interferes with subsequent analysis.

The long-term storage of urine samples is not advisable. The frozen samples are generally bulky and inadequate data exist on the stability of mercury in frozen samples over long periods of time. Freeze drying of the urine sample might result in substantial loss of mercury by volatilization although this aspect has not been the subject of any careful study. The addition of thymol as a preservative is a common procedure in preserving urine for a variety of determinations. However, it should not be used in the case of mercury as thymol may interfere with some atomic absorption procedures.

In summary, urine and blood samples may be collected and transported over long distances without serious difficulty and without including serious errors in the final determination. However, both urine and blood present serious problems with respect to long-term storage.

METHYLMERCURY COMPOUNDS IN FOOD

(a) Rationale for choice of indicator media

The metabolic model for the uptake, distribution, and excretion of methylmercury compounds in man and animals is far better understood than in the case of inhaled mercury vapor. In general, methylmercury moves within body compartments at rates much faster than the excretion rate of methylmercury. As a result, the elimination from the whole body can be accurately described by a single elimination half-time with value averaging about 70 days. Clearance from blood, brain, and other tissues, roughly parallels clearance from the whole body. Animal observations as well as tracer observations on humanslend support to the idea that concentrations of methylmercury in blood reasonably well reflect concentrations in the critical organ, i.e., the central nervous system (for full discussion, see TGMA 1973, Subcommittee on Toxic Metals, 1976 ; Nordberg and Skervfing, 1972). However a question has been raised by Berlin (1976) that when blood concentrations attain a toxic range (100 ng/ml) the simple proportionality seen at lower exposures may disappear. However, for most actual conditions of human exposure the linearity of the metabolic model appears to hold, and the conclusion that blood is a suitable indicator medium seems to be well founded. Close correlations have also been seen between long-term methylmercury intake in food and steady state blood concentration.

The concentration of methylmercury in red cells is about ten times the simultaneous concentration in plasma. Consequently, the concentration of methylmercury in the whole blood sample is influenced by changes in haematocrit. The latter should always be determined wherever possible when samples are collected for methylmercury analysis. It has been customary in some surveys to express methylmercury concentrations per unit weight of red cells so that collection procedures should take into account this possibility.

A considerable body of evidence now exists for both people in steady state and non steady state exposures that the concentration of mercury in samples of hair closely parallels the concentration in blood at the time of formation of the hair sample. A knowledge of the growth rate of hair (approximately 1 cm/month) would allow, therefore, a recapitulation of previous blood levels of methylmercury. An illustration of this is given in Figure 1 which describes concentrations of mercury in one centimeter segments of two hair samples collected at different times from a person in Iraq who had been exposed to high dietary intake of methylmercury for a period of one or two months. The mercury concentration in each centimeter is plotted as a function of distance from the scalp of the individual. It may be seen that at the farthest distances from the scalp, the methylmercury concentration in the hair sample was very low, of the order of about 1 ppm. As one approaches the scalp, i.e., moving forward in time, the point is reached where there is a very rapid rise in the mercury concentration in the hair segment reaching a peak value after which a decline occurs. The rising phase corresponds to the period of intake of methylmercury in the diet and the falling phase corresponds to the clearance of methylmercury from blood. The two samples of hair were collected approximately six months apart and it may be seen that the peak positions, as measured from the scalp, differ by approximately six centimeters, corresponding to a growth rate of approximately one centimeter per month. Blood samples were also collected from this same person and knowing the growth rate of the hair and allowing approximately a one month's period between incorporation of mercury into the growing hair filaments and the appearance in the one centimeter next to the scalp, it is possible to directly compare blood concentrations with simultaneous concentrations in hair. An excellent correlation is seen in this individual (Figure 2). The hair concentration is approximately 300 times a simultaneous concentration in blood.

Under circumstances where the individual has received a pulsed exposure as described in Figure 1 and Figure 2, great care has to be exercised in the collection of the hair sample itself. If displacement of the individual strands of hair takes place during collection, transport, or storage, the past history of exposure may become blurred. An example of the relationship between the concentration profile in a single strand of hair versus the bundle of hair strands from the same person is indicated in Figure 3. It may be seen that the peak hair concentration and the area under the peak is approximately the same both in the bundle (50-100 strands) and in the individual strands. However, the concentration profile is much sharper in the individual strand, particularly with respect to the peak concentration. Furthermore, the peak concentration tends to be significantly higher than that seen in the bundle. In general, current analytical methods are not sufficiently sensitive to determine amounts of mercury in one centimeter segments in single strands of hair so that it is necessary to resort to the measurement of relatively large numbers of strands of hair, usually between 50 and 100. If lateral misalignment takes place in these strands, a blurring effect will occur with respect to the peak concentrations and with respect to the initial rising phase. This effect is illustrated in Figure 4. The upper figure diagrammatically represents a number of single strands of hair in a bundle showing lateral misalignment of each strand. Although the concentration profile in each strand is sharp (upper figure), when the group is measured a blurring effect occurs (lower figure). If the information required from the hair sample is the maximum blood concentration, or the precise measurement of the period of exposure to mercury, considerable care has to be taken to avoid misalignment of samples. Some misalignment is bound to occur due to differential rates of growth of individual strands of hair which cannot be avoided. This problem has been discussed in detail by Giovanoli and Berg (1974) who find that differences in growth rate for an individual strand has a standard deviation of about 15.

Opinions differ as to the importance of washing the hair sample prior to analysis for methylmercury. In general, individuals exposed to methylmercury from the diet would not normally experience any atmospheric contamination. However considerable care has to be exercised with regard to the possibility of the use of hair lotions or washes that may be contaminated by mercury. Some workers wash their hair sample prior to analysis with organic solvents such as acetone which results in a slight decrease in weight of the hair sample with a consequent increase in the observed concentration of mercury in the washed hair sample. In most situations a small change in concentration due to washing of the order of 10 % is of little practical importance. The separate determination of methyl and inorganic mercury in the hair sample may be useful as a possible index of external contamination since in most cases external contamination will be from inorganic mercury.

The concentration of total mercury in human milk in individuals exposed to methylmercury shows a close proportionality to the simultaneous blood concentrations (Figure 5).   The concentration in milk is usually between 5 and 10 % of the concentration in whole blood although studies on fish eating populations in Sweden indicate that this percentage may be higher at the lower levels of exposure (Skerfving 1974). Methylmercury in milk from mother to infant was an important source of exposure in the Iraqi outbreak and despite the low concentration in milk, the continued ingestion leads to accumulation in the suckling infant and to a more prolonged exposure than in the case of the mother. Milk samples, therefore, may be of considerable importance in assessing exposure of suckling infants in the event that their mothers have high blood levels of methylmercury.

Urine samples are not suitable for determination of exposure or body burdens of methylmercury.   Determination of total mercury in urine has no correlation with simultaneous blood levels with the Iraqi outbreak (Table 2).   In part, this is due to the fact that very little mercury is excreted in the urine and that most is in the inorganic form.   It is possible that methylmercury measured in urine by gas chromatography might correlate with blood levels but no studies have been done on this question.

Measurements of mercury in faeces of individuals exposed to methylmercury may be useful in assessing average daily intakes.   This would apply to individuals who have attained a balance with regard to methylmercury where faecal excretion would roughly balance daily intake.   Extensive studies on humans given radioisotopes, and on animals, indicate that faecal excretion accounts for about 90 % of total elimination from the body.

(b) Collection, Transport, and Storage

Blood samples for methylmercury analysis should be collected as described in the section for elemental mercury vapor.   However, in this case it is often more important to determine the haematocrit at the time of collection and also to separate plasma so that plasma-red cell concentrations may be determined.   The methods for transport and storage of the blood specimens are the same as that already described for metallic mercury vapor.   In addition, it should be noted that bacterial contamination of blood samples containing methylmercury   result in the conversion of some of the metal to inorganic mercury.

As large a sample as possible of milk should be collected since the concentration in milk is only 5 to 10 % of that in maternal blood.   Usually the sample is frozen immediately after collection and transported in this form to the site of analysis.   The same caveats with regard to cleanliness of the glassware, absence of bacterial contamination, apply to milk as already discussed above.   Some workers prefer to determine the protein and fat content of milk to see if there is any correlation between methylmercury and these parameters.   A major problem in interpreting methylmercury concentrations in milk is the large fluctuations in the concentration of the milk sample.   Inadequate information is available on what would be a suitable correction factor although it may be that the relation of the mercury concentration to the protein content of the milk might be a useful procedure.

Wherever possible a hair sample should be collected from the individual.   The procedure is to identify a suitable bundle of hair strands from the head hair, preferably the longest strands available.   These strands usually numbering 50 and 100 are held between finger and thumb, then clamped usually by a haemostat.   The hair is then cut with surgical scissors as close as possible to the scalp.   The hair sample may now be tied with cotton thread, usually about 1 to 2 cm away from the cut end.   Alternatively, the samples may be placed directly into a plastic bag, still held by haemostat, and fastened to the sides of the bag using a paper stapler with three staples usually placed about 2 cm away from the cut end.   Only after the hair sample has been tied, or secured to the sides of the bag with staples, should the haemostat be released.   The bag, usually a polyethylene plastic bag is closed and placed in an envelope for storage.   The bag should be labelled with a suitable marker pen.   The collection and packaging of the hair sample in this way allows convenient transport.   Storage is also easy in that the envelopes containing the hair sample are easily labelled and held in office files where they are readily identified for future analysis. Hair samples can be stored in this way for several years without any loss of mercury from the sample.

SUMMARY

Samples of blood and urine are the most suitable for assessing exposure to metallic mercury vapor. With suitable care, the samples may be collected and transported without serious problems. They do not lend themselves readily to long-term storage. There is some question as to how well mercury levels in urine and blood truly represent the concentration of mercury in the critical organ following exposure to mercury vapor.

Mercury concentrations in samples of whole blood or red cells are believed to reasonably reflect the concentration of methylmercury in the critical organ (i.e. the brain). This conclusion appears to hold well in both steady state and the non steady state exposures. The hair sample, when suitably collected and stored prior to analysis, represents an ideal means of recapitulating past exposures to methylmercury. Hair to blood ratios are about 300 but may vary from one individual to another. Thus it is always preferable to obtain at least one blood sample as well as a hair sample from an individual so as to determine the blood to hair ratio for that particular person. Determination of the concentration of mercury in milk may be important in situations where the mother of the suckling infant has had a substantial exposure to methylmercury.

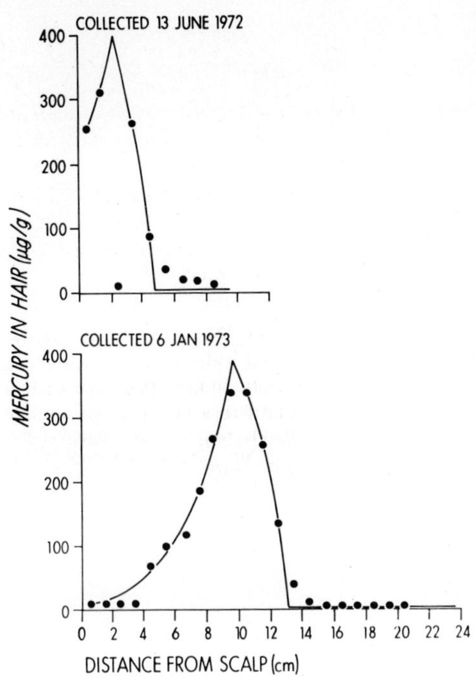

Fig. 1
The concentration of total mercury plotted according to the centimeter segment from the scalp. The two hair samples were collected from an Iraqi patient who had been exposed to methylmercury from contaminated homemade bread. One sample was collected in the summer of 1972 and the other in the winter of 1973.

Fig. 2
The correlation of simultaneous concentrations of total mercury in blood and corresponding centimeter segments in hair in the Iraqi patient described in figure 1. Altogether four hair samples were collected, two of which are depicted in figure 2.

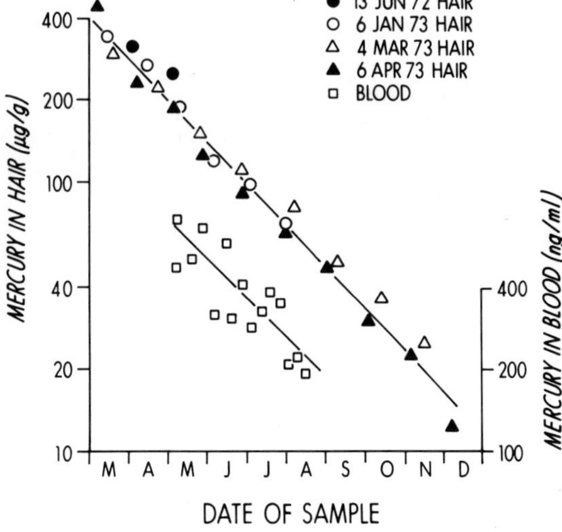

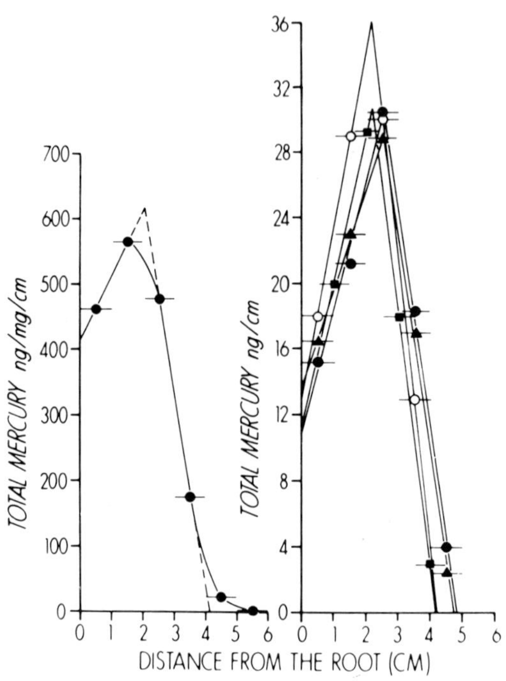

Fig. 3
The distribution of total mercury in hair from an Iraqi subject in a bundle of hair, (left) and in four individual hairs from an adjacent bundle, (right). This figure is taken from the publication Giovanoli and Berg (1974).

Fig. 4
A diagrammatic representation of the longitudinal distribution of mercury in individual strands of hair (upper figure) and in a bundle of hair (lower figure). The figures are intended to depict the consequences of lateral displacement or misalignment of individual hair strands (upper figure) showing a blurring of concentrations in a bundle of the same strands (lower figure).

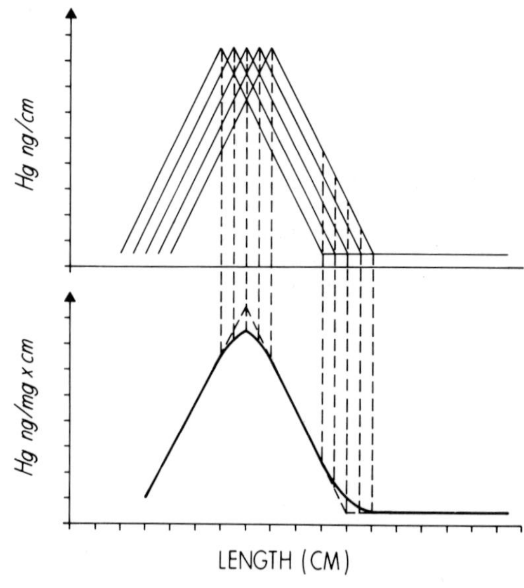

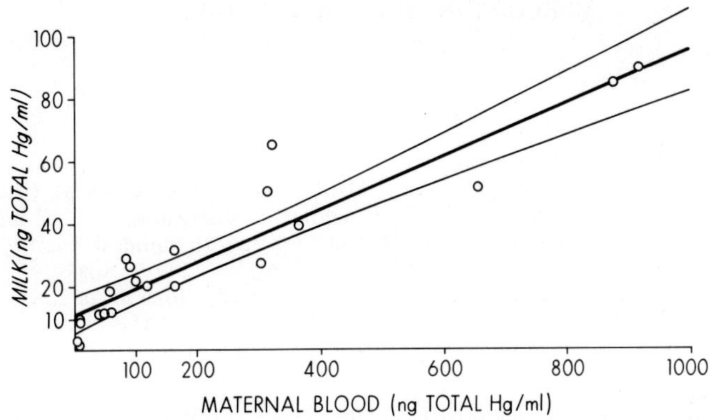

Fig. 5
The relationship between concentrations of total mercury in milk and in simultaneous concentrations in blood samples taken from an Iraqi mother who had been exposed to methylmercury during pregnancy. This figure is taken from Amin-Zaki et al , (1976).

TABLE 1

SOURCES OF ERROR DURING COLLECTION, TRANSPORT, STORAGE AND ANALYSIS

Sampling and collection . . . . E_s

Transportation and storage . . . . E_t

Preparation . . . . E_p

Analysis (machine error) . . . . E_a

Accidental event . . . . e

$$E_t^2 = E_s^2 + E_t^2 + E_p^2 + E_a^2 + e^2$$

TABLE 2

MERCURY IN BIOLOGICAL FLUIDS

Biological Fluid	N	MERCURY IN BIOLOGICAL FLUID		
		% whole* blood	Correlation with blood	% inorganic
Blood	224	100	1.0	7
Plasma	14	18	0.8	22
Milk	44	5	0.9	39
Urine	21	6	0.1	73
Cerebrospinal	5	6	**	**
Amniotic	1	2	**	**

(From Table 3 in Bakir et al 1973)

*   Figures based on the concentration of total mercury in the biological fluid and heparinized samples of whole blood.

**   Not determined

REFERENCES

AMIN-ZAKI, L., S. HASSANI, M.A. MAJEED, T.W. CLARKSON, R.A. DOHERTY and M.G. GREENWOOD (1976). Am. J. Dis. Child, **130**.

BERLIN, M. (1976). In : 'Effects and Dose-Response Relationships of Toxic Metals', Ed. G.F. Nordberg, pp.31, Elsevier, Amsterdam.

GIOVANOLI-JAKUBCZAK, T. and G.G. BERG (1974), Arch. Environ. Health **28**, 139-144.

GREENWOOD, M.G. and T.W. CLARKSON (1970). Amer. Ind. Hyg. Assoc. J., **31**, 250-251.

HURSCH, J.B., G. CHERIAN, T.W. CLARKSON and J.J. VOSTAL (1976). Archiv. Environ. Health (In press).

MAGOS, L., A. TUFFERY and T.W. CLARKSON (1964). Brit. J. Ind. Med. **21**: 294.

MAGOS, L. and A.A. CERNIK (1969). Brit. J. Ind. Med. **26**.

NORDBERG, G.F. and S. SKERFVING (1972). In : 'Mercury in the Environment', Eds. L. Friberg and J. Vostal, pp.29-91, CRC Press, Cleveland.

SKERFVING, S. (1974). Toxicol. 2:3.

SMITH, R.G., A.J. VORWALD, L.S. PATIL and T.F. MOONEY (1970). Amer. Ind. Hyg. Assoc. J. **31**, 687-700.

Subcommittee on the Toxicology of Metals (1976). In : 'Effects and Dose-Response Relationship of Toxic Metals', Ed. G.F. Nordberg, pp.31, Elsevier, Amsterdam.

TGMA (1973). Task Group on Metal Accumulation, Environ. Physiol. Biochem. **3** : 65-70.

THE ANALYSIS OF URINE SAMPLES AS A MEANS OF DETECTING EXPOSURE TO ENVIRONMENTAL ORGANIC CARCINOGENS

B. Commoner and A. Vithayathil
Center for the Biology of Natural Systems
Washington University
Saint Louis, Missouri

I. INTRODUCTION

This paper considers a relatively specific problem : the possibility of using stored urine as a means of determining the risk of cancer in human populations due to exposure to organic chemical carcinogens. The importance of such a procedure if it should be practicable, is evident from the following considerations :

1) At least in highly industrialized countries, a very large proportion of the incidence of cancer is due to environmental agents, most of which are organic chemical compounds, usually synthetic.

2) Efforts to control exposure to such chemical carcinogens require epidemiological analysis of the incidence of cancer, relative to body burden.

3) The occurrence of cancer is usually delayed by a number of years following exposure to a carcinogen ; hence stored samples capable of yielding data on body burden are important for retrospective epidemiological analyses.

4) As a result of the activities of the synthetic chemical industry new organic carcinogens are being continually introduced into the environment, many of which are not known to be carcinogens until long after they are introduced. For this reason, and because of the lag-time inherent in the carcinogenic process, it is likely that in future years it will become necessary to learn, retrospectively, whether populations have been exposed to substances not now known to occur, as carcinogens, in the environment.

5) Most organic carcinogens are active only after metabolic conversion in the body to metabolites, which may be excreted in the urine. Hence the detection of a substance which is **inherently** carcinogenic in urine may be taken as evidence not only that an individual has been exposed to the precursor of this metabolite, but also that the substance is likely to act as a carcinogen **in that individual**. (Evidence relative to this point is presented below).

Thus, there would be value in the storage of urine samples for the purpose of concurrent or later analysis to determine the presence of metabolically transformed (or, in some cases, untransformed) compounds that, on the grounds of epidemiological or animal studies, are believed to act as carcinogens.

To achieve this goal, there is an initial prerequisite : achieving a capability for the analysis of numerous samples, each likely to contain a number of compounds, some of which are carcinogenic (but not all of them as yet identified as such). The method must also be sufficiently rapid and inexpensive to enable the numerous analyses that are required in epidemiological studies.

Until recently, the methods for detecting carcinogens were not suitable to the attainment of these goals. One possible strategy is to use conventional fractionation and analytical methods (e.g., GC/MS) to identify **all** the synthetic organic compounds that occur in a sample. However, such methods would require analyses so detailed as to demand very large samples ; they would also be so expensive as to preclude the large numbers of analyses needed for epidemiological studies.

Another complicating factor is that present tests do not determine, unambiguously, that a substance is carcinogenic toward people. Present determinations of carcinogenicity involve long-term observations of two or more species of laboratory animals, which may respond to exposure to a given carcinogen in different ways depending on the route of administration and other factors such as diet and the sex of the animal. Such studies often show that a given substance is highly carcinogenic toward some species and wholly inactive toward others.

Therefore, the demonstration that a given substance is an active carcinogen toward one or more laboratory species does not always signify that it is also carcinogenic toward people, but only that it **may** be. Relative to people, then, such a substance should be regarded as a **presumptive** carcinogen. (Accordingly, in this paper the term 'carcinogen' will be reserved for those substances known to cause cancer in people, and the term 'presumptive carcinogen' will be used to designate a substance shown to cause cancer in one or more species of laboratory animals, but not as yet in human beings.)

Fortunately, as a result of certain recent studies, it is now possible to develop a more effective strategy. Samples can be rapidly screened for **bacterial mutagenesis**-- an activity which, it can now be shown, correlates closely with the capability of synthetic organic compounds to induce cancers in laboratory animals. Thus the method is an effective screening technique for **presumptive** carcinogens. At the same time, a further development of the technique also offers the possibility of determining which presumptive carcinogens are in fact carcinogenic toward people.

This approach has its origin in recent developments in research on the biochemistry of carcinogenesis. Among the very considerable mass of data produced by such studies, two areas are most relevant to the problem under consideration here : the metabolic fate of carcinogenic agents in the body, and the relation between carcinogenesis and mutagenesis.

It is now known that most carcinogenic substances must be converted, metabolically, into an active substance before cancer is induced. (For example, 2-acetylaminofluorene, AAF, must be converted to a proximal carcinogen, such as N-hydroxy AAF, before carcinogenesis occurs.) Such observations have helped to resolve ambiguities regarding variations in the carcinogenicity of a given substance toward different species. Thus, when fed, AAF is a powerful hepatocarcinogen in the rat, but is totally inactive in the guinea pig because, unlike the rat, the guinea pig does not convert AAF to N-hydroxy AAF metabolically. On the other hand, N-hydroxy AAF causes cancer in both animals. Metabolic activation is usually due to hydroxylase enzyme systems localized in the microsomal fraction of liver and other tissues.

On theoretical grounds there is reason to expect a close connection between carcinogenesis and mutagenesis, based on the hypothesis that both processes originate in the cell's genetic apparatus. This led to the simple idea that any substance that is carcinogenic should also be mutagenic and **vice versa**. However, it has been found that there are many exceptions to this expectation. For example, while AAF is a powerful carcinogen, it is not mutagenic.

However, the foregoing results regarding the formation of active carcinogen metabolites suggested the solution to the ambiguity–that the active substance produced by metabolic conversions of the original carcinogenic substance is **both** the proximal cancer-producing agent and the mutagen. Thus, it has been found that, while AAF is not a mutagen, N-hydroxy AAF **is**. Another result of these studies was the observation that derivatives of the active metabolites may appear in the urine of carcinogen-fed animals.

Based on such results an effective system for measuring the mutagenic activity of microsome-activated carcinogens, using specially developed strains of **Salmonella typhimurium**, has been developed by Ames, et al.[1] As will be shown below, this method provides the basis for the sought-for urine test, capable of assessing exposure to synthetic organic carcinogens that occur in the environment.

The Ames test has been validated by comparing the responses, in this test, of compounds which have been previously shown to be active carcinogens toward laboratory animals (usually rat and/or mouse) and compounds which are non-carcinogenic. Such comparisons, of organic compounds covering a wide range spectrum of structures ranging from aliphatic compounds to polycyclic hydrocarbons, show that the test can distinguish between the two classes of compounds with a reliability of the order of 80-90 percent.[2,3] Accordingly, in the terminology adopted above, the Ames test is capable of detecting, with a satisfactory degree of reliability, organic compounds that are **presumptive** carcinogens.

As already indicated, exposure of a human being to a presumptive carcinogen (i.e. a substance which is known to cause cancer in one or more species of laboratory animals) does not **necessarily** mean that there is a risk that cancer will actually develop. However, it is possible to use the mutagenesis test to answer this question as well–i.e., to determine whether or not a given species is likely to respond positively to exposure to a substance which has been shown to be carcinogenic toward some other species.

On the basis of the considerations discussed earlier, one can formulate, as an hypothesis, that those species in which a given substance produces tumors are capable of metabolizing that substance to the **intrinsically** active form, whereas a species in which the substance does not produce cancer is unable to carry out this metabolic process.   The Ames test is readily able to distinguish between a substance such as AAF, which is **not** intrinsically active, and a substance such as N-hydroxy-AAF, which is.   AAF will produce mutant bacterial colonies only if a microsomal preparation is present, whereas N-hydroxy-AAF will produce mutant colonies even in the absence of the microsomal preparation.   Hence, if in a carcinogen-fed animal, an active metabolite were to become stabilized (for example, by conjugation to form a glycoside) and excreted in the urine, its presence could be detected by a mutagenic response in the test system in the absence of a microsomal preparation.   Such evidence would indicate that the particular species is likely to develop tumors when exposed to that carcinogen.   Conversely, if the urine of an animal exposed to a presumptive carcinogen does not contain mutagenic material that is active in the absence of a microsomal preparation, this would suggest that the metabolic conversion of the carcinogen does not occur in that species which is therefore not likely to develop tumors. We have carried out a test of this hypothesis by studying the mutagenic activity of urine from rats and guinea pigs after feeding with AAF.   The results are reported in Table I, from which it is evident that, in keeping with the foregoing hypothesis, inherently active mutagens are present in the rat urine, but not in the guinea pig urine.

These results indicate that, at least as an heuristic hypothesis, there is merit in determining by means of the **Salmonella** test, whether metabolites of carcinogens to which people may be fortuitously exposed occur in urine.

II.   THE OCCURRENCE OF ORGANIC CARCINOGENS IN THE ENVIRONMENT

Some of the very large amounts of synthetic organic compounds that are now manufactured enter the environment as a necessary outcome of their use (for example : pesticides and solvents used in inks and paints which evaporate into the air as these products dry).   Many of them escape into the workplace environment, and may affect those who work in it.   Others are disseminated into the environment as wastes, either intentionally or by accident, from industrial plants.   In addition, various industrial combustion processes inadvertently produce organic compounds--some of which are carcinogenically active--that are disseminated into the environment.

These considerations suggest that the environment, in particular air and surface waters, must contain some numbers of synthetic organic compounds which are responsible for a considerable part of the incidence of cancer in the populations of industrialized countries.   However, thus far only a few substances have been identified as environmental carcinogenic agents because they have caused actual cases of cancer in people exposed to them.   The earliest example is exposure to substances in coal tar.   In 1775 Sir Percival Pott observed that cancer of the scrotum was characteristic of the chimney sweeps, and it was later shown that this was due to polycyclic hydrocarbon carcinogens such as benzo(a)pyrene, present in coal tar.   Coke oven workers are still, today, exposed to these same carcinogens and experience a considerably elevated cancer incidence.   The latest example of an environmental carcinogen that remained undetected until it caused cancer in people, is vinylchloride.   More general evidence of the impact of environmental agents on the incidence of cancer is a recent study by the National Cancer Institute, which shows that cancer mortality is most pronounced in urban and industrialized areas, and particularly where the regional density of the petrochemical industry is high.[4]

There is reason, therefore, to regard the commercial production and use of synthetic organic chemicals as a major source of environmental carcinogens.   The total production of synthetic organic chemical in the U.S. has increased exponentially in the last 30 years at an average annual rate of increase in 1962-1971 of 11 percent.   Large-scale production of synthetic organic compounds is a postwar phenomenon ; annual production increased tenfold between 1946 and 1966.   This fact, plus the lag-time that is expected between exposure to a carcinogen and the appearance of cancers (generally of the order of 16-25 years) suggests that the actual effect of such substances on the incidence of cancer in industrialized countries may just now begin to appear.

From these considerations it is apparent that human populations may be exposed to organic carcinogenic compounds through many routes : ambient air, water supplies, food, and contact with industrial products.

124

The occurrence of a carcinogen, benzo(a)pyrene, in urban air has been known for some time. More recently, in collaboration with the City of Chicago Department of Environmental Control, we have begun to carry out Ames tests on particulate samples ($4cm^2$ of filter papers) from different regions of the City. Mutagenic activity of **hexane-isopropanol** extracts of these air particulates is shown in Figure 1. The amount of mutagenic activity is roughly proportional to the amount of air particulates in the sample. Chromatographic fractionation of such particulate extracts indicates that at least two, and probably more, constituents are present which are mutagenic and are therefore likely to be presumptive carcinogens (see Figure 2). Recent analyses of U.S. water supplies reveal the presence of a number of presumptive carcinogens, apparently originating in industrial effluents[5]. As shown in Table II, our own analyses of effluents from chemical plants near Houston, Texas, reveal the presence of presumptive carcinogens in certain effluents. Certain commonly used food additives have been shown to be presumptive carcinogens[6]. The most notable instance which has occurred in the general population are hair dyes[7]. Much more numerous instances are known among industrial workers, especially in the chemical industry.

Except for relatively specific industrial situations, the available data regarding the nature of organic carcinogens to which human populations are exposed, and the intensities of exposure, are far too limited to provide useful generalizations. However, the epidemiological evidence indicates that exposures to certain substances must be sufficiently high to appreciably affect the incidence of cancer, and the continuing expansion of the petrochemical industry indicates that these levels will increase in the future.

III. ANALYTICAL PROCEDURES

The foregoing considerations suggest the value and feasibility of using the analysis of urine for substances capable of elevating the rate of mutation in the **Salmonella** (Ames) test as a means of assessing the exposure of human populations to presumptive carcinogens. Since the method is relatively new and experience with human populations is relatively limited, the analytical procedures must be regarded as subject to improvement and suggestions regarding the collection of human samples must be regarded as highly preliminary.

The basic procedure for detecting mutagenic activity has been described by Ames and others[2, 8, 9, 10]. Specially developed strains of **Salmonella typhimurium** are used. These strains have a histidine negative genome (and are therefore unable to grow unless histidine is present in the culture medium) and include other genetic factors that render them specially sensitive to chemical mutagenesis. One of Ames' strains (TA 1535) is designed to detect mutations due to base-pair substitutions and therefore tends to respond selectively to mutagens such as alkylating agents. Two strains (TA 1538 and TA 1537) detect frameshift mutations ; TA 1538 responds particularly well to a number of carcinogens such as 2-nitrofluorene ; TA 1537 responds to carcinogens such as 9-aminoacridine. Each strain also includes in its genome mutations that greatly increase its overall sensitivity to mutagens. One of these causes loss of DNA excision repair system and the other the loss of the lipopolysaccharide barrier that coats the surface of the bacteria (thus enhancing the penetration of the large molecules).

Mutation causes the bacteria to revert to a histidine-positive genome (i.e., the mutant bacteria can now synthetize histidine). Mutant colonies can therefore be detected by their growth on a nutrient medium that lacks histidine. In practice, nutrient plates are seeded with a suitable **Salmonella** strain ; the substance to be tested is added, together with an aliquot of a microsomal preparation. Substances are usually also tested in the absence of the microsomal preparation to determine whether they are, themselves, proximal carcinogens that are active without metabolic transformation. After 48 hours of incubation the mutant colonies are counted (on replicate plates) and compared with controls lacking the substance or sample being tested.

Using this standard Ames technique, we have previously shown that mutagenic metabolites can be found in the urine of rats after the feeding of certain chemical carcinogens[11]. Results of this type are shown in Table III. However, such urine analyses involve certain methodological difficulties : (a) The compounds of interest are likely to occur as water-soluble conjugates of water-insoluble constituents. Since the conjugates are usually mutagenically inactive it is necessary to split off the added group, such as a glucuronate moiety, by incubating with β-glucuronidase.

(b) Since the active substances may be present in urine at low concentrations, there may be insufficient numbers of mutant colonies produced in the **Salmonella** test unless relatively large amounts of urine are used.   However, this induces problems due to the possible presence of histidine in the urine, which stimulates the growth of the histidine-less test strains, giving false indication of enhanced mutation.   (c) Since the urine is aqueous, and the foregoing steps occur in an aqueous medium, it is feasible to concentrate the active agents (once split off from the conjugated groups) by extraction in a suitable organic solvent.   Although this step also reduces possible interference from histidine, it is time-consuming.

The procedure which we have described earlier overcame some of these difficulties and was able to yield data regarding the presence of mutagenic metabolites produced from at least two well-known carcinogens, 2-acetylaminofluorene (AAF) and N, N-dimethylaminoazobenzene (DAB), although in the latter case the number of mutant colonies was rather low.   As shown below, we have also used this technique in a preliminary way, to test human urine samples.   However, the procedure involves several complex steps and is so slow as to be unsuitable for the large numbers of analyses that would be required in any field test, which is the ultimate aim of developing this technique.

Accordingly, we have now adopted the alternative approach of carrying out the entire procedure (i.e., enzymatic hydrolysis of the active materials, treatment with the microsome preparation and the mutagenic step) in liquid medium rather than on the nutrient plate.   This has the advantage of eliminating the time-consuming extraction steps, but it has certain disadvantages associated with the low concentration of active materials expected in urine samples.   However, by incubating the preparation for extended periods of time, revertant bacteria formed as a result of contact with the mutagen may multiply sufficiently so that a small aliquot of the incubation mixture contains sufficient numbers to yield a satisfactory colony count.   This approach also makes it possible to overcome the problems created by the presence of histidine in the urine ; by using only a small aliquot of the original sample for plating purposes, the histidine content of the urine is sufficiently diluted to have no effect on the plate.

After a number of trials based on this approach the following procedure was adopted : A 5 ml sample of urine to which   β-glucuronidase is added (1,200 units/ml of urine) is sterilized by millipore filtration.   A 0.1-3.0 ml aliquot of the urine sample is placed in a 50 ml Erlenmeyer flask with 1 ml of standard rat liver microsome preparation (prepared from rat liver after induction with either PCB or sodium phenobarbital) together with 2 ml of a complete nutrient medium (i.e., containing histidine).   The entire mixture, amounting to a total of 3-6 ml forms a thin layer (about 5 mm thick) on the bottom of the flask, so that aeration--which is essential for the activity of the microsomal oxidase enzymes--is effective.   An inoculum of an appropriate **Salmonella** strain is then added and the flask is incubated at 37°C for 16 hours.   At that time a 0.1 ml aliquot of the incubation mixture is transferred into 2 ml of melted top agar (45° C) containing a small amount of biotin but lacking histidine (in this procedure it is not necessary to add a small amount of histidine to the plate to facilitate sufficient growth to allow mutation to occur--this phase having already been accomplished in the incubated solution) and plated out on a standard **Salmonella** test plate containing minimal medium.   The plate is then incubated at 37° C for 48 hours and the number of revertant colonies counted in the usual way.

Results comparing the above procedure with the conventional one using a standard AAF solution (in place of urine), are shown in Figure 3.   It is evident that the new procedure yields values that are comparable to those obtained with the standard procedure, and in fact is significantly better at very low concentrations of AAF.   Table IV shows typical results yielding by the new methods from urine obtained from a rat injected with 10 mgm of AAF (the urine sample collected for a 24-hour period immediately following injection), as compared with urine from a control rat not treated with AAF.   The results show that (a) when the procedure is carried out in the presence of β-glucuronidase, a very significant, easily counted number of revertant colonies is observed ; (b) in the absence of the enzyme the number of revertant colonies is significantly reduced, indicating that most of the active material is in the form of glycosides, but that some intrinsically active material (i.e., not requiring microsomal activation) is present ; (c) analyses of urine from the control animal give no evidence of activity.

A test of the capability of the method for detecting mutagenic metabolites in the urine of DAB-fed rats (0.06 % DAB, 19 days) is shown in Figure 4.   It is evident that the method is capable of detecting active material in as little as 0.1 ml of urine with colony counts that differ considerably from the background values obtained with urine from an animal on a control diet.

These results indicate that the liquid incubation method outlined above may be successfully employed to detect mutagenically active materials in very small amounts of urine from carcinogen-fed rats (0.1-0.2 ml as compared with approximately 1 ml required for the conventional method).

As indicated earlier, it may be possible by means of analysis of human urine for mutagens to determine whether an individual is exposed to a carcinogen which is capable of being metabolized and therefore, in accordance with the foregoing hypothesis, likely to induce tumors in that species. As an initial step in this strategy we began preliminary analyses of human urine samples by means of the extraction technique originally described.[11] Figure 5 summarizes these results. The data include analyses of urine samples from a group of research laboratory workers ; a group of individuals including some exposed in the workplace to a variety of synthetic organic compounds (analysed blind) ; a group of workers exposed to possible carcinogens in the workplace. The urines were fractionated, according to the method described earlier[11] following enzymatic and acid hydrolysis and the mutagenic activity ratios* of material occurring as glycosides (Fraction I) and as sulfate esters (Fraction II) were determined separately. However, because of the large amount of urine needed for analyses carried out by this method, it was possible only to carry out analyses in the presence of the microsomal preparation.

It should be emphasized that the results described in Figure 5 are not intended to provide evidence regarding the relative occurrence of urinary mutagens in chemical workers and others. The numbers involved in this preliminary population of samples are clearly too small to support such a determination. Rather, what is pertinent about these results is that they show the range of values of mutagenic activity that occurs in the human urine samples. It is evident that most of the values center around a ratio indicative of the absence of mutagenic activity, with only a small fraction of the individuals exhibiting ratios in the range of 2.5-5.0. This suggests that the range of 'normal background' values of urinary mutagenic activity rations is sufficiently narrow so that the occurrence of samples with values above 5.0 can be regarded as positive. Figure 5 shows that six urine samples fell in this elevated range ; four of them happen to be chemical workers and two non-chemical workers.

The ultimate aim of the urine test is to provide a rapid and inexpensive method of analysing human urine in order to determine whether an individual is exposed to (and metabolizing) an environmental carcinogen. Because of its complexity, this original plate method would probably be too slow and expensive to be used in large-scale epidemiological studies. However, the liquid system described above simplifies the procedure significantly. We have now begun initial tests of urine from our own laboratory workers by means of the new liquid method in order to begin to establish a baseline for the further use of this method. The initial results are shown in Table V, together with comparative analyses of several samples by means of the original plate method.

Table V shows, first, that with one possible exception all the samples are negative with respect to mutagenic activity. The variation among the samples is about the same in the two methods. Thus, the liquid method gave values, with TA 1538 in the presence of microsomes, ranging from 16 to 63 colonies, with a control value of 45, while the plate method, under the same conditions, gave values ranging from 13 to 32, with a control value of 13. It is of interest that the one value which, according to the liquid test, may be positive (No. M-0-5, with 18 colonies, against a control of 1, in the absence of microsomes) was not positive, under these conditions in the plate test.

On the basis of these results, we are now prepared to apply the new, more rapid (and apparently more sensitive) liquid technique to initial screening of human urine samples from different environmental conditions.

---

*Mutagenic activity ratio is defined as $E - C/\bar{C}$ where E is the number of mutant colonies per plate when the compound is present, C is the corresponding value for the control, with the compound absent (obtained on the same day), and $\bar{C}$ is the historical average control value for all the tests done in our laboratory for the bacterial strain in the presence of the particular microsome preparation.

IV.   OTHER CONSIDERATIONS

Because the procedure described above has been applied to samples of human urine in only a very limited way, little can be said as yet about logistic, organizational and related problems.   However, on the basis of current experience the following relevant observations can be made :

1) Samples :

Urine samples should be chilled immediately and frozen as soon as possible in order to prevent bacterial action or other processes that might degrade the sought-for metabolites. In our experience the activity of urine samples from carcinogen-treated rats is stable for at least six months, in the frozen condition.   This suggests that long-term storage is feasible.   It is possible that analyses might be carried out on samples of blood ; studies on this problem are now underway in this laboratory.

2) Interpretation of results :

In interpreting the raw data yielded by the **Salmonella** test careful consideration must be given to methods of computing the influence of control, or blank values.   We have prepared a method based on the computation of a 'mutagenic activity ratio'.   This procedure yields a numerical value which, on the basis of results obtained with known non-carcinogens and presumptive carcinogens, can be used to determine to which of these classes of compounds an unknown sample should be assigned, and with what precision this can be done.[2]   Thus, the end result is a **qualitative** distinction between a non-carcinogen and a presumptive carcinogen.   It is important to recognize that a numerical value--i.e., the number of mutant colonies observed-- derived from the **Salmonella** test cannot be regarded as a quantitative measure of the degree of mutagenicity or carcinogenicity.

3) Programme design :

It is obvious that the use of the proposed analytical technique must be carefully guided by environmental and epidemiological considerations.   In general, the following sequence of steps seems indicated:

(a)   Analysis of environmental samples (air, dust, water, soil, food) should be carried out, using the Ames test, in order to assess the environmental levels of presumptive carcinogens, and to trace their origins and movement in the environment.

(b)   Fractionation of the foregoing samples, and mutagenic analyses of the fractions, should be carried out with the ultimate aim of identifying the substances responsible for their mutagenic activity.

(c)   'Biological monitoring' of populations exposed to various levels of presumptive carcinogens can then be carried out by means of urine analyses.   Where samples are active they can be fractionated, so that the mutagenic metabolites present in the urine can be compared with the active agents found in environmental samples.

(d)   'Collections for future reference' of urine samples can then be organized in connection with the establishment of epidemiological studies of the affected populations.

4) Cost of analyses :

The cost of urine analysis depends on the degree of detail desired--i.e., the number of **Salmonella** strains and sample concentrations used in the test.   For the plate test each plate counted is likely to cost on the order of $ 2.00 at present.   With multiple strains and concentrations the total cost of analysing a sample might amount to $ 100-200.00 under ordinary laboratory conditions.   This cost might be reduced significantly in a laboratory solely devoted to this analysis, as a routine.   The liquid system involves similar costs at present.   However, in this case it would be possible to automate the analysis by using optical absorbency as a measure of bacterial growth.   This might reduce the cost considerably.

REFERENCES

1. AMES, B.N., W.E. DURSTON, E. YAMASAKI, and F.D. LEE, **Proc. Nat. Acad. Sci., 70,** 2281 (1973).

2. COMMONER, B, 'Reliability of Bacterial Mutagenesis Techniques to Distinguish Carcinogenic Chemicals' Final Report to the U.S. Environmental Protection Agency, EPA-600/1-76-022 (April, 1976)

3. McCANN, J., E. CHOI, E. YAMASAKI, and B.N. AMES, **Proc. Nat. Acad. Sci., 72,** 5135 (1975).

4. HOOVER, R., and J.F. FRAUMENI Jr., **Environmental Research, 9,** 196 (1975)

5. KEITH, L.H., A.W. GARRISON, F.R. ALLEN, M.H. CARTER, T.L. FLOYD, J.D. POPE, and A.D. THRUSTON Jr., in 'Identification and Analysis of Organic Pollutants in Water' pp. 329-373, edited by Laurence H. KEITH, Ann Arbor Science Publishers, Inc., Ann Arbor, Mich. (1976).

6. YAHAGI, T., T. MATSUSHIMA, M. NAGAO, Y. SEINO, T. SUGIMURA, and G.T. BRIAN, **Mutation Research, 40,** 9 (1976).

7. AMES, B.N., H.O. KAMMEN, and E. YAMASAKI, **Proc Nat. Acad. Sci., 72,** 2423 (1975)

8. AMES, B.N., J. McCANN, and E. YAMASAKI, **Mutation Research, 31,** 347 (1975)

9. BARTSCH, H., C. MALAVEILLE, R. MONTESANO, **Cancer Research, 35,** 644 (1975)

10. FRANTZ, C.N., and H.V. MALLING, **Mutation Research, 31,** 365 (1975)

11. COMMONER, B., A.J. VITHAYATHIL, and J.I. HENRY, **Nature, 249,** 850 (1974).

TABLE I

METABOLITES OF AAF IN RAT AND GUINEA PIG URINE

Urine Sample	Diet	No. of Days on Diet	Equivalent Amount of Urine/Plate	Number of Colonies per Plate (TA 1538)	
				Without Liver Microsomes	With Liver Microsomes
Rat Urine I (before hydrolysis)	0.06% AAF	7 days	4 ml	76	1,820
Rat Urine II (after β-glucuronidase hydrolysis)	0.06% AAF	7 days	4.2 ml	696	1,624
Rat Urine III (after acid hydrolysis)	0.06% AAF	7 days	5.25 ml	292	319
Guinea Pig Urine I	0.06% AAF	13 days	4 ml	24	287
Guinea Pig Urine II	0.06% AAF	13 days	4 ml	16	330
Guinea Pig Urine III	0.06% AAF	13 days	4 ml	7	22

TABLE 11

MUTAGENIC ACTIVITY OF AQUEOUS EFFLUENT SAMPLES FROM

INDUSTRIAL SOURCES AT THE HOUSTON SHIP CHANNEL

SAMPLE NUMBER	EFFLUENT SOURCE	TYPE OF SAMPLE	DATE OF COLLECTION	EQUIVALENT AMOUNT OF SAMPLE PER TEST (ml)	NO. OF COLONIES/ PLATE*		MUTAGENIC ACTIVITY RATIO**
					Control	Experimental	
1	Pulp Mill	Black Liquor	10-3-75	1	31	36	0.2
2	Pulp Mill	Outflow Water	10-3-75	50	41	32	-0.4
	Pulp Mill	Outflow Water	10-3-75	125	41	47	0.3
	Pulp Mill	Outflow Water	10-3-75	250	41	63	1.0
3	Steel Mill	Outflow Water	9-5-75	25	42	41	0
	Steel Mill	Outflow Water	9-5-75	62.5	42	64	1.0
	Steel Mill	Outflow Water	9-5-75	125	42	17	-1.1
4	Petrochemical Plant A	Outflow Water	9-23-75	125	26	86	2.6
	Petrochemical Plant A	Outflow Water	9-23-75	250	26	82	2.4
5	Petrochemical Plant B	Return Sludge	6-26-75	5	17	35	0.8
6	Chemical Plant A	Outflow Water	6-26-75	100	42	41	0
7	Chemical Plant B	Outflow Water	6-26-75	25	22	11	0.5
8	Indust. Waste Treatment Plant A	Outflow Water	9-23-75	50	36	53	0.7
	Indust. Waste Treatment Plant A	Outflow Water	9-23-75	125	36	58	1.0
	Indust. Waste Treatment Plant A	Outflow Water	9-23-75	250	36	83	2.0
9	Indust. Waste Treatment Plant B	Outflow Water	9-23-75	50	31	127	4.2
	Indust. Waste Treatment Plant B	Outflow Water	9-23-75	125	31	182	6.6
10	Indust. Waste Treatment Plant B	Outflow Water	1-5-76	100	17***	259***	24.2

*   Tested on Strain TA 1538 in the presence of rat liver microsomes (phenobarbital-induced).

**   Mutagenic Activity Ratio $= \dfrac{E - C}{C_{Av.}}$, where

E is the number of colonies per experimental plate (i.e. with sample present); average of two plates.

C is the number of colonies per control plate (i.e. identical to experimental plate except that sample is not included; carried out on the same day); average of two plates.

$C_{Av.}$ is the historic control value for the indicated strain and microsome preparation (i.e. the average of daily controls over an extended period of time).

***   In the absence of liver microsomes.

TABLE III

MUTAGENIC ACTIVITY OF URINE OF
CONTROL AND CARCINOGEN TREATED RATS

Compound	Class*	Route & Dose of Administration	Fraction**	Equivalent Amount of Urine/ Plate (ml.)	Number of Revertant Colonies/Plate							
					TA 1535		TA 1537		TA 1538		TA 100	
					No Micro-somes	With Micro-somes	No Micro-somes	With Micro-somes	No Micro-somes	With Micro-somes	No Micro-somes	With Micro-somes
Control	---	---	I	1.25	7	9	6	15	10	25	118	208
	---	---	II	"	11	5	10	5	25	20	289	343
	---	---	III	"	6	6	10	11	8	15	275	300
Acetylaminofluorene	C-1	0.06% In diet (2 weeks)	I	1.25	11	9	10	73	32	2359	--	--
			II	"	15	18	15	67	115	7000	--	--
			III	"	7	8	15	153	219	1470	--	--
6-Aminochrysene	C-1	0.06% In diet (2 weeks)	I	1.25	1	6	4	53	17	31	--	--
			II	"	1	3	8	421	10	1845	--	--
			III	"	0	7	7	143	15	1026	--	--
o-Tolylazotoluidine	C-1	0.06% In diet (2 weeks)	I	1.25	5	8	4	12	9	196	--	--
			II	"	0	5	2	29	11	650	--	--
			III	"	2	7	8	21	39	3910	--	--
3,3'-Dichlorobenzidine	C-1	0.06% In diet (2 weeks)	I	1.25	--	--	--	--	--	58	--	--
			II	"	--	--	--	--	--	405	--	--
			III	"	--	--	--	--	--	207	--	--
1,2,5,6-Dibenzanthracene	C-1	50 mg. I.P.	I	1.3	--	--	--	--	19	77	--	--
			II	"	--	--	--	--	15	19	--	--
			III	"	--	--	--	--	20	28	--	--
N,N-Dimethylamino-azobenzene	C-2	0.06% In diet (2 weeks)	I	1.25	12	21	8	--	4	600	--	--
			II	"	11	22	1	--	9	275	--	--
			III	"	14	19	4	--	10	75	--	--
3'-Methyl-N,N-dimethyl-aminoazobenzene	C-2	0.06% In diet (2 weeks)	I	1.25	17	21	2	--	5	115	--	--
			II	"	9	17	4	--	9	55	--	--
			III	"	5	25	2	--	4	60	--	--
N-Nitrosodiethylamine	C-2	50 mg. I.P.	I	1.2	7	8	11	10	28	45	312	377
			II	"	6	10	17	11	21	50	298	345
			III	"	7	14	15	17	22	37	311	339
N-Nitrosodimethylamine	C-2	25 mg. I.P.	I	2.3	10	12	8	5	32	48	296	299
			II	"	11	13	9	13	41	40	332	409
			III	"	14	18	11	11	34	40	333	353
Thioacetamide	C-3	50 mg. I.P.	I	3.0	9	9	14	8	32	42	355	484
			II	"	9	13	9	8	43	24	291	402
			III	"	22	16	6	14	38	42	408	324
Auramine O	C-3	25 mg. I.P.	I	1.3	1	8	6	9	11	15	118	173
			II	"	7	7	6	9	40	24	139	220
			III	"	6	10	4	13	17	39	138	191
Safrole	C-3	0.05 ml. I.P.	I	1.1	7	6	3	5	12	30	249	319
			II	"	10	9	7	9	25	40	276	430
			III	"	19	16	5	16	6	31	408	343

*   Class C-1 represents compounds which yield a positive response in the standard _in vitro_ Salmonella test,
Class C-2 represents compounds which are negative in the standard _Salmonella_ test but become positive in the absence of DMSO after preincubation with PCB-induced liver microsomes,
Class C-3 represents compounds which have yielded negative results in all _in vitro_ tests thus far.

** Fractions I, II and III represent sequential ether extracts of straight urine, β-glucuronidase hydrolysed urine and acid hydrolysed urine respectively. For details of the extraction and the bacterial test procedure see reference 2.

TABLE IV

MUTAGENIC ACTIVITY OF URINE
OF RATS INJECTED WITH AAF

Sample	Equivalent Amount of Urine/Flask	β-Glucuronidase Treatment	No. of Colonies/Plate (TA 1538)	
			Without Liver Microsomes	With Liver Microsomes
Urine from Control Diet	3	—	14	13
Urine from Control Diet	3	+	19	23
Urine from AAF-Injected Rat	3	—	30	255
Urine from AAF-Injected Rat	3	+	48	1073

TABLE V

Mutagenic Activity of Human Urine Samples

Sample No.***	Type****	Volume of urine/5 ml medium (ml)	Liquid Culture Method*					Standard Plate Method**					
				No. of Revertants/0.1 ml of Culture Medium				Equivalent amount of urine/ plate (ml)		No. of Revertants/Plate			
			Date of Analysis	TA 1535		TA 1538			Date of Analysis	TA 1535		TA 1538	
				No microsomes	With microsomes	No microsomes	With microsomes			No microsomes	With microsomes	No microsomes	With microsomes
Control (no urine)			10/27/76	1	2	1	45		11/3/76	1	5	9	13
M-0-5	N	2	10/27/76	4	4	18	25	1	11/3/76	2	5	6	29
M-0-5		0.5	10/27/76	1	2	5	76						
M-0-10	N	2	10/27/76	2	3	3	46	1	11/3/76	1	4	9	13
M-0-10		0.5	10/27/76	1	3	3	49						
F-0-15	N	2	10/27/76	2	3	3	50	1	11/3/76	2	4	8	20
F-0-15		0.5	10/27/76	3	4	3	41						
M-0-15	N	2	10/27/76	3	7	6	16	1	11/3/76	1	2	6	13
M-0-15		0.5	10/27/76	0	3	2	63						
Control (no urine)			11/3/76	2	4	2	24		11/5/76			11	17
M-1-2	S	2	11/3/76	2	2	3	35	2	11/5/76			14	32
M-1-2		0.5	11/3/76	2	3	4	47	0.5	11/5/76			20	24
M-1-4	S	2	11/3/76	2	7	1	23	2	11/5/76			6	16
M-1-4		0.5	11/3/76	1	3	5	23	0.5	11/5/76			14	20
M-0-6	N	2	11/3/76	4	2	5	38	2	11/5/76			6	24
M-0-6		0.5	11/3/76	3	3	4	24	0.5	11/5/76			18	22
M-0-8	N	2	11/3/76	3	3	5	44	2	11/5/76			12	18
M-0-8		0.5	11/3/76	2	2	2	25	0.5	11/5/76			12	18
Control (no urine)			11/15/76			1	32						
F-1-18	S	2	11/15/76			0	24						
F-1-18		0.5	11/15/76			1	55						
F-0-14	N	2	11/15/76			0	33						
F-0-14		0.5	11/15/76			1	29						
M-0-12	N	2	11/15/76			4	30						
M-0-12		0.5	11/15/76			1	32						
F-0-16	N	2	11/15/76			1	49						
F-0-16		0.5	11/15/76			1	18						

*After adding β-glucuronidase the urine sample was sterilized by millipore-filtration. Samples were incubated in nutrient broth; see note, Table I, for counting procedure.

**After incubation overnight with β-glucuronidase the urine was extracted with a mixture of benzene/isopropanol (80:20).
The extract was evaporated to dryness and taken up in DMSO, and aliquots were tested against the bacteria by the standard plate method.

***Sample numbers beginning with letters M and F represent males and females respectively.

****Letters S and N represent smokers and nonsmokers respectively.

Figure I

Mutagenic Activity of Chicago Air Particulate Samples
240
200
160
120
80
40
0
Number of Mutant Colonies/Plate
0
100
200
300
400
Concentration of Air Particulates (μgm/M³)

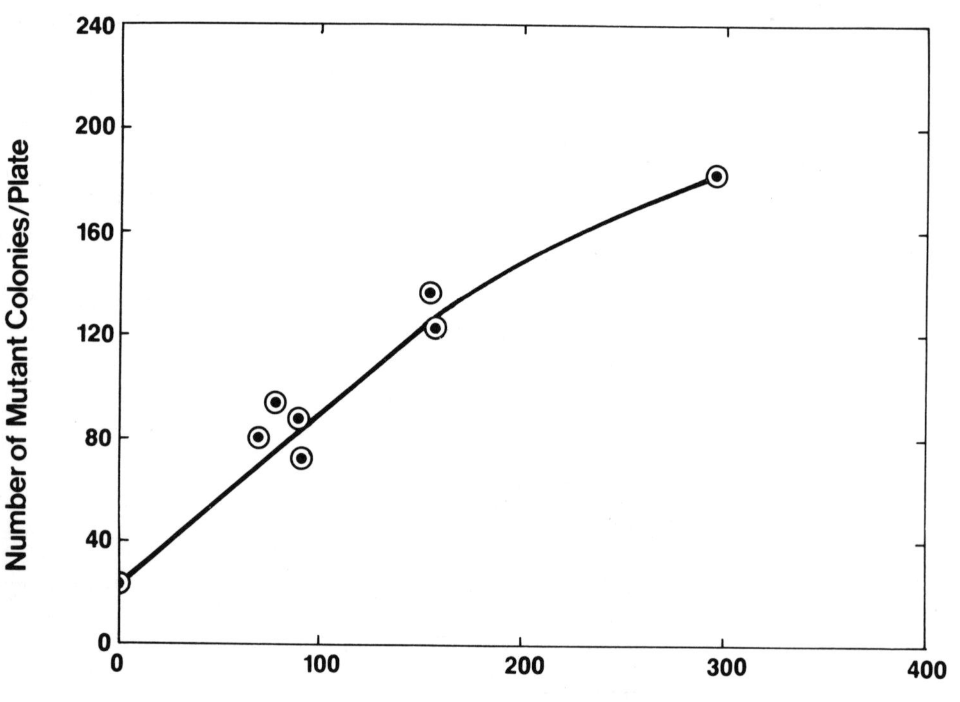

Figure 2

TLC Fractionation of
Chicago Air Particulate Samples
Number of Mutant Colonies/Plate
300
250
200
150
100
50
Sample No. 44195
Particulate Conc:
298 µg/M³
Control Value
Sample No. 01167
Particulate Conc: 241 µg/M³
100
50
Control Value
Sample No. 01166
Particulate Conc: 228 µg/M³
100
50
Control Value
-1 0 1 2 3 4 5 6 7 8 9 10 11 12
Chromatographic Zone (cm. from origin)

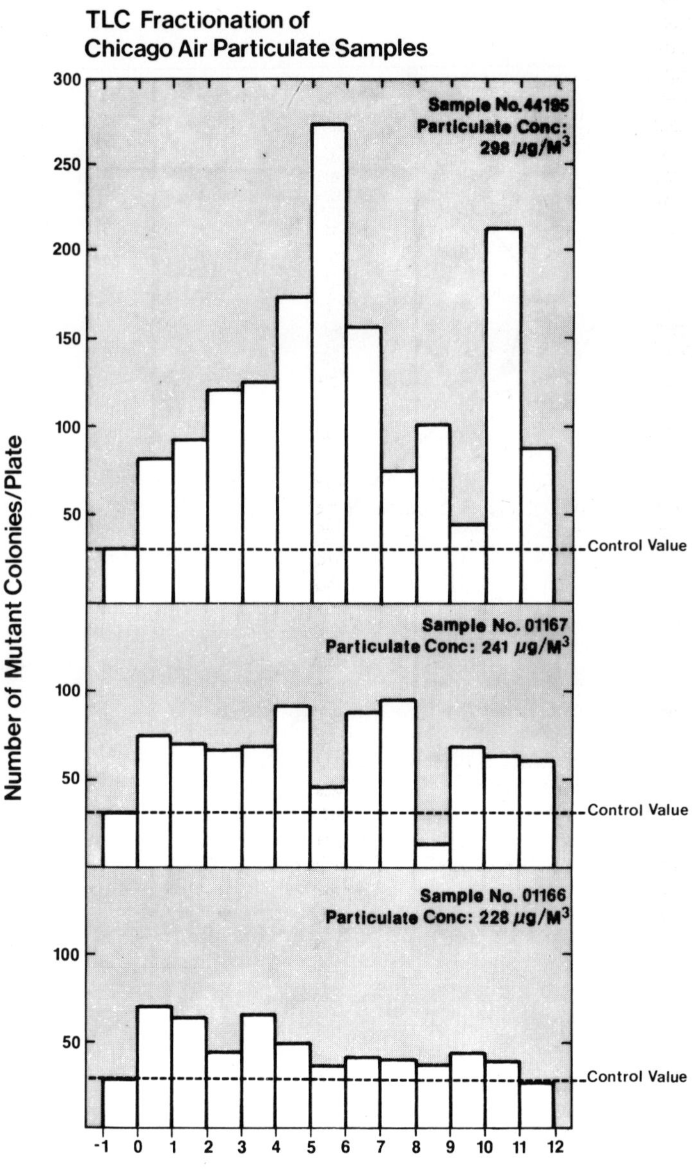

Figure 3

Salmonella Test of AAF by the
Liquid Culture and the Standard Plate Method.

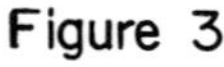

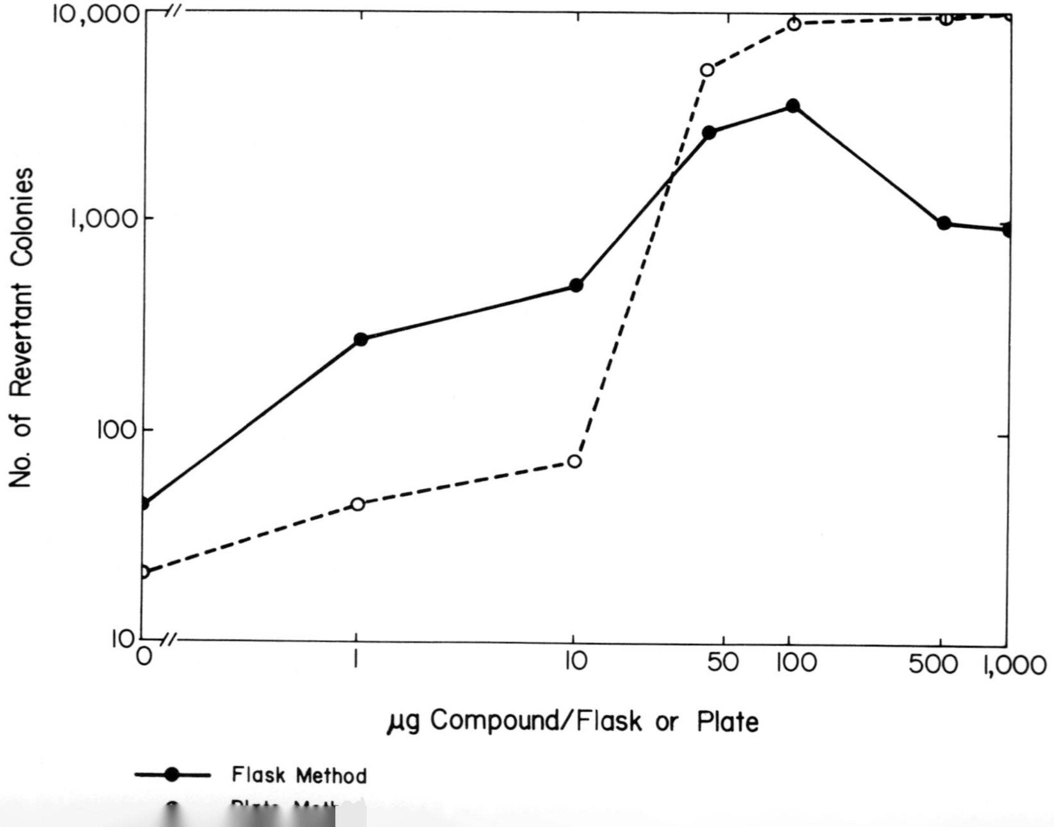

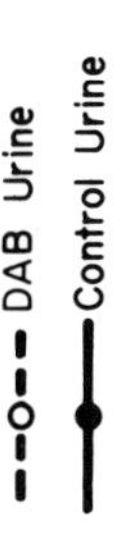
Figure 4
Mutagenic Activity of Urine of Rats Fed Control and DAB Diets (19 days).
TA 1538
No. of Revertant Colonies
400
300
200
100
0
.1
.2
.5
.75
1.0
1.5
2.0
Amount of Urine/Flask (ml)
DAB Urine
Control Urine

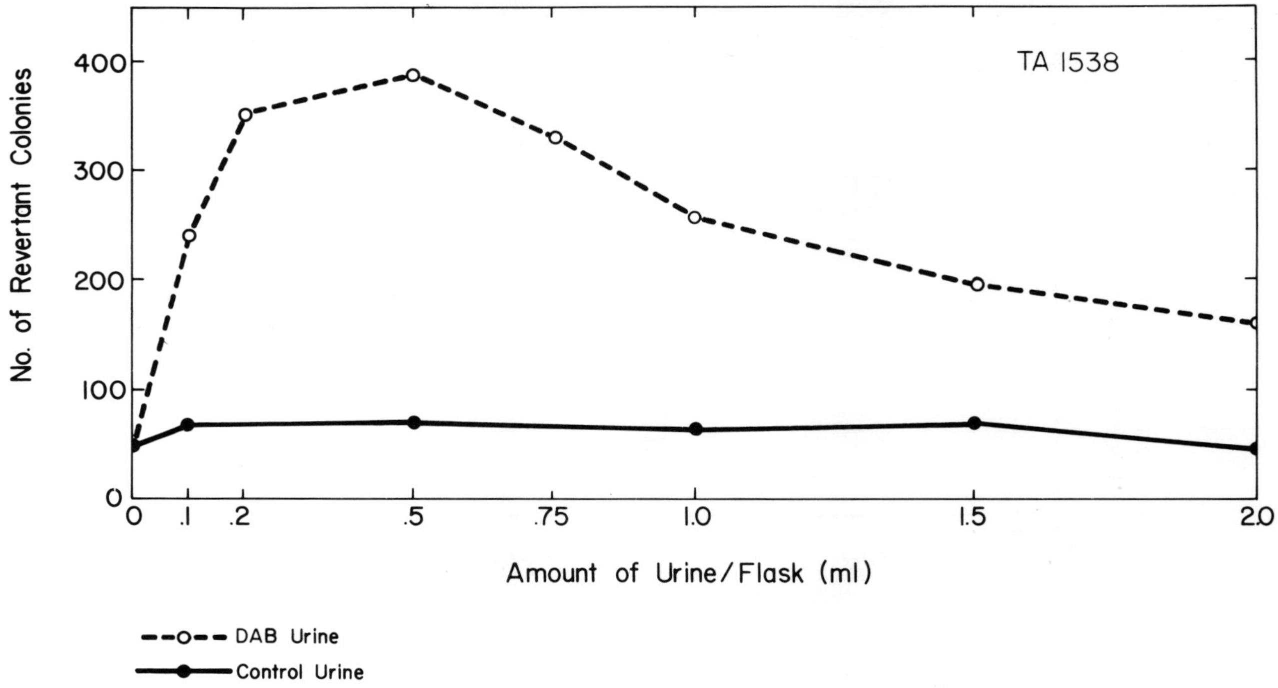

Figure 5

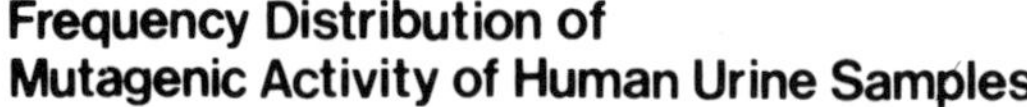

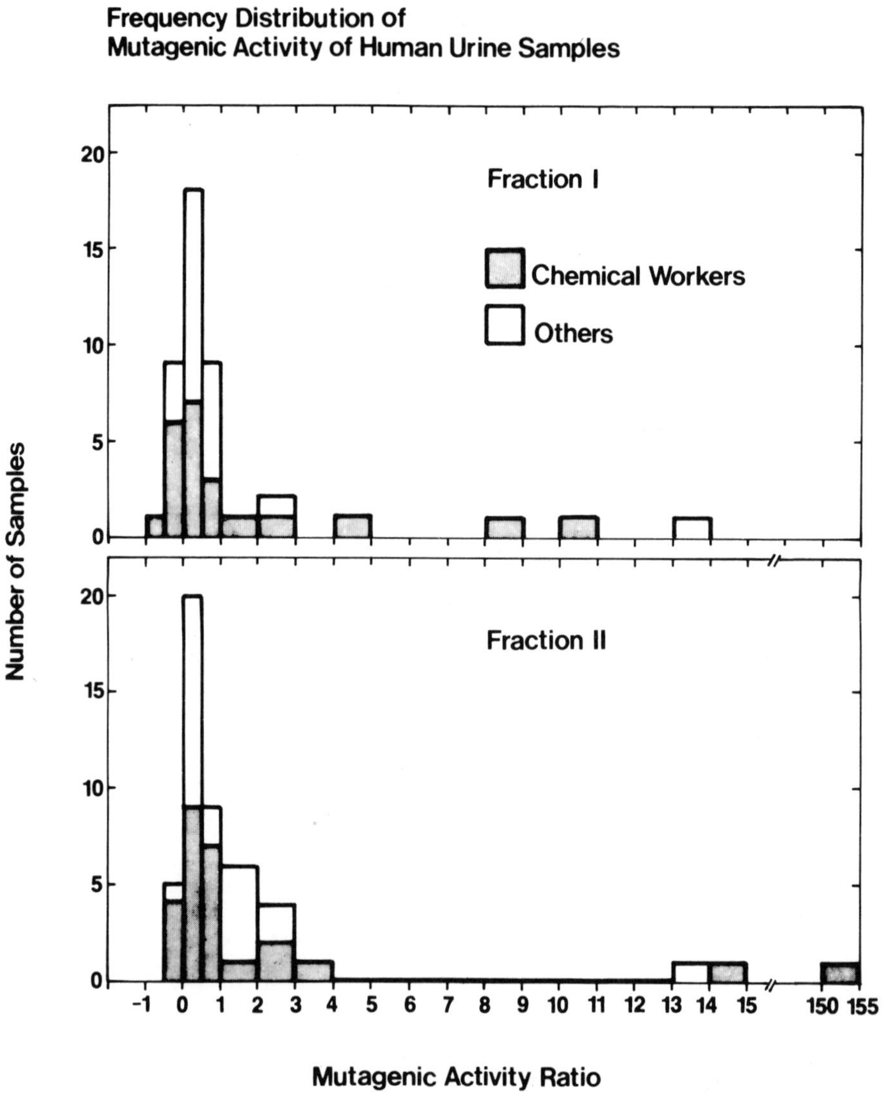
Frequency Distribution of
Mutagenic Activity of Human Urine Samples
Fraction I
Chemical Workers
Others
Fraction II
Number of Samples
0
5
10
15
20
-1 0 1 2 3 4 5 6 7 8 9 10 11 12 13 14 15 150 155
Mutagenic Activity Ratio

ORGANIC AND INORGANIC COMPOUNDS: ANALYTICAL ASPECTS

H. Egan
Laboratory of the Government Chemist, London

In reviewing analytical aspects of the assessment of exposure to environmental pollution of human populations there are a number of variables which must be taken into account. One feature is general however: the interest is virtually exclusively confined to trace analysis. To begin with it is necessary to distinguish between analyses for various purposes such as routine health screening, screening for regulatory control, screening in emergency circumstances following accidental over-exposure and reference measurements for research purposes, perhaps at subclinical levels.

Physiological responses to exposure to environmental pollutants vary widely in character and this fact has a substantial influence on the type of sample which is of interest. Toxicity problems which are obviously acute in character will first involve the examination of the normal range of physiological fluid and other biopsy samples; this may extend to environmental media to which the populace may be exposed including the atmosphere and the dietary intake. Chronic situations may be relatively well characterized by analytical parameters, though there is still room for considerable discussion even in some areas which have been studied for many years, such as the relative significance (and the levels concerned) of lead in blood and urine. On the other hand for chronic exposure situations the analytical interest may in practice be more meaningful in relation to the source of exposure rather than to human tissue. This is notably the case for the carcinogens or potential carcinogens such as mycotoxins, polynuclear aromatic hydrocarbons and N-nitrosamines. The analytical methods now in use for these are among the most sensitive in regular use today; but this is not to say that there may not be an interest in developing yet more sensitive methods which could, for research purposes, be applied to human tissue including physiological fluids. In considering pollutants I will try for each group to give a brief understanding of the analytical approach, the levels of interest and the limits of detection involved; but it is important to realise that in most cases there is relatively little point in following day to day levels in human tissues.

The general range of sample substrates of environmental interest thus varies with the pollutant. Blood and urine levels may be of interest for trace metal pollutants such as lead, cadmium or mercury and subcutaneous fat for organochlorine pesticide residues and certain other persistent compounds including the polychlorobiphenyls (PCBs). Whether these substrates are of interest for carcinogens such as polynuclear aromatic hydrocarbons is not yet known, the presumption being that if they are, then the levels concerned are below — perhaps substantially below — the normal current limits of detection. For such pollutants (if that is the right word in this context) the amount in the environmental media to which man is exposed — air, water, food — is at present of greater interest. And whilst it would be wrong not to recognize that current trace methods of analysis can be improved as regards sensitivity, specificity and accuracy, any substantially lower levels of special significance might be associated with new and as yet undiscovered species. To preserve biological tissue in storage for long periods against the possibility of the discovery later of better methods of examination for factors significant in this way has the added difficulty that (by the nature of the exercise) the storage characteristics of the substances involved are unknown. It is perhaps appropriate in this context to consider what materials, appropriately preserved a century (or a millennium) ago, one would wish now to examine using present-day trace analytical methods. Whilst this does not provide a full answer to the possibility that something completely new, as yet undiscovered, might not emerge later, the essential difficulty of not being able in advance to ensure that the unknown factors remain unaffected in long storage now is still daunting.

In the present context, the pollutants of interest tend to be chronic in their action rather than acute. This is to some extent reflected in their relation to biological, chemical or physical stability to degradation, which varies among the synthetic hormones, antibiotics, so-called persistent organochlorine pesticides, mycotoxins, nitrosamines, polynuclear aromatic hydrocarbons, trace metals and asbestos fibres. Whilst the short-term stability afforded biological samples by simple chemical preservation or anticoagulant treatment in general may have no significant effect on any of these pollutants which may also be present, such treatments are not appropriate to longer-term storage. The latter calls for the lyophilization (freeze drying) of tissue or fluid samples; and freeze storage. However many contaminants, including pesticides, mycotoxins and industrial chemicals, are not stable indefinitely. There is evidence of solid state reactions even when stored at very low temperatures: thus unsaturated fats may oxidize in freeze-dried samples. Such measures therefore may not provide stability over periods longer than a few months for the less stable of the pollutants and further work on storage stability over longer terms than a year or so is needed. There is no short cut to this: and there are some complications, notably the question of the standardization of analytical methods and the need in many areas for reliable biological standard reference materials for analysis.

The question of the standardization of analytical methods has given rise to considerable discussion in recent years. The International Federation of Clinical Chemists among others, have given the matter particular attention, to the extent that there are currently proposals for international definitions for types of method, a distinction being drawn between a method which after exhaustive investigation is found to have no known source of inaccuracy or ambiguity (definitive method), one that can be accomplished with generally available equipment and which after exhaustive investigation has been shown to have acceptable, known inaccuracy in comparison with a definitive method (reference method) and other less demanding types of method (1). The development of even a reference method is a major exercise, that conducted by the American Association of Clinical Chemists also illustrating the reference material problem: in this, diacetone glucose (1,2:5,6-di-0-isopropylidene-D-glucofuranose) was selected as a standard for glucose because of ease of preparation and its simple, well characterized mass fragmentation behaviour (2).

Instability on long-term storage is a limitation in the interest in analysis of samples treated in this way, except insofar as analysis is itself a measure of the instability: at the same time, there is considerable interest in the standardization (perhaps the term 'stabilization' also would not be appropriate) of analytical methods themselves. Whilst long-term storage thus presents some difficulty, it is doubtful whether in view of the high sensitivity of the methods now available it would be worthwhile holding such samples (even if this were feasible) for long periods of time against the later development of more sensitive methods. The methods at present available in general offer adequate sensitivity although there may be some scope, as indicated above for the improvement of reproducibility between laboratories. It seems likely that storage of tissue samples to await the recognition of new factors and the development of analytical methods for their determination will also be of limited value, since the question of the stability of the new factors and the significance of results from the stored samples will also arise. It is difficult enough to ensure that the trace environmental factors at present recognized are stable during long-term storage and more work is necessary here if this is considered to be a desirable objective. But, as already indicated, it is impossible to design long-term conditions such that factors as yet undiscovered will remain unchanged during storage.

Biological Specimens and Individual Pollutants

The type of human biological specimen of interest in context of exposure to environmental pollutants can differ for different pollutants. For some there is uncertainty as to the relevance of human specimens, the main substrate of interest being the medium for the ingestion of the pollutant (air, water, food for example). The main substrates of interest are blood, urine and other physiological fluids (trace metals and possibly nitrosamines, toxic gases, polynuclear aromatic hydrocarbons and other hydrocarbons) muscle tissue (antibiotics, synthetic hormones), various organs including kidney and liver (trace metals, some pesticides, asbestos) and subcutaneous or other fatty tissue (organochlorine compounds). The relevance of biological samples, particularly in the long-storage context, is unclear for mycotoxins, nitrosamines and a number of organic materials including polynuclear aromatic hydrocarbons and vinyl chloride. There are other complications such as the relative stability of sample substrate and trace pollutant and the long-term relevance of subclinical levels of significance. For these reasons it is the most convenient to deal with individual pollutants. The analytical aspects of these are considered in the following paragraphs with indications for each of the limits of detection and stability on long-term storage (6, 7). The picture is far from complete and there is something of a need to define the long-term storage problem — what substrates, what levels of pollutants and for how long.

Nitrosamines

Trace Nitrosamine analysis has been the subject of considerable attention in recent years, mainly in relation to foods in the preparation of which nitrates or nitrites may have been used. Like most other procedures for trace analysis this involves a preliminary extraction or separation stage, a detection and estimation stage (which is the basic analytical observation) and a stage in which the identity of the species is confirmed. The latter is of particular importance in trace nitrosamines work because of the wide variety of possible interferences; and usually calls for the use of a mass spectrometer coupled to a gas chromatograph. Nitrosamine work is thus expensive. It is also relatively slow since the sensitivity requirement is high and the gas chromatographic analytical stage may have to be used near to the limit of detection; the gas chromatographic method is normally successful only if selective detection systems are used. For these reasons it is usual also to insert a concentration stage into the analytical procedure, so that the trace nitrosamines extracted or otherwise separated from the food sample at the beginning of the analysis are concentrated into approximately 0.5 ml of an appropriate solvent before gas chromatographic examination. The initial extraction stage, normally steam distillation or solvent extraction is the most time-consuming usually taking 2 to 3 h per sample. The length of the gas chromatography and mass spectrometry stages depends on the number and molecular weight of the nitrosamines sought. If a range of C_1 to C_4 and heterocyclic nitrosamines are included, chromatography may take 1-2 h but this can be shortened by the use of pressure programming and programmed elution techniques.

Samples of greatest interest are cured meats and fish and some cheeses. In some cases, for example fried bacon, formation takes place during the cooking of bacon. Some of these foods may contain 1-10 microgram/kg of nitrosodimethylamine or certain other nitrosamines, the lower limit of detection being about 0.1 microgram/kg. Nitrosamines are decomposed by ultraviolet irradiation, initially to nitramines. Sample extracts in the course of examination are therefore stored (where necessary) in the dark at 5-10°C, preferably in a sealed container: extracts held in this way are stable for several months.

Pesticide Residues

The principal area of interest has for many years been the organochlorine compounds, mainly dieldrin, HCH, DDT and its immediate degradation products. The interest has also extended to a number of other more-or-less persistent organochlorine compounds, notably the polychlorobiphenyls (PCBs) which have a variety of industrial uses. Analytical methods based on gas-liquid, thin-layer and more recently high-pressure liquid chromatography, supported as necessary by other techniques including high-resolution mass spectrometry, are now in regular and routine service. When used in conjunction with suitable extraction and clean-up techniques (of which the chromatographic processes themselves may form part), limits of detection down to about 0.05 mg/kg are possible with thin-layer chromatography. With gas-liquid chromatography limits of detection vary slightly with the retention time but levels down to 0.001 mg/kg (1 μg/kg) are usually attainable though for most purposes levels as low as this are not always appropriate. Hexachlorobenzene residues may be significant in some countries and have on occasion been confused with isomers of hexachlorocyclohexane (HCH) on account of similar retention times on some stationary phases commonly used in gas chromatography.

Abbott et al have described a gas-chromatographic procedure for the estimation of organochlorine compound residues in human fat based on the use of diethylene glycol succinate on silanized Chromosorb P and a cyanosilicone column (9, 10). Samples may be held in deep-freeze storage for several months pending examination. They are then first freed from non-fatty tissue and dried with cellulose tissue, extracted with hexane and the extract cleaned up by dimethylformamide solvent partition followed by alumina column chromatography. An electron capture detector is used in the subsequent gas chromatographic examination; the identity of the residues found may be confirmed by thin layer chromatography (11). These aspects were also discussed at an earlier European Colloquium in Luxembourg (12). Although this is usually regarded as a satisfactory means of preserving samples for residue analysis, it may not always be convenient or practicable. Moreover it may not fully inhibit the break-down of some compounds; pp'-DDT has been reported as breaking down to pp'-TDE in liver (4). 4 per cent formaldehyde solution has been suggested as a preservative for tissue samples; 10 per cent phenol is also effective (5).

The PCB compounds are of interest for their ability to interfere with trace organochlorine pesticide residue analyses but at the same time they may be a convenient index of pollution (or potential pollution) situations. The methods of estimating levels differs from that used for pesticides since it is necessary to refer to some convenient standard mixture of material rather than to a single standard reference material: one approach has been to measure the total chromatographic peak area on the chart record and interpret this in terms of the weight of pp-DDE (which is not a PCB compound) which gives the same response. The limit of analytical detection for PCBs in biological media is of the order of 0.01 mg/kg or 0.002 mg/l for milk.

Organophosphorus pesticide residues, for the most part much less persistent, can also be estimated by similar methods but detection limits in routine work tend to be somewhat higher, of the order of 0.003 mg/kg, but it is seldom necessary to work down to such levels. It is not normally appropriate to consider long storage for samples. Increasing attention is being paid to residues of other pesticides including triazine and chlorophenoxy compounds and a wide range of analytical techniques is used to cope with these, mainly in water and plant tissue. Determination limits depend on the particular combination of compound and method, but normally fall between 0.1 and 0.01 mg/kg.

As regards the stability of pesticide residues in biological tissue during storage, experience relates mainly to organochlorine residues in human and fats such as dieldrin, DDT and DDE isomers, HCH isomers in deep freeze storage: no significant changes are found on re-examination at intervals of up to a year. The general review of stability published by Kanar, de Batista and Gunther (17) deals with the cold storage of foods and extracts of both organochlorine and organophosphorus compounds: stability is influenced by temperature, substrate and duration.

Vinyl Chloride Monomer

Vinyl chloride (vinyl chloride monomer, VCM) is a gas at normal temperatures and pressures but traces may be occluded in polyvinyl plastics materials and subsequently leached from these. The monomer polymerizes on exposure to light or under the influence of certain catalysts; and whilst relatively stable at room temperature, traces, where they occur in biological tissue, cannot be considered as stable indefinitely even when the tissue is held in deep freeze. The analytical approach is gas chromatographic, using a solvent extract (for example butan-Z-one) of the sample material followed by direct injection, or headspace gas analysis. Levels of interest are below 1 mg/kg, the detection limit in food being of the order of 0.05 mg/kg or 0.005 mg/l for liquids.

Antibiotic Residues

Antibiotic residues may occur in meats, including poultry meats, following the veterinary use of these materials, usually as injections or as additives to feeds. Veterinary usage currently permitted within the Community is confined to a few selected antibiotics at low levels as growth promoting feed additives. The methods of analysis available have mainly been used to establish that residues in food, where these occur, are so low as to be of no practical significance. Residues in muscle tissue are detected by direct application of the sample to seeded agar plates; using an agar-gel diffusion technique, the limits of detection vary depending on the potency of the antibiotic relative to the test organism used but are of the order of 0.1 to 0.5 µg/g. Antibiotic residues arising from the treatment of farm animals may also occur in milk, due in most instances to failure to observe the recommended withdrawal periods between treatment of the cow and resumption of marketing the milk. Samples should be examined as quickly as possible. If storage is necessary chemical preservatives may not be used. Low temperature or drying can be considered but antibiotic activity may diminish. Freeze-drying followed by cold storage is to be preferred but frozen tissue samples may if subsequently transmitted unfrozen give 'false positive' reactions after a day or two, owing to the formation by normal spoilage microflora of natural bacterial inhibitory substances, perhaps including a C18 unsaturated fatty acid. Deep-frozen milk retains penicillin activity for a few months; dried milk powder shows a variable loss, possibly depending on the moisture content.

Synthetic Hormones

Synthetic hormones such as hexoestrol, diethylstilbestrol (DES) and methyl testerone may be used in beef cattle and poultry meat production either by implantation in vivo or by incorporation in feeds. Both chemical and biochemical methods are available for residue detection. In biochemical testing, the uterine method depends on the increase in weight of immature female rats or mice after the ingestion of oestrogens; this assay is sensitive but not specific. An alternative method depends on the change in the histological character of vaginal smears after oestrogen treatment. This test is specific but not sensitive but in combination with the uterine method it can detect 2 to 10µg/kg of oestrogen. Both gas-liquid and thin layer chromatographic chemical techniques are available with similar limits of detection.

Radio-immunological methods are both specific and sensitive, being capable of detecting down to 2-10 ng/kg. They use a specific radio-labelled antigen for each hormone to be detected but, on account of their high sensitivity, are also liable to interference by hormones naturally present.

Mycotoxins

Toxic mould metabolites may arise as a result of the growth of spoilage moulds on foods and feeding stuffs. The aflatoxins result from a limited number of strains of Aspergillus and Penicillium species, and eight compounds of related molecular configuration are now recognized, aflatoxins B_1, B_2, B_{2a}, G_1, G_{2a}, M_1 and M_2. Over 100 mycotoxins are known in all, including also zearalenone, patulin and ochratoxin; these are potent carcinogens to many animal, piscean and avian species.

Analytical methods employed are generally based on chromatographic procedures, principally TLC, for the purification and separation of the individual compounds. Mixtures of chloroform and methanol in various proportions, together and with acetic acid, have been used as development solvents with silica gel as a support. Detection and semi-quantitative estimation have generally been achieved by the use of visual fluorescence techniques under illumination by UV radiation, the limits of detection and the relative fluorescence intensities of the various aflatoxins depending on whether the fluorescence is observed on a solid support or in solution. In methanol for example the detection limits for aflatoxins B_1 and G_1 are respectively $2 \cdot 10^{-2}$ and $5 \cdot 10^{-4}$ µg/ml, but on solid TLC supports about 0.2µg per spot of aflatoxin B_1 (blue fluorescence) and 0.1µg per spot of aflatoxin G_1 (green fluorescence) may be detected. The presence of non-characteristic pale-white fluorescence may be used to reduce the detection limits of TLC plates by approximately one order of magnitude. For confirmation of aflatoxin B_1, adduct reactions using formic acid-thionyl chloride, acetic acid-thionyl chloride and trifluoroacetic acid have been proposed, fluorescent spots with modified R_f values being obtained with the adducts formed. Irradiation degradation of the aflatoxins B_1 and G_1 on silica gel has also been used as a means of confirmation, three products with reduced R_f values being revealed by UV irradiation for each. Other methods used include paper and partition column chromatography, but the limits of detection of silica gel have been found to be superior to those obtained on other supports. Similar analytical methods are used for other mycotoxins but gas chromatographic methods have also been used for zearalenone as the tri-dimethylsilyl ether derivative with a limit of detection of about 0.5µg.

Substrates usually examined are foods, notably cereals, for which partition methods, both liquid/liquid and liquid/solid have been used as a means of preparing extracts. Column systems using Celite, Florisil and silica gel have been described following extraction with methanol-water or aqueous acetone-hexane. Pigments and other interfering materials can be removed with hexane, tetrahydrofuran or diethylether. Solvents for desorption of aflatoxins include chloroform-hexane and chloroform-methanol. Aflatoxin M_1 has been detected in milk at a level of 0.3 mg/l and has been directly related to the ingestion of approx. 1 mg of aflatoxin B_1 by a 500 kg cow. Aflatoxin M_1 has been detected in human urine from subjects known to have ingested contaminated peanut butter.

Asbestos Fibres

Asbestos is a mixture of silicates of iron, magnesium, calcium, sodium and aluminium. It occurs naturally as a fibre in various forms, the three most important being chrysotile, crocidolite and amosite. These are normally characterized and counted by purely physical means. Physical or chemical methods may be used for the preliminary removal of extraneous matter from the sample. Tissue counting techniques have been described by Oldham (21) and Pooley (22): the latter concludes that no single method of preparation for electron microscopy examination is yet available. Optical microscopy is normally used for identification, supported where necessary by X-ray diffraction spectrometry or scanning electron microscopy. The examination involves the measurement of fibre size (length to breadth ratio) and count, the latter normally being restricted to fibres of length greater than a specified minimum (say 5µm) and exceeding a specified length to breadth ratio (say 3), and a diameter less than 3µm. The limit of detection (length) by visual optical means is about 0.5µm. The stability of the fibres is characteristic and any question of long storage of samples is a matter of the preservation of the substrate.

Trace Metals

Many methods have been developed over the past 50 years for the detection and estimation of traces of arsenic and such metals of environmental interest as copper, mercury, lead and cadmium. These have been principally colorimetric or spectrophotometric in nature, often based on the use of selective (if not specific) organic reagents especially developed for the purpose; but the methods also extend to almost every other technique in analytical chemistry, including for example coulometry, polarography, gravimetry and chromatography. The technique which has become the general method choice in most control laboratories is atomic absorption spectroscopy. The usual method for biological tissue involves preliminary oxidative destruction of organic matter, either by wet oxidation with nitric and sulphuric acids or by dry ashing in a platinum dish, although some fluids, for example, can be examined with no preliminary treatment at all. Where the highest sensitivity is required, the trace element from the sample or sample digest can be concentrated into a small volume by extraction with a suitable organic complexing agent, ammonium pyrrolidine dithiocarbamate being widely used in conjunction with 4-methyl-pentan-2-one solvent extraction for cadmium, lead and nickel. In this way lead and cadmium levels down to about 0.05 mg/kg and 0.01 mg/kg respectively can be measured in most tissues (15) and 0.002 mg/l for cadmium and 0.01 mg/kg for lead in fluids. Special interest attaches to the analyses of blood and other biological fluids for lead and their delta-aminolevulinic acid dehydratase (ALAD) activity as an indicative or supplementary test for this, both of which (for blood) are the subject of a current draft Directive. Heparinized blood may be stored at 4° if necessary before ALAD estimation, but not for longer than 24 h.

Trace mercury analyses are also most conveniently done by atomic absorption spectrophotometry, special attention being necessary at the initial oxidation or digestion stage to avoid losses of mercury by volatilization. Following oxidation (which converts all of the mercury present into the mercuric form) excess of reducing agent is added to liberate elemental mercury, which by a stream of air is then carried through the cell of a flameless atomic absorption spectrophotometer. Levels down to 0.005 mg/kg can be detected (16). Special attention attaches to certain food fish, notably tuna, for the ability to concentrate mercury in an organically bound form (methylmercury compounds) regarded as distinctly more toxic to man than inorganically bound mercury. Methylmercury compounds are extracted from the sample with benzene, then extracted into aqueous cysteine solution, acidified and back extracted into benzene for gas chromatographic examination. Levels down to about 0.02 mg/kg may be estimated in this way. Atomic absorption techniques have also been applied to the estimation of selenium, arsenic and antimony. This involves the evolution of the element as the hydride from an acid digest with sodium borohydride. The hydride is swept by a flow of argon into an argon-hydrogen entrained air flame, or decomposed in a heated silica tube followed by atomic absorption spectrophotometry. Useful working ranges are 0.2-30 ng/ml for selenium and 0.7-50 ng/ml for arsenic. Another application of atomic absorption spectroscopy involves the use of the heated graphite furnace flameless technique which is of particular value for the estimation of trace elements where sample size is limited.

Selenium may also be detected and estimated at levels down to between 0.01 and 0.03 mg/kg. The sample to be examined is digested with nitric and perchloric acids under strongly oxidising conditions; following this a fluorescent selenium complex is formed with 2,3-diaminonaphthalene (naphtho-{2,3-d}-2-selena-1,3-diazole), which is extracted into cyclohexane, back extracted into 0.1M hydrochloric acid and compacted spectrofluorimetrically with standard selenium solution under similar conditions.

Multi-element analysis methods such as neutron activation analysis, spark source mass spectrometry and emission spectrometry may also be used. With the development of very high temperature plasma emission sources, matrix effects can be largely eliminated and emission spectrometry offers considerable promise for a cheap and reliable multi-element analysis.

Great importance attaches to the avoidance of contamination during sampling, particularly for such metals as iron, chromium, cobalt and manganese. Anticoagulant measures for blood involving heparin may also introduce trace metals and Folg has discussed the special care needed to avoid contamination from the laboratory environment itself (20). Tissue samples for trace metal analysis can be stored by most normally accepted methods although some migration can occur between phases and, in the case of mercury in particular, the balance between organically bound and inorganically bound metal may change with time. Few systems have been studied systematically with stability in storage in mind, however, and there is scope for further work in this field.

A number of possible variable factors have to be taken into account if long-term storage is to be considered. These may include the oxidation state of the metal if in solution or the relationship between particle size and dissolution if in micron or submicron particulate form. The effect of microorganisms should be eliminated by heat sterilization or lyophilization. Contaminants can occur due to absorption of trace metals from the surface of the container or leaching of metal-containing additives from the materials from which the containers are made. Zinc, or occasionally cadmium, calcium or tin, may be present in some plastics compositions. A study of borosilicate glass or polypropylene shows that these materials are suitable for samples frozen at pH 2 to reduce interaction between metal ions and the container surface. On the other hand, adsorption from the sample solution of trace pollutant onto the walls of the vessel containing the sample may be a hazard, even in short-term storage. Adsorption onto a borosilicate glass surface of some trace metals can be prevented by acidification to pH 2 but it may not be possible to use polypropylene or other plastic materials (3). The long-term storage problem is illustrated by Hamilton in a review of strategies and tactics in relation to trace elemental analysis in biological tissue (18). He points out that the significance of the levels of most environmental contaminants is not clearly known and many contaminants have not even been identified. Whilst these conclusions can be justified, they must be interpreted with some caution since it is only too easy to postulate a problem the solution of which is beyond the reach of methodology without the means of either proving or disproving it (19). Tölg has made a special study of the calibration problems involved in the determination of trace metals and other elements in various substrates and has concluded that these are simplified by the use of dissolution techniques (20). These could obviously also simplify the problem of long-term storage, provided the species to be measured is known with certainty and steps are taken that the solution process takes these into account.

Polynuclear Aromatic Hydrocarbons

Some of the polynuclear aromatic hydrocarbons have been shown to possess carcinogenic activity and synergism between compounds may occur. One of the major problems confronting the analyst in this field is that it is the exception rather than the rule to find contamination by a single compound and since levels of the order of µg/kg are of interest it has been necessary to develop multi-component methods of analysis. Methods for the simultaneous determination of 13 compounds are available and have been studied on a collaborative basis. General procedures for food, sensitive to about 2 µg/kg, are based on solubilization of the sample with methanolic potassium hydroxide solution followed by solvent extraction and partition between dimethyl sulphoxide and an aliphatic solvent. Column chromatography on Florisil followed by paper chromatography and thin-layer chromatography is used for removing interfering substances and for semi-quantitative analysis by fluorescence techniques, a general method being available for a number of hydrocarbons including benzo(a)pyrene, benzo(g,h,i)perylene, benzo (a)anthracene, benzo(e)pyrene, pyrene, fluoranthene and benzo(k)fluoranthrene (13) and a specific method for benzo(a)pyrene (14). If evidence of the presence or otherwise of a single indicator compound (usually benzo(a)pyrene) is sought, a shortened procedure may be used. Solution techniques, UV and fluorescence spectrometry and mass spectroscopy have been used as confirmatory methods and a method based on gas liquid chromatography with flame ionization detection has also been used.

Other Hydrocarbons

Minute traces of aliphatic and aromatic hydrocarbons, of the order of 1 µg/kg or less, may occur in foods from the natural decomposition of lipids, proteins, steroids and other organic substances (8). The normal analytical approach is gas chromatographic, with a limit of detection varying down to 1 µg/kg or less. Although for the most part relatively stable substances, particularly at deep-freeze storage temperatures, insufficient work has been done on the stability of the very large range of straight and branched chain aliphatic and benzenoid compounds concerned to know whether significant changes occur in periods of time of the order of 1-10 years or more.

REFERENCES

1.   MITCHELL, F.L., Pure Appl. Chem. 1976, **45**, 59-62.
2.   SCHAFFER, R., Pure Appl. Chem. 1976, **45**, 75-79.
3.   STRUEMPLER, A.W., Anal. Chem. 1973, **45**, 2251-2254.
4.   JEFFERIES, D.J. and C.H. WALKER, Nature 1966, **212**, 533-534.
5.   FRENCH, M.C. and D.J. JEFFERIES, Bull. Environ. Contam. Toxicol. 1971, **6**, 460-463.
6.   EGAN, H. Food Cosmetic Toxicol. 1971, **9**, 81-90.
7.   EGAN, H. and R. SAWYER, Toxicology 1975, **4**, 245-252.
8.   JOHNSON, A.E., H.E. NURSTEN and R. SELF, Chem. Industry, 1969, 10-11.
9.   ABBOTT, D.C., J.O'G. TATTON and R. GOULDING, Brit. Med. J. 1968, **3**, 146-149.
10.   ABBOTT, D.C., G.B. COLLINS and R. GOULDING, Brit. Med. J. 1972, **2**, 553-556.
11.   ABBOTT, D.C., H. EGAN and J. THOMSON, J. Chromatog. 1964, **16**, 481.
12.   WESTON, R.E., 'Problems Raised by the Contamination of Man by Persistent Pesticides', pp 355-362, European Economic Community, Luxembourg 1975.
13.   HOWARD, J.W., R.T. TEAGUE, R.H. WHITE and B.E. FRY, J. Assoc. Office. Anal. Chem. 1966, **49**, 595.
14.   HOWARD, J.W., R.H. WHITE, B.E. FRY and E.W. TURICCHI, J. Assoc. Offic. Anal. Chem. 1966, **49**, 611.
15.   'Environmental Pollutants: Selected Methods of Analysis', pp 180-183, SCOPE, Paris 1975.
16.   'Environmental Pollutants: Selected Methods of Analysis', pp 174-176, SCOPE, Paris 1975.
17.   KAWAR, N.S., G.C. de BATISTA and F.A. GUNTHER, Residue Reviews 1973, **48**, 45-77.
18.   HAMILTON, E.I., Science of Total Envir. 1976, **5**, 1-62.
19.   EGAN, H., Chem & Ind. 1975, 814-820.
20.   TOELG, G., Talanta, 1972, **19**, 1489-1521.
21.   OLDHAM, P.D., 'Biological Effects of Asbestos', p. 45, IARC Scientific Publication No. 8, Lyon 1973.
22.   POOLEY, F.D., idem, p. 50.

GENERAL WORKING PAPER

F.A. Fairweather
Department of Health and Social Security
Alexander Fleming House
Elephant and Castle
London SE1

The effects of exposure on an individual from a pollutant depend on a number of factors which include the size and duration of the exposure-dose, the port of entry into the body, and the biological characteristics of the particular compound including its half life in the body. Consideration of these points is a necessary introduction to this subject.

Extent of Exposure

The significance of the effects of a substance on the body is related to the biological changes it causes. We are not concerned in this paper with acute toxicity, but chronic toxicity, teratogenicity, mutagenicity and carcinogenicity are within its remit. These last three are likely to be of importance when considering biological sampling though, since the exposure required to initiate the cytological disturbances may have taken place at a much earlier period and have left minimal tissue residue. An example of this would be a volatile compound such as bis-chloromethyl ether which is carcinogenic at low concentrations and there is little body storage. It is therefore necessary to acquire data on each individual pollutant with respect to the length of exposure and the concentration before any conclusions can be drawn. The physico-chemical form of the substance is a further factor, as with a relatively insoluble compound there may be a smaller uptake than with soluble one. This has been shown with lead, where compounds containing comparable amounts of lead were absorbed to varying extents from the gut of the test animals. A similar set of circumstances occurs in soil where the uptake by plants and animals of trace metals varies depending on the 'availability' of the salts. The availability depends on solubility and fixation of the compound with protein or other organic material. This is of importance in relation to cadmium in soil, where the availability is affected by the soil pH so that the addition of lime reduces the availability.

Port of Entry

Environmental exposure is by inhalation or by ingestion, and absorption through the skin is rarely of significance. The mechanisms involved and in consequence the rates of absorption tend to be very different in view of the functional differences at the sites of entry. Lead for example when absorbed from the gut in adults is taken up to the extent of 8-10 per cent (Kehoe, 1961) as compared with 45 per cent from the lung (Chamberlain et al , 1975). The toxic effects are also very different, and using cadmium as an example, a pulmonary emphysema-like state is seen in the lung, and a chronic form of gastro-enteritis in the alimentary tract. There may be local occurrences of malignancy at the sites of entry, and as with asbestos this may be observed in the lung with prolonged inhalation or in the gut with ingestion. But with other pollutants entering by either route, the target organ may be elsewhere in the body, such as the liver where angiosarcoma may result from exposure to vinyl chloride monomer. The characteristics of the individual substances are therefore important and must be taken into account in a particular situation.

Biological Characteristics

The level of pollutants found in tissue samples is not only dependent on exposure levels so that it is essential to obtain controls by careful matching. The following are some of the factors which require consideration in this respect :

i.   Sex differences
ii.   Age differences
iii.   Ethnic origin
iv.   Nutritional state
v.   Nature of employment
vi   Residential environment

When a pollutant is taken into the body, it may remain locally and not be transported to any great extent. An example of this is asbestos which may be seen in the sputum for many years. The identification at the transport stage of lead, cadmium or mercury is possible by blood estimations when the metal is attached to the red blood cells or to the plasma proteins. This is sometimes useful as a measure of the exposure when the half life in the blood is reasonably long, so that lead exposure may be usefully assessed in this way. From the blood, these substances are deposited for storage at various sites, and target organs may then be identified. Most trace metals can be found in the liver, and some also in the kidney (e.g. cadmium). Arsenic is found in the nails and hair, and organic compounds such as PCBs can be determined in the subcutaneous fat.

Many pollutants are only stored in the body to a limited extent under environmental conditions, which assumes that the intake is small and the biological half life is short. This means that the excretion is relatively complete over the period of time and allows no increase in the body burden. It is obvious that the biological effects of the substance are characteristic of the pollutant and that body burden measurements and means of assessing it must be considered individually. In consequence the techniques of biological sampling and the value of such specimens must be looked at for each compound and generalizations must be made only after careful scrutiny.

a. Review of Past and Current Programmes

The custom in the United Kingdom is to show conclusively first that there is a health risk before undertaking any biological sampling which may establish that excessive exposure of the population has taken place.

Such a demonstration may be made by measurements of air pollution, water analysis or data derived from the composition of food and the estimation of the dietary intake. Each of these will be discussed below.

Air Monitoring

Studies in this area are undertaken by the Department of the Environment and where there are people exposed to levels which are thought to be raised and the possibility of their receiving excessive quantities of the pollutant exists, the situation is brought to our attention and the question of the health risk associated with such levels is put to us.

Sources of such air pollution are derived mainly from factory and vehicle emissions. There are a number of different techniques available for studying the population exposure to these. One method is to look at people residing near the factory and compare them with individuals in another town or in part of the same town. A more satisfactory procedure is to group the population around the factory, so that those living less than 300 metres from it are compared with those 300-600 metres away, and 600-900 metres from it. In this way the expected reduction of exposure with increasing distance from the factory allows a built-in system of controls which makes the assessment of the findings an easier exercise. A third technique is to compare the population living around the factory with newcomers to the area. This is only a possibility where there is a marked turnover of house residents in the neighbourhood.

These procedures have been used in considering the health risk around lead factories. The second method is probably one of the most useful. A similar study using such a method and carried out near a lead source gave the results set out in Table 1.

These findings may be expressed more convincingly in terms of frequency distribution curves. Figure 1 shows results from lead workers' children compared with a control population presented as a histogram, and indicating that the blood lead figures in the exposed group are shifted to the right.

Water Analysis

With respect to chemical analysis of the water supply, water as delivered to the house in nearly all instances in the UK is free from levels of pollutants thought to be associated with health risk. The statutory requirement is for water to be 'wholesome' and legal definitions of the chemical composition do not exist.

However the plumbing in some areas with old housing and with plumbo-solvent water, results in delivery at the tap of increased levels of lead in the water at some time during the day. It has been considered prudent to carry out biological sampling on the residents in such areas. The problems associated with these studies are discussed below.

A large and complex investigation is also being undertaken into the relationship of cardio-vascular disease and hardness of water, which would be inappropriate to discuss in detail here. It could be noted though that this is thought to be associated with trace metal content of the water, or a protective one in the hard water.

Food studies

The Ministry of Agriculture, Fisheries and Food undertake surveillance of food and from time to time report on the content of dietary constituents with respect to certain elements in particular lead, cadmium and mercury. (These are attached in Appendices 1, 2 and 3). Since these metals are particularly taken up and stored by shell-fish it seemed appropriate for us to seek out heavy eaters of this article of diet and investigate them. Because of the seasonal avail-ability of fresh shell-fish and the relatively small numbers of heavy eaters of them, the study was not conclusive but no evidence was found of excessive intake of noxious substances from this source.

The question was asked as to whether people whose diet came from live-stock living on land heavily treated with sewage sludge and vegetables grown on such land would be at risk since sewage sludge contains such a high concentration of trace metals. It was possible to sample the sludge, the soil treated with sludge and vegetation grown on it and show the serial fall in lead and cadmium from the sludge to the vegetation. The live-stock were found to have no increase in the muscle content of trace metals, and the liver changes were not statistically significant. The figures which were obtained are shown in Tables 2 and 3 and Appendix 4.

Although there is continued watch on the Pesticide Residues, hormones and antimicrobial content of foods, no study has been appropriate on the human population as no health risk has been identified in these connections.

b. Programme Design

The study must be set up to solve a specific problem, so it is essential to state this clearly so that the objective is appreciated. Secondly in order to achieve this objective an appropriate population must be identified. In order to obtain a sample population with controls, the inde-pendent variables of sex, (since women tend to be biologically different from men), age (since child-ren have many metabolic features different from adults), and ethnic origin must be taken into ac-count. Socio-economic variations have to be considered, which would be relevant in terms of nutritional state and patterns of behaviour. There must be a random selection of this population to avoid a selection basis such as occurs when people are asked to volunteer, and this is the first part of the statistical contribution to the exercise. The statistician should advise on the neces-sary size of the sample, and take into account the errors involved in the sampling and analytical techniques.

When the study is planned, there may be sampling problems which require attention. Some biological parameters have variations with time, so that diurnal and seasonal rhythms must be catered for in order that comparability in the results is obtained. With some pollutant such as lead, it is necessary to check the lead levels in the equipment as the soap for cleaning the skin, spirit for the antiseptic swabs, the syringes and sample bottles. Where the levels of lead in air are high, particular care has to be taken that contamination does not occur during the sampling pro-cedures.

The choice of the biological sample will depend on the pollutant which is being investi-gated. The problems related to this were mentioned briefly above, but it is fair to say that there is still need for further enquiry into the best means of assessing the body burden of pollutants, and it can only be stated that in our present state of knowledge the choice in a particular set of circumstances has to be determined by factors based on the pollutant in question.

The method of assessment as for the planning must depend on the use of the most suit-able statistical technique, and expert advice in this area is an essential part of the programme.

c. Organisational Aspects

The theoretical background to a study may well be used repeatedly in subsequent surveys but there will always be a need for modifications to fit the conditions of a situation. Furthermore practical considerations may often mean reconsideration of the details of a survey. There is no point in needlessly duplicating surveys which have been carried out before, so it is necessary to bring up to date the background knowledge before mounting further studies. In this way the reason for undertaking the study can be clearly phrased and the objectives set out. The structure of the survey will then be specific to obtain the information desired.

There are two points which are particularly relevant here. First when setting up a study the preliminary work in relation to the analyses and planning is essential and failure to undertake and complete this adequately may result in invalidation of the entire survey. Secondly if the first study is carried out satisfactorily there is no point in repeating this simply with a view to checking the findings. Consideration must be given to the time scale over which events are likely to take place and influence the body burden. For example if a study indicates high levels of cadmium in air round a factory, remedial measures will be required to reduce these. Such measures must be planned and then implemented before any biological changes can be observed, and these effects will not be measurable over a short period as the half life of cadmium is long. Such factors must be borne in mind when planning in the long term.

There is a single organisational point which could be added to this. When carrying out original work, it is easy to think of minutiae which could be tacked on to the original project, with the feeling that while the study is going through it would be a pity to miss the chance of collecting a little more information. This temptation if not resisted tends to disturb the balance of the study and reduce the status of the results from which the conclusions are drawn.

d. Ethical and Legal Considerations

All information about an individual's health in the UK must be considered confidential, and not divulged to a person or organisation without his or her written agreement. It is accepted that if an adverse finding is obtained, it will be transmitted to the individual's family doctor with advice where this is appropriate. The decision on whether to act on this advice rests with the doctor in consultation with the individual himself.

When the form of survey has been planned, it must be accepted that all sampling is on a voluntary basis. Where there is a health risk provided that good publicity is carried out, a high attendance rate may well be obtained. This assumes that the sampling is no more than a blood sample. The failure rate is commonly higher in the control group, and it is necessary to pay considerable attention to this to ensure an adequate response. In general this is a public relations exercise rather than a medical or scientific one.

Voluntary attendance at sampling centres for adults is commonly accepted as permission to take blood, though a signature on a form is an additional safe-guard which many feel is desirable. Children provide quite a different problem. If there is a health risk, it is desireable that a parent or guardian gives permission for the blood sampling. To obtain a control sample in a child is more difficult. This has legal connotations and brings to attention the way in which UK law differentiates individual from communal health matters. If the sampling necessitates more than a blood sample, such as a subcutaneous fat specimen, a piece of skin, or a liver biopsy, it is essential to explain fully the extent of the procedure and to obtain written permission before starting the technique.

TABLE 1

(for explanation see text)

BLOOD LEAD VALUES IN µg/100 ml			
Distance from source	0 - 100 m	100 - 300 m	Greater than 300 m
Males	20.7	19.4	18.9
Females	17.1	16.6	16.6

TABLE 2

(for explanation see text)

	Sewage Sludge (dry matter ppm)	Soil (dry matter ppm)	Herbage (dry matter ppm)	
			autumn-winter	summer
Lead	400	170	30-90	20-30
Cadmium	170	29	5-10	4-5

TABLE 3

(for explanation see text)

CATTLE		
SEWAGE FARM	**CADMIUM**	**LEAD**
Liver average	0.95	1.2
range	0.50-1.20	0.6-1.7
Muscle average	0.50	0.2
range	0.05-0.05	-
Blood average	0.47	13.3
range	0.40-0.50	12.0-15.0
UNTREATED PASTURES		
Liver average	0.05	0.20
range	0.05	0.20
Muscle average	0.05	0.20
range	0.05	0.20
Blood average	-	-
range	-	-

REFERENCES

CHAMBERLAIN, A.C., W.S. CLOUGH, M.J. HEARD, D. NEWTON, A.N.B. STOTT and A.C. WELLS (1975). Proc. Roy. Soc. B. **192** : 77.

KEHOE, R.A., (1961). J. Roy. Instit. Pub. Hlth. Hyg. **24** : 81.

154

Number
of children
20
15
10
5
0
20 Leadworkers' children
18 Control children
0
10
20
30
40
50
60
70
BLOOD LEAD values in µg/100 mls.

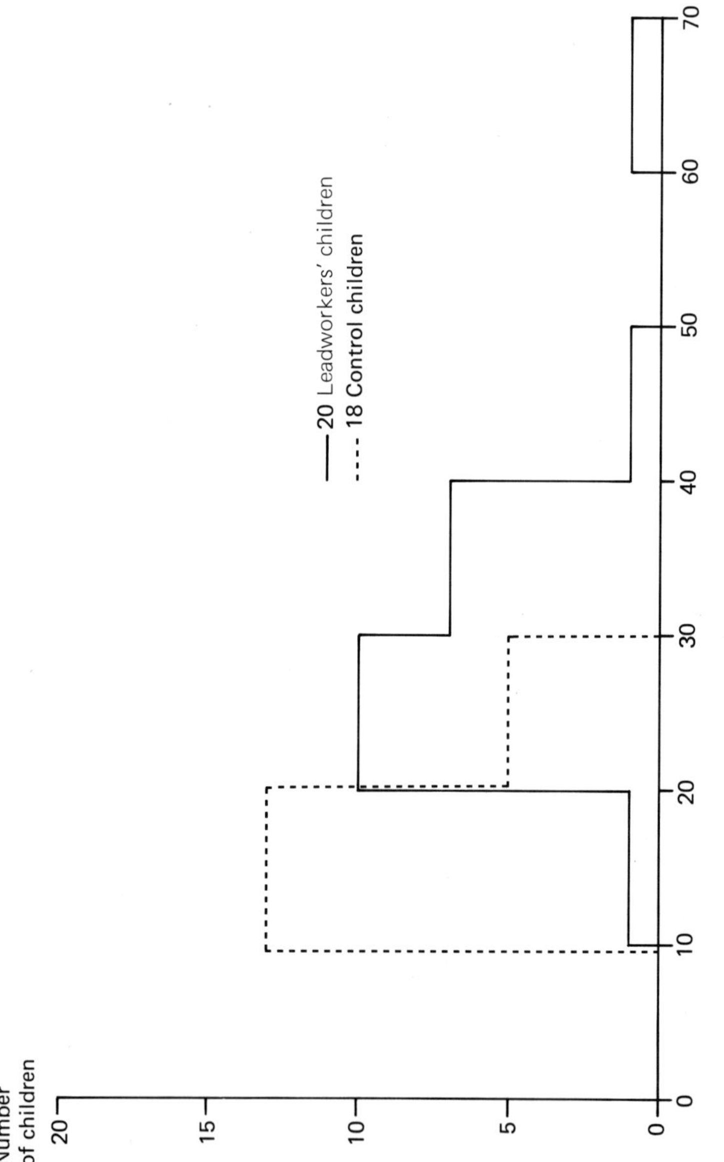

COLLECTION OF HUMAN BIOLOGICAL SPECIMENS IN DEVELOPING COUNTRIES FOR MONITORING ORGANOCHLORINE COMPOUNDS

M. Taghi Farvar*, PhD
Vice-Rector for Environmental Sciences, Bu-Ali Sina University, Hamadan, Iran

Introduction

This paper reviews the current knowledge and the problems associated with the collection and storage of biological specimens from human populations in developing countries for the assessment of exposure to Organochlorine Compounds (OCC). It also contains recommendations for studies designed to evaluate the extent of occurrence and impact of these pollutants on human health. Special consideration is given to the relatively unexplored problem of OCI (particularly DDT) compounds in human milk in developing countries because of the possible direct deleterious effect of these compounds on the developing infant.

I. Review of past and current programmes

Although the most intensive uses of pesticides have been in both agricultural and public health programmes in the developing countries, yet studies evaluating the impact of these compounds on human health and the environment are very rare. One must conclude that after a quarter of a century of pesticide use and only a few biological monitoring programmes and impact studies, an enormous empirical experiment has been conducted with no experimental design to assess the outcome, and little care as to its deleterious effect on the people of the developing countries. In fact, the most comprehensive survey published so far on OCC in human tissues (Wassermann, Tomatis and Wassermann, 1975) lists only four references which deal with OCC in mother's milk in developing countries (Lofröth, 1971; Olszyna-Marzys et al, 1973; Hornabrook et al, 1972; and Gejvall et al, 1972). Of these, one (Gejvall, Jensen, and Lofröth, 1972) is a personal communication to Wassermann et al, and two others (Lofröth, 1971; Olszyna-Marzys et al, 1973) refer to the same data based on informal and partial reporting of early results in an unrefereed journal (CBNS Notes, 1971)! The latter results refer to data from a collection of 47 samples of human milk from rural Guatemala which was carried out by this author and his colleagues. The complete results have been reported fully elsewhere by Farvar (1972), and summarized later by Farvar et al (1975).

Since the review by Wassermann et al, mentioned above, a further study was initiated in Guatemala by the author and his colleagues (Farvar, Winter, and Thomas, 1975; Winter, Thomas Wernick, Levin, and Farvar, 1976) and in Iran (Ahmed, Södergren, Farvar, Manuchehri, and Vojdani, 1976).

All these results are summarized in Table 1.

II Rationale for interest and concern

An examination of Table 1 makes possible the following observations:

1. Published data on occurrence of OCC in human milk from developing countries are very rare, and essentially limited to two countries (Guatemala and Papua-New Guinea). Two other countries have reported information but as yet the results are not published (Iran and Ghana). In the case of Ghana, no information was given as to the number of samples, the techniques of analysis, nor where the laboratory analysis was performed. The Iranian data, analysed in the University of Lund laboratories, will be published in the near future and are summarized in Table 1.

2. The quantities of total DDT in human milk have ranged from an average of 0.011 ppm in unsprayed areas of Papua-New Guinea (PNG) to an average of 4.07 ppm in Cerro Colorado (Escuintla, Guatemala) which is an intensively sprayed area, and from a minimum of 0.0 ppm in unsprayed areas of PNG to a maximum of 12.21 ppm in Cerro Colorado (Escuintla, Guatemala). These levels are two orders of magnitude greater than anything reported from industrialized countries of North America, East and West Europe.

---

*   The author is grateful to Drs. Wasif Ahmed and Richard Garcia for help in correcting the manuscript, and to W. Ahmed, A. Södergren, M. Winter, A. Olszyna-Marzys, M. Thomas, and J. Schirmer for earlier work in sample collection and/or analysis.

3.   Compared with the maximum Acceptable Daily Intake (ADI) in humans established by WHO/FAO (1969) for DDT (0.005 mg/kg body weight) the averages in Table 1 range from about 1/2 ADI value in unsprayed areas of PNG to 488 times more than ADI in Guatemala.   This is assuming that a neonate in these countries weighs about 3.0 kg and consumes about 0.6 liter of mother's milk per day.   Thus, the average values ingested in PNG range from about 1/2 ADI to almost 10 times ADI.   In Guatemala, according to the latest results, the ingested amounts of DDT range from an average of 1.4 ADI in Nebaj (highland area with little spraying) to about 35 ADI in Livingston, a Caribbean coastal settlement with continued biennial indoor spraying by anti-malaria teams.   In Ghana the value given corresponds to about 16 percent above ADI.   In Iran the infants, whose mother's milk was tested, were ingesting an average of 55 times more DDT each day than the maximum permissible by international standards.   The range in the 17 Iranian samples was from about 15 times to 101 times more than the ADI.

4.   The high amount of DDE in human milk (Table 1) is usually an indication of prolonged exposure to DDT.   However, it is not known how much of the DDE is truly the result of breakdown in the human body and how much, if any, happens during storage and/or analysis.   More investigations are needed to answer these questions.

5.   There are also other insecticides than DDT in most of the samples, as can be seen from Table 1.   BHC was found in amounts ranging from 0.0 to 0.101 ppm in Guatemala which is the highest so far reported anywhere.   The "practical residue limit" established for BHC is 0.004 ppm for gamma-BHC in milk (WHO/FAO, 1969).   In the case of heptachlor epoxide, the values range from 0.0 to 0.021 ppm, an order of magnitude higher than the "practical residue limit" of 0.002 ppm.   Other OCIs, such as dieldrin and HCB, have been reported in some specimens and in the case of Ghana PCB (Wassermann et al , 1975).

The occurrence of these compounds shows that there are several routes of exposure for humans which include agricultural and private domestic uses in addition to intradomiciliary spraying by malaria eradication teams.

6.   Most of the data favour the hypothesis that the main cause of the unprecedentedly high accumulation of DDT in human milk in these areas is indoor spraying of the compound for malaria eradication programmes.   For example, in the 1970-71 survey of La Bomba, Cerro Colorado, and El Rosario, Guatemala, it was shown that at the P < 0.01 confidence level there was no significant difference among the DDT levels of the three communities, all of which had received about 13 years of DDT spraying for malaria control (without much success).   Yet La Bomba has not been subjected to the heavy agricultural spraying on cotton plantations, while the other two communities have received very heavy and regular applications of OCI on cotton plantations.   The subsequent study in 1974 supports this hypothesis.   Agricultural uses form a secondary (although important) source of human milk contamination, as shown by the presence of other insecticides than DDT which are not used domestically. A recent study by Davies, Edmundson, and Raffonelli (1975) indicates that contamination of house dust by domestic spraying of DDT is primarily responsible for human serum residues.   The Davies et al study therefore lends support to our hypothesis that the anti-malaria use of DDT is primarily responsible for excessive accumulation of this insecticide in human milk in developing countries.

7.   The follow-up study in Guatemala in 1974 shows that when DDT spraying for malaria control stopped in some of the communities in Guatemala because of insecticide resistance to OCI, there was a moderately rapid drop in the concentration of DDT in human milk (Table 1).   This information supports the necessity of alternative strategies and methodologies of malaria control.

8.   Because of the limited information on OCC in human milk in developing countries, there is an urgent need for further studies in more countries of the developing world to ascertain the extent and level of this source of contamination.

9.   There are no standardized analytical procedures used in the reported results in Table 1, which indicated a need to develop standardized techniques.   Such techniques exist for cow's milk, but human milk presents a different set of problems from collection to storage, analysis and interpretation.

III. Biological effects of organochlorine compounds

Application rate of DDT in malarial spraying operations is approximatively $2mg/m^2$ applied twice per year.   When compared to agricultural rates, this is equivalent to 40 kg/hectare of technical DDT, which is one order of magnitude greater than any agricultural applications.   OCI in agricultural uses are dissipated in the environment and enter the ecological food chains.   While this fact presents a new set of problems, the process also results in the dilution and breakdown of the pesticides before they reach the human body.   On the contrary, intradomiciliary applications of OCI remain in the immediate environment of human beings, where they come into daily contact with these products.   The OCIs remain on walls, household goods, and house dust (Davies et al , 1975).   They are thus absorbed through inhalation and ingestion, and result in greater rates of accumulation.   The human infant thus becomes the final consumer.

We shall now briefly review the known biological effects of the accumulation of OCC in the body with special reference to humans.

1.   Unfortunately, little is known about the basic mechanisms of OCC action in humans.   This is partly due to difficulties (ethical and other) of performing controlled toxicological experiments in people.   The studies done by Hayes, Jr. and associates (1956 and 1971) on healthy adult male prisoners in southern United States, in which the subjects were fed measured doses of DDT are irrelevant and must be rejected as any proof of the innocuousness of these compounds in humans. This is both because the study did not cover effects on enzymatic systems, and more importantly because the effect on the human foetus and neonate, when the nervous and enzymatic systems, etc., have not yet developed into their final stable state, is likely to be a different matter altogether and cannot be judged from clinical studies on healthy adults.

2.   In addition, it is likely that subjects (particularly neonates) living in the less developed, protein deficient areas may be more susceptible to physiological effects of pesticides than those who live in areas with a higher living standard and better nutrition.   This is already known in animal populations.   For example, it has been determined that rats obtaining 1/7 the optimal amount of protein in the diet suffered significantly greater toxic effects from 16 different pesticides than those with optimal protein intake (Boyd and Taylor, 1970, in Boyd and Krupa, 1970). (See Table 2).

3.   It has been found that growth rates significantly decrease and mortality rates increase in suckling neonate offspring of rats fed on a low-protein diet beginning immediately after parturition.   Offspring of the group receiving 10 ppm DDT with low protein showed significantly greater intensity of these factors than those feeding on low protein without DDT.   Mortality in the offspring was similarly significantly higher in the protein-deficient DDT-exposed group. Ten ppm DDT in the rat food correspond to some 05 - 1.0 mg/kg body weight - an amount reached or exceeded by many infants in our study (Fahim, 1970).

4.   In the Guatemalan study, the infant mortality rate among the population studied in La Bomba and Cerro Colorado was 162 per 1,000 reported for Guatemala in 1968 (Farvar, 1972; United Nations, 1970).   Although the sample size should be considered insufficient for obtaining overall infant mortality rates, yet the finding indicates an urgent need for further investigation of such a relationship in view of the information given in paragraph 3 above.

5.   The residues in mother's milk are considered by some to be high enough to cause further biological effects (inhibition of corticoids synthesis, gluconeogenic enzyme activity, and the interference with calcium, vitamin D and sex hormone metabolism. See Adamovic et al , 1971, in Wassermann et al , 1975).

6.   It is also possible that neurological disorders may occur in infants exposed to such high levels of pesticides.   Accumulated pesticides in the adipose tissue due to continuous daily exposure would be flushed into the circulatory system during times of starvation, such as at weaning or during attacks of diarrhoeal diseases.

7.   The use of newly developed approaches to the metabolism of these compounds in the fields of epidemiological toxicology and ecology have resulted in a better understanding of impact on defense mechanisms of the body.   Thus DDT has been shown to decrease the half-life of some drugs in the body by interfering with enzymatic activity of drugs detoxication (Hart and Fouts, 1963, in Wassermann et al 1975).

8.   OCIs are believed to induce an increase of cholesterol synthesis in the over 45 year age group (Wassermann et al , 1975).   Serum PBI was found to be significantly lower in workers occupationally exposed to OCI in comparison with non-occupationally exposed workers (D. Wassermann, 1972) and rats (D. Wassermann, 1973; M. Wassermann, 1973).   An accelerated degradation of thyroid hormones in the presence of high level of OCC as powerful inducers of non-specific metabolizing enzymes, leads to hyperactivity of the thyroid gland as a negative feed-back reaction (D. Wassermann, 1973).
9.   There is evidence that DDT impairs the immunological response in rabbits by decreasing total gamma-globulins (M. Wassermann, 1969, 1971).   In fact, there may be a bidirectional relationship between a detoxication process and an immunological response to antigens.
10.   Other observed effects in animals include thymus atrophy in rabbits, increased mortality from hepatitis virus in ducklings, serum gamma-globulin lowering and serum albumin increase in rabbits due to action of PCBs (Vos and Beems, 1971; Vos and de Roij, 1972; M. Wassermann, 1973;   and Friend and Trainer, 1970, in Wassermann et al , 1975), an increased lethal effect of tumour cells in the presence of DDT in mice (M. Wassermann et al , 1975) as well as increased serum albumin levels in rabbits receiving OCI (ibid).
11.   There have also been reports of mutagenesis due to the action of OCI.   DDT, DDD, DDA, and Dieldrin have been found to have induced genetic mutations in rats, mice, mallard ducks, **Salmonella typhimurium** and **Drosophyla melanogaster** (Buselmaier et al , 1972, 1973; Vogel, 1972; Johnson and Yalal, 1973; Legater, 1969; and Bunch, 1973, in Wassermann et al , 1975).

The above brief review (for a more detailed review see bibliography, particularly Wassermann et al , 1975) shows the reasons for concern regarding OCC residues in the human environment, particularly DDT and its metabolites and other OCI in human milk from rural areas of developing countries.   There have been few studies carried out so far.   It is therefore urgent to organize scientific investigations of the occurrence, diffusion, causes and effects of OCI in human milk from the rural Third World to assess the extent of their impact and to help provide alternative preventive and curative measures.

IV.   CONSIDERATIONS FOR HUMAN SAMPLE SELECTION, COLLECTION, CONTAIN-MENT, SHIPMENT AND STORAGE

As mentioned above, it is primarily human milk which carries the OCI load to infants.   Thus, this is the specimen that should be collected with greater insistence.   Much is known about concentrations in human milk from developed countries (Wassermann et al , 1975; Farvar, 1972; Gatti, 1974), but even in these countries most collections are from urban areas, due to ease of access to lactating women in urban hospitals and clinics.   But it would be advisable to collect milk from women in rural areas.   For example, it is known that people living in the rural southern United States are exposed to much more intensive uses of OCI (which probably explains why North American Blacks have more OCI residues in the adipose tissues than Whites since many live or have migrated from cotton-growing areas where OCI are used intensively).   To date there are no known milk samples from rural farm workers reported there.

The **collection** of milk samples presents certain difficulties.   First, access with equipment to rural areas is sometimes difficult, particularly in less developed countries.   Secondly, proper containers for milk samples are not usually available.   We have found that the best containers are about 25 cc wide-mouthed metal (particularly aluminium) flasks.   Glass is not preferred because it is breakable under hard field conditions of storage and transport.   Another serious problem is the pre-cleaning procedures, as the appropriate chemicals (e.g., par pesticide-grade acetone and/or hexane) are frequently unavailable in most less developed countries.   The unavailability of dry ice is another problem.   Sometimes breweries make dry ice as a by-product of fermentation, but even if available, the time involved for collection and return of the specimens may be too long for its use.   Alternative procedures for preservation have not yet been satisfactorily worked out and tried on human milk.   Liquid nitrogen is awkward and dangerous, and centrifuging is almost impossible under field conditions.   It may be possible to modify drying techniques such as by use of sodium sulphate anhydrous, but this may introduce new impurities.   It also has the dis-advantage of virtually eliminating the aqueous portion of milk, which should be preserved and stored in the laboratory for future reference.   In reference to introducing impurities, it should be noted that the use of plastic containers, caps, and corks should be avoided.

Manual expression of breasts by the donors of milk has in our experience proved the best means of obtaining milk. Pumps are not convenient since they cannot be cleaned chemically in the field after each use. Perhaps the worst disadvantage is that pumps introduce an artificial element into the already difficult field worker-donor relationship. The issue of cultural problems sometimes arises. For example, the population of a Guatemalan indigenous village escaped from the field workers soliciting milk (even though the latter were **women** anthropologists) which was apparently due to possible fear of witchcraft. Their village priest was contacted who then convinced the villagers of the necessity of this work. The problem of embarrassment due to exposure of breasts, however, is usually not a factor in less developed countries because, fortunately, the breast has not yet lost its primary function as a means for feeding the new-born child.

It is nevertheless important to have female field workers and researchers involved. They should be carefully instructed to make sure that neither the hands, clothes, and skin of the donor, nor those of the field worker, should come in contact with the collection flask. Contamination of the samples must be avoided at all times. After collection, the flasks should be covered with clean aluminium foil or with a cap dressed in aluminium foil and immediately placed on dry ice.

We have found that it helps to combine milk collection with other on-going work or study in rural areas. In the case of Guatemala, the collection exercises were a part of a much larger study of the environmental impact of insecticides, and were particularly integrated into an anthropological investigation of use patterns, diffusion and attitudes regarding pesticides. Therefore, there were usually field workers who had been living in an area before attempting collection of milk. The result was that in such communities we had a zero refusal rate amongst lactating women, as there had already been a good deal of mutual trust generated. In the case of Iran, the milk collections were made in connection with an entomological study of plant pests and resistant anophelines in the rural area in question.

The problems associated with **shipment** of samples are serious, since dry ice is bulky and cumbersome. It is not possible to depend on unaccompanied freight being delivered on time (before the speciments thaw out) to the right country, city and laboratory. If possible, it is better to transport the collected samples as accompanied baggage to the laboratory for analysis.

Storage should be done under deep freeze conditions (at least -20°C). The major difficulty is when the samples thaw and refreeze in the process of transport or storage as a result of insufficient dry ice or interruptions in the electrical current.

V. ANALYTICAL PROCEDURES

These procedures are in general well-known. In addition, advances in gas chromatography over the past few years have simplified and automated them considerably. However, the preparation still presents problems primarily because there are no standardized procedures among the various laboratories conducting the analyses. In the case of refrozen samples, there are problems of determination of exact fat percentage as well as clean-up procedures. The techniques in general are described in Olszyna-Marzys et al (1973) and Winter et al (1976) and are usually based on EPA analytical procedures manuals (Thompson, J.F., ed., **Analysis of Pesticide Residues in Human and Environmental Samples**. Environmental Protection Agency, Research Triangle Park, N.C., USA, continuously revised and updated). There is a need for inter-laboratory collaboration for standardizing procedures for both collection, transport, storage and analysis of residues, with special attention to the conditions in less developed countries.

VI. PROGRAMME DESIGN

In order to advance knowledge of the occurrence, distribution and significance of OCC in human specimens with particular reference to human milk from less developed parts of the world, a proposal was made by us to the United Nations Environment Programme, involving the collaboration of the Environmental Pollution and Hazards Unit of WHO and the Pesticide Analysis Laboratory, Ecology Institute of the University of Lund, Sweden. The proposal, which has been accepted in principle but not yet approved for financial support, is briefly described in the Appendix.

TABLE 1

Residues of Organochlorine Compounds Reported in Human Milk Samples
from Developing Countries, in Parts per Million

Place	Ref.	No.	Total DDT	Total DDE	Total BHC	Dieldrin	Heptachlor Epoxide
Papua-New Guinea							
7 districts	11	74	0.242	Average where DDT used for malaria			
			0.011	Average where DDT not used for malaria			
Ghana (a)	8		0.029		0.030		
Iran							
(Fars)	1	17	1.384	0.476			
			(0.384-	(0.171-			
			2.521)	0.846)			
Guatemala							
El Rosario	5	27	1.84	0.933	0.007	0.003	0.002
(Retalhuleu)			(0.342-	(0.285-	(TR-	(TR-	(TR-
(1970) (b,c)			4.97)	3.104)	0.069)	0.010)	0.008)
El Rosario	6	31	0.276	0.180	0.001		
(1974)			(0.050-	(0.033-	(0.0-		
			0.912)	0.661)	0.011)		
La Bomba	5	11	2.232	1.121	0.029	TR	0.003
(Santa Rosa)			(0.411-	(0.124-	(0.009-	(0.0-	(0.0-
(1970)			11.50)	6.360)	0.101)	0.003)	0.021)
La Bomba	6	31	0.587	0.240	0.003		
(1974)			(0.089-	(0.035-	(0.0-		
			1.764)	0.996)	0.009)		
Cerro Colorado	5	9	4.073	2.101	0.015		TR
(Escuintla)			(1.567-	(0.604-	(0.0-		
(1971)(d)			12.211)	6.130	0.057)		
Cerro Colorado	6	31	0.466	0.306	0.002		
(1974)			(0.041-	(0.022-	(0.0-		
			2.193)	1.603	0.007)		
Livingston	6	30	0.864	0.427	0.001		
(Izabal)			(0.140-	(0.058-	(0.0-		
(1974)			5.686)	2.964)	0.014)		
Asunciòn Mita	6	31	0.490	0.345	0.015		
(Jutiapa)			(0.051-	(0.033-	(0.0-		
(1974)			2.506)	1.872)	0.018)		
Nebaj	6	28	0.035	0.019	0.005	0.034	
(Quiché)			(0.005-	(0.002-	(0.0-	(1 sample)	
(1974)			0.183)	0.115)	0.018)		
Guatemala City	6	78	0.233	0.176	0.011		
(1974)			(0.015-	(0.013-	(0.0-		
			1.01)	0.874)	0.070)		
San Pedro Carchà	6	30	0.273				
(Alta Verapaz)			(0.003-				
(1974)			1.310)				

(a)   Also PCBs (<0.005) and HCB (0.086)
(b)   Also aldrin (0.0-0.005) and endrin (0.0-0.001)
(c)   TR : trace amounts (<0.001)
(d)   Also heptachlor (TR)

TABLE 2

The Acute Oral LD_{50} of Sixteen Pesticides in Male Albino Rats for
28 days from Weaning on a Diet Deficient in Protein Compared with Values
in Controls Fed Normal Amounts of Protein as Casein or as Laboratory Chow[a]

Pesticides	Protein-Deficient (3.5 % Casein) Diet Group I[b]		Normal Protein (26 % Casein) Diet Group II [c]			Laboratory Chow Diet Group III	
Captan	480 ± 110	(26)	12600 ± 2100		(1.0)	12500 ± 3500	
Cabaryl	89 ± 11	(6)	575 ± 51		(1.3)	744 ± 40	
Chlordane	137 ± 30	(2)	267 ± 44		(1.2)	311 ± 44	
Chlorpropham	2590 ± 480	(4)	10390 ± 1580		(0.4)	4440 ± 480	
Demeton	2.13 ± 0.37	(4)	7.62 ± 0.22		(1.4)	10.40 ± 0.77	
Diazinon	215 ± 26	(2)	415 ± 39		(1.1)	466 ± 87	
Dicophane (DDT)	165 ± 34	(3)	481 ± 13		(0.8)	368 ± 38	
Dimethoate	147 ± 29	(2)	152 ± 22		(2.4)	358 ± 9	
Diuron	437 ± 139	(5)	2390 ± 1440		(0.4)	1017 ± 222	
Endosulfan	24 ± 10	(4)	102 ± 16		(1.2)	121 ± 16	
Endrin	6.69 ± 0.80	(2)	16.60 ± 3.01		(1.6)	27.24 ± 6.54	
Lindane	95 ± 33	(2)	184 ± 16		(0.9)	157 ± 37	
Malathion	559 ± 138	(2)	1401 ± 99		(0.8)	1090 ± 83	
Monuron	950 ± 240	(3)	2880 ± 310		(0.5)	1480 ± 310	
Parathion	4.86 ± 1.31	(8)	37.1 ± 4.9		(0.6)	23.4 ± 5.4	
Toxaphen	80 ± 19	(4)	293 ± 31		(0.8)	220 ± 33	

(a) The LD_{50} is expressed as mg/kg ± standard error; the data are from publications cited by Boyd and Taylor (1970).

(b) In parenthesis is the value obtained by dividing the LD_{50} in group II by that in group I.

(c) In parenthesis is the value obtained by dividing the LD_{50} in group III by that in group II.

REFERENCES

1. Ahmed, W., A. Södergren, M.T. Farvar, S. Manuchehri and M. Vojdani. Unpublished results 1976.
2. Boyd, E.M. and V. Kupra. Protein deficient diet and diurin toxicity. **Journal of Agricultural Food Chemistry, 18** (6).
3. Davies, J.E., W.F. Edmundson, and A. Raffonelli. The role of house dust in human DDT pollution. **American Journal of Public Health, 65** (1) 53-57 (1975).
4. Fahim, M.S., R. Bennett and D.G. Hall. Effects of DDT in the nursing neonate. **Nature,** 228 (5277). 19 December (1970).
5. Farvar, M.T., **Ecological Implications of Insect Control in Central America: Agriculture, Public Health and Development.** Ann Arbor, Michigan: University Microfilms (1972).
6. Farvar, M.T., M. Winter and M.L. Thomas. Pesticides in Developing Countries: significance of chlorinated hydrocarbon residues in human milk from Central America. In **Proceedings of the International Conference on Environmental Sensing and Assessment.** New York: Institute of Electrical and Electronics Engineers, Inc. Document No. 75CH 1004-1 ICESA (1975).
7. Gatti, G.L. Pesticide Residues in Human Fat and Human Milk in the Nine Member States of the European Community. Luxembourg: Commission of the European Communities (Directorate of Health Protection, Directorate General of Social Affairs) (May 1974).
8. Gejvall, T., S. Jensen, and G. Lofröth. Personal communication 1972 to Wassermann et al. 1975.
9. Hayes, Jr., W.J., W.F. Durham and C. Cueto, Jr. The effect of known repeated oral doses of chlorophenothane (DDT) in man. **Journal of the American Medical Association, 162:-** 890-897 (1956).
10. Hayes, Jr., W.J. La inocuidad del DDT en el hombre demostrada en el control de la malaria. **Boletin de la Oficina Sanitaria Panamericana, 7:** 481-499 (1971).
11. Hornabrook, R.W., P.G. Dyment, E.D. Gomes and J.S. Wieseman. DDT residues in human milk from New Guinea natives. **Medical Journal of Australia, 25** (1): 1297-1300 (1972).
12. Lofröth, G. **Ecologist, 1** : 8 (1971).
13. Olszyna-Marzys, A.E., M. de Campos, M.T. Farvar and M.L. Thomas. Residuos de plaguicidas clorados en leche humana y de vaca de Guatemala. **Boletin de la Oficina Sanitaria Panamericana, 75:** (February 1973).
14. Wasserman, D. et al. **Bulletin of Environmental Contamination and Toxicology, 6:** 85 (1971).
15. Wassermann, D. et al. **8th International Conference of Toxic. Occup. Med.** (8-11 July 1973).
16. Wassermann, M. et al. **Annals NY Acad. Sci. Biological Effects of Pesticides.** 160: 393 (1969).
17. Wassermann, M. et al. **Bull. Env. Contam. Toxic.** 6: 426 (1971).
18. Wassermann, M. et al. **Bull. Env. Contam. Toxic.** 8: 177 (1972).
19. Wassermann, M. et al. **Bull. Env. Contam Toxic.** 10: 42 (1973).
20. Wassermann, M., L. Tomatis and Dora Wassermann. Organochlorine compounds in the general population of the seventies and some of their biological effects (in man and animals). **Pure and Applied Chemistry, 42:** No. 1-2 (1975).
21. Winter, M., M. Thomas, S. Wernick, S. Levin and M.T. Farvar. Analysis of pesticide residues in 290 samples of Guatemalan mother's milk. **Bulletin of Environmental Contamination and Toxicology, 16:** No. 6 (1976).
22. World Health Organization/Food and Agriculture Organization. **Report of Joint Expert Committee on Pesticide Residues.** WHO Technical Report Series NO. 417 (1969).

APPENDIX

Summary of Project Proposal on the 'Global monitoring of DDT and other organochlorine compound residues in human milk and food chains due to pesticide applications to the environment'.

This proposal was made to the Global Environmental Monitoring Systems (GEMS) of the United Nations Environment Programme in 1976.   It was made by the Environmental Sciences and Ecodevelopment Cluster of the newly established Bu-Ali Sina University in Hamadan, Iran, in collaboration with the Pesticide Analysis Laboratory of the Ecology Institute at the University of Lund, Sweden, and the Environmental Pollution and Hazards Unit of the World Health Organization.

The project would last about twenty months and cost about U.S. $140,000 to be met by UNEP and the two universities.

The proposed project will enable the collection and dissemination of data on the extent of accumulation of DDT and other chlorinated hydrocarbon compounds in human milk from a number of carefully selected developing countries.   It will also make it possible to evaluate the relative contribution of various sources of pesticide application (such as agricultural, public health, and personal domestic uses).   It is expected that the information thus obtained will be used for decision making and more rational policy formulation regarding the important question of pesticide use in the developing countries.

About five to six developing countries in each of Africa, Asia and Latin America will be carefully selected for study based on the primary criterion of their known history and patterns of insecticide use in agriculture and public health.   In each country several areas will be selected in consultation with local scientists, authorities and WHO based on local patterns of insecticide use with particular emphasis on DDT.   At least three areas will be selected for study in each country: (1) areas with no known insecticide use, (2) areas with a history of agricultural uses of insecticides, and (3) areas with a history of intradomiciliary use, particularly of DDT for public health protection.   Finally, where both conditions (2) and (3) prevail will also be included where appropriate.

An effort will be made to obtain about 30 samples of human milk under carefully controlled conditions and in pre-cleaned receptacles from each area of communities in question.   Background data on patterns of insecticide use as well as other relevant factors (such as age of mother and neonates, number of dead and live children born to each donor, major dietary habits, length of residence in the area, etc.) will be collected and recorded.   Samples will be placed under deep-freeze immediately after collection and transported to the laboratory in Hamadan as soon as possible.

The samples will be analysed using advanced gas chromatography techniques and the results will be analysed attempting to correlate each case with the major insecticide use patterns.   Some samples of major items in the diet will also be collected for analysis in order to determine its possible role in pesticide accumulation.

It is expected that WHO will aid the project staff in facilitating access to relevant information on intradomiciliary insecticide use patterns and local arrangements and advice in each country.   The Lund laboratory will provide methodological assistance and will also analyse paired samples for quality control purposes.

The Intergovernmental Monitoring Meeting of UNEP (1974), the Expert Group Meeting of the Environmental Health Monitoring Programme of WHO (1974), as well as the recent UNEP/WHO meeting on Bio-Environmental Methods of Control of Malaria have all emphasized the importance of urgently undertaking detailed studies of the accumulation of DDT in human milk from developing countries in order to assess its importance and causes.

The results of the study will be published in the scientific literature and will also be disseminated widely to all concerned bodies.   It is expected that these reports and their recommendations will lead to a revision of current insecticide use patterns in agriculture and public health and will result in new epidemiological investigations.   A project for long-term epidemiological investigation will be devised during this study to investigate the health effects of such exposures, never before studied in human populations.   The Health Sciences Cluster of the University of Hamadan will collaborate in this stage of the studies.

THE NATIONAL ENVIRONMENTAL SPECIMEN BANK –
ITS CONCEPTS, ITS HISTORY AND ITS OBJECTIVES

G. Goldstein
U.S. Environmental Protection Agency, Health Effects Research Laboratory
Research Triangle Park, North Carolina

Abstract

A specimen bank will enable scientists to identify geographic variations in pollutant burdens and to distinguish natural background pollution levels from increments attributable to manmade pollution. This is useful in determining whether or not present pollution control techniques are adequate to prevent increased body burdens. Such burdens must be regarded with concern. The specimen bank will have a dual function. First, it will serve as an environmental warning system by providing real time analysis of a fraction of the collected specimens. This would permit the identification of pollutant problems in specific parts of the world as they first emerge. Second, it permits the use of tomorrow's more sensitive and more specific methods of chemical analysis upon today's specimens. This retrospective capability will allow tissue burden patterns to be more confidently compared with fluctuations in morbidity and mortality to test hypotheses dealing with the inception and aggravation of disease.

Making this specimen bank a reality has been the subject of concerted efforts by the U.S. Environmental Protection Agency (EPA) in cooperation with the National Bureau of Standards as well as other Federal Agencies. EPA's present efforts in specimen banking are a logical extension of the Health Effects Research Laboratories' population studies of the late 1960's and early 1970's. These studies involved short-term tissue banking, aerometry measurements, tissue trace element analysis and epidemiological studies.

I.   CONCEPTS

Chemicals are an important part of our daily lives. Like many things, however, chemicals have both good and bad effects. Thus, while some chemicals in 'trace' amounts are essential to human life, others can be deadly.

For example, scientists recently discovered that asbestos and vinyl chloride, two chemicals commonly used to make a variety of consumer goods, caused cancer in workers some 20 to 30 years after they were exposed to the substances. And recently, consumers learned that chlorine, which is routinely added to drinking water in many municipalities to kill disease-causing bacteria, apparently reacts with chemical pollutants in the water to form barely detectable, but potentially dangerous, amounts of carcinogenic agents.

These examples are only two of the discoveries made possible in part because scientists have developed more sensitive, accurate ways of detecting and measuring trace chemicals present in very low concentrations in food, tissues, water and air. Now people are beginning to wonder which of the apparently harmless chemicals in our present-day environment might prove to be health hazards.

Finding an answer to this question is the major reason that the Environmental Protection Agency (EPA), the National Bureau of Standards (NBS) and the National Science Foundation (NSF) are studying the feasibility of a National Environmental Specimen Bank (NESB).

The basic idea of this bank is that from time to time scientists will encounter new chemicals in the environment – new because measurement technology has improved to the point where they can be detected or new because they have shown up in the environment for the first time. These chemicals may be significant pollutants or health hazards. EPA expects that if the capability exists to select and store certain tissues and other environmental samples, then when these new chemicals are encountered, scientists could go back in time and measure their 'baseline' concentrations in the stored samples, using the latest analytical methods. By comparing the concentrations of the chemicals in samples taken many years apart, scientists could determine how significant a health problem the chemical represents.

The purpose of the bank would be twofold; to provide these retrospective capabilities, and equally important, to serve as an 'ecological indicator' or real time monitoring system, with pollutant trends reflecting the dynamics of specific pollutants in the environment. This information is a valuable resource for environmental standards setting and is essential to detect potentially new health hazards as well as to assess the effectiveness of pollution control measures (1).

II.   HISTORY

A.   Environmental Protection Agency

The storage of tissue for analytical measurements is a natural outgrowth of an environmental monitoring system.   This need for such a monitoring system was realized in the late 1960's by the National Air Pollution Control Administration, the predecessor to the U.S. Environmental Protection Agency with the initiation of human population studies (2).

The objectives of these studies, (i) to evaluate existing environmental standards, (ii) to quantitate pollutant burdens in exposed populations and, (iii) to quantitate health benefits of pollutant control, were addressed by coupling sensitive health indicators to comprehensive environmental monitoring in communities representing a pollutant exposure gradient, thus allowing replicated dose response studies over time.

Environmental monitoring was divided into two separate aspects, exposure monitoring and tissue pollutant burdens monitoring.   Exposure monitoring consisted of ambient air monitoring, (Appendix A), whereas pollutant burdens, levels of environmental residues greater than that required of optimal growth and development, were measured in selected tissues (Appendix B and D).   Exposure monitoring was then correlated with health indicators and covariates to assess the health impact of the various classes of air pollutants (Appendix C).

From the very onset of the human pollutant burden studies, short-term tissue banking became an integral part of this program.   A tissue or group of tissues were collected to test a specific hypothesis.   These tissues were stored until they could be analysed, and were then discarded.   As the pollutant burden program expanded, the need for a fully developed tissue banking systeme became more apparent.

During the period between 1970 and 1971, tissue collections consisting of autopsy sets, maternal-foetal sets, and hair were being collected at a rate 50-75 per cent faster than the required analysis could be performed.   As a result, it became necessary to store these samples by the most readily available mechanism — freezing.   This extension of short-term storage into long-term banking raised many questions.   Does tissue storage by freezing alter specific trace substances determined by destructive and nondestructive analytical techniques? Is freezing the best method of storage? What tissues do we collect? How much tissue do you collect? The questions continued, but the answers were not readily available.

In the fall of 1971, the need for a National Tissue Bank was addressed by the Epidemiology Staff at EPA.   The epidemiologists reported that a plan to establish a National Tissue Bank should be formulated.   It was suggested that an advisory panel be convened, composed of experts in areas of interest to the bank, to supplement in-house expertise.   This program was estimated to cost approximately $100,000, exclusive of in-house personnel and require two years to complete.

B.   National Academy of Science/National Research Council

Many millions of dollars have been spent in numerous programs by components of Federal and State government, private industry and academic institutions to collect, store and analyse specimens of environmental interest.   These programs lack coordination and the information derived from them was accessible to only a very few individuals.

In an effort to upgrade the availability and long-term protection of environmental samples and to make the information gathered with each collection readily available, the Subcommittee on the Geochemical Environment in relation to Health and Disease (GERHD) of the National Committee for Geochemistry, National Academy of Sciences/National Research Council (NAS/NRC) at their Asilomar workshop in California (1972), recommended that a group of specialists be convened to study this problem at its Capon Springs Workshop in May 1973 .

C.   National Environmental Specimen Bank System Workshop

In EPA's continuing effort to establish a National Tissue Banking System, a two day working session was held in February 1973 at EPA's National Environmental Research Center, Research Triangle Park, North Carolina to discuss and propose plans for the establishment of a National Environmental Specimen Bank System.   This meeting of thirty-one scientists represented eight Federal agencies, three EPA research centers, two universities and one private research laboratory.

The broad objectives of this working session were:
1.   Establish current trends in human pollutant burdens (short-term banking).
2.   Creating a specimen bank that would provide adequate specimens for future analysis (long-term banking).

The establishment of current trends in human pollutant burdens was a function of the population studies program. In 1973, over 250,000 persons in the U.S. participated in this national program. Although this program was primarily concerned with air pollutants, the health effects of exposure from multi-media sources were constantly being included. Short- and long-term health indicators were employed in surveys of selected populations such as frequency and aggravation of asthma attacks and other evidence of illness or mortality that could be linked to pollutant exposure.

Pilot studies were underway at EPA for the collection of human tissue specimens from biopsies and autopsies with the objective of systematically determining baseline pollutant levels in different organs as a function of age, race, smoking status, residence history and occupational exposure. This determination of baseline temporal and geographic patterns of selected pollutant burdens would enable the measurement of the impact of these environmentally harmful substances upon the health and body burdens of populations at risk.

In addition to EPA's efforts in tissue banking, other efforts were underway to survey exposure problems of a particular nature (Appendix E).

The remainder of the meeting covered topics relating to the formulation of a NESBS. The following comments and recommendations were offered:

The object of the program is to establish a tissue banking system at the national level that will cross all agency lines and provide human tissue representative of the period in which the sample was taken. The proper storage of these tissues would permit retrospective analysis using improved methods that are likely to be available.

These improved methods are expected to be incremental, i.e. development of currently known scientific principles rather than significant new breakthroughs. Analytical methods of present interest that apply to tissue elemental analysis include:

1. Atomic absorption spectrophotometry — flame, graphite furnace
2. Spark source mass spectrometry — isotope dilution
3. Neutron activation analysis — radiochemical and instrument
4. Polarography
5. Anodic stripping voltometry

Optical emission spectrometry, x-ray fluorescence and specific colorimetric techniques may also play an important part in elemental analysis. Eleven elements were given current priority as potential health hazards. These include cadmium, lead, mercury, arsenic, copper, nickel, vanadium, selenium, beryllium, chromium and manganese. With the present technology, accuracy for these priority elements in the range of 5-10 percent was viewed as a reasonable goal. The preparation of protocols for analytical techniques and developing interlaboratory control capability was regarded as essential.

Attention was also given to environmental organic pollutants. The need was stressed for further investigation in the areas of sample collection, preparation and storage to insure that the integrity of the sample remains intact.

A NESB will require a continuing source of specimens collected in a systematic fashion. The generation of sampling protocols would be a step toward assuring the compatibility of tissue samples obtained by participating hospitals and pathologists. It is expected that biopsies and autopsies would be the source of these specimens.

In a limited banking system, it was the general consensus of opinion that the age groups of the collected samples should be: (1) children, 7-10 years old and, (2) adults, 35-40 years old. The minimum number of samples collected per year should be 1000. The rate of sampling, intensively at periodic intervals, or steady rate was discussed. It was pointed out that sampling intensively between long time intervals would tend to reduce uniformity and increase cost. This results from continual start-up problems. No legal difficulties or permit problems were anticipated in collecting tissue specimens through pathologists.

The myriad of substances that would be sampled for analysis at a future date would require a multiple approach to the preparation and storage of tissue specimens. A variety of approaches were presented. (Appendix F).

D. GERHD

The concepts from the EPA Specimen Bank Conference were reinforced by the Capon Springs Workshops (May 6-12, 1973). This workshop was under the auspices of the Subcommittee on the GERHD/NAS/NRC.

The workshop recognized the need for a NESBS to ensure the continuing availability of a comprehensive collection of scientifically selected environmental specimens and information.

The GERHD proposal envisioned the NESBS as a central coordinating institution, relying on specimens collected from a combination of currently existing single-purpose collections and materials banked under its own collection program.   A strict quality control methods standardization program would ensure that items needed for future environmental studies are acquired, validated and properly preserved.

The NESBS could be the mechanism used to continually monitor the environment and assess the effectiveness of control practices.   To accomplish this task, the GERHD Workshop set forth the following objectives:

1.   Establish mandatory criteria for the sampling, storage, and measurement of the various types of specimens that are to be accepted into the System.

2.   Provide historical specimens for: (a) the measurement of contaminants not previously investigated, (b) re-evaluation as analytical methods are improved, and (c) measurements of trends.

3.   Make samples available for use in measuring rates of changes of persistent environmental substances (both natural and man-made), through a program of systematic sampling and careful storage of specimens for retrospective examination.

4.   Establish a centralized data and information storage and retrieval system appropriate to the selected specimens.   This system would be available to the scientific community, and to other interested users.

5.   Provide samples that can be used in assessing the long-term environmental effects of new industries and technologies, or of other activities.

6.   Provide information useful for the assessment of current environmental policies, and for the establishment of revised environmental policies.

7.   Establish a framework for national coordination of current and future specimen banks and collection activities to minimize duplication of efforts.

8.   Foster cooperation and establish working arrangements for the international exchange of information and specimens.

The GERHD subcommittee concluded that the U.S. Government should establish, on a permanent basis, a National Environmental Specimen Banking System.   Initial coordinating and funding of the multi agency system should be considered by the National Science Foundation. The Environmental Protection Agency should be considered as the most logical organization to establish the system.

Four tasks were proposed to begin development of the NESBS.

Task I.   Conduct an inventory and assessment of the value of existing specimen collections as potential candidates for participation in the NESBS.

Task II.   Establish a steering committee composed of representatives from a variety of concerned groups that are providing funds, participating in specimen collection, and operating monitoring programs.   This committee would be responsible for:

1.   Developing the organizational and managerial structure of the NESBS.

2.   Identifying the types of specimens and information to be stored in the Banking System.

3.   Developing interim protocols for sampling, sample handling, and storage of specimens to be included in the bank.

4.   Planning for a data handling, storage, and retrieval system.

Task III.   Identify research needs as determined during the implementation of the NESBS. Areas already identified are:

1.   Sampling strategies

2.   Sample processing procedures

3.   Measurement strategy

Task IV.   Conduct meetings at national and international level, of user and research groups, to exchange current information that would be relevant to the NESBS.

III.   OBJECTIVES

In December, 1973, meetings were held between the NSF and EPA to formulate plans for the development of a National Environmental Specimen Bank System.   A four point proposal was put forth, with joint funding being provided by the NSF, EPA and NBS.   The four point proposal was designed to set the ground work for establishing a specimen bank, meeting the requirements of both Federal and State Governments and of the academic community.

A.   Four Point Proposal

1.   Specimen Collection Survey.

The initial phase of the specimen bank program is to establish a broad data base on the various aspects of specimen banking.   This data base would subsequently be utilized in developing guidelines for the NESBS.   Oak Ridge National Laboratory, working through an interagency agreement with EPA, has conducted a national survey of existing specimen collections, the purpose of which was to attempt to identify those places in the Continental United States that are currently, or have been storing material collected in either research or monitoring activities.   The survey objectives were to identify, (1) where collections were located, (2) who maintained the collections, (3) what the collections consisted of, (4) what analysis had been performed on the material in the collections, (5) how the sample collections had been preserved and stored, and (6) the accessibility of the stored materials and associated data to both research and regulatory personnel.   The survey was designed to include collections in the following areas: geological, atmospheric, human tissues, plant and animal tissues and water samples.   The survey began in May, 1974 and was completed in August, 1975.   Of the 4506 letters of survey intent that were mailed, 649 positive responses were compiled into the data base.   The classification of collection is shown in Appendix G.

2.   Specimen Collection Evaluation.

NBS has critically evaluated the results of the survey as to their utility and applicability to the NESBS.   Few of the survey respondents answered the questions in sufficient detail to give a definite answer, but most of the collections should be of use for taxonomical purposes.

In developing guidelines for the evaluation of this survey, a large portion of the recent literature concerning sampling and storage of environmental specimens has been examined.   In addition, the advice and opinions of workers in various aspects of the field has been obtained.

3.   Protocol Development.

NBS, working through an interagency agreement with EPA, is generating state-of-the-art methodology for sample collection, preparation, storage and analysis.   This task is envisioned as a continuing function for the life of the specimen bank.   This approach would allow for the continued updating of methodology to meet the needs of the bank, of regulatory agencies, and of members of the scientific community.

4.   Planning Document for the Organization and Management of the NESB.

The formulation of a plan for the development and operation of the bank will be undertaken in a series of interrelated tasks.   These tasks include:

a.   Review of the Problem:

An identification and description of the issues which create the need for an NESB will be developed.   The kinds of environmental insults and dangers which could be better managed and the kinds of analyses required to assess the magnitude and trends of such dangers will be described.   In addition, the contribution that such a bank could make to better environmental management, will be estimated.   The result of this task will be a statement of need, including the types of information that would be generated, their various applications as well as a thoroughly documented rationale for the bank.

b.   Development of Specific Bank Objectives:

Based on the rationale and need, a set of specific objectives will be developed to identify just what functions the NESB will be expected to perform and how it will meet the needs specified in Task a.

c.   Identify and Specify Sample Type:

The types of specimens that will be collected for the bank, the areas of collection and trophic levels to be sampled will be based upon existing and anticipated future needs and objectives as stated in Task b.   Specifications of the kinds of demographic and technological data which must accompany the samples will be developed.

d.   Evaluate and Formulate Methods of Analysis:

Analytical procedures applicable to the NESB will be evaluated.   Preferred methodology will be specified along with the amount and condition of sample required to perform such an analysis.

e.   Analysis of Specimen Collection, Preparation and Storage Requirements:

Based upon the kinds and amounts of specimens and the required storage condition of samples, so as to maintain their usefulness, the procedures available for collection, preparation and storage will be analysed and the preferred methods and procedures will be identified. In addition, the total amounts of specimens to be stored will be estimated.

    f.   Analysis of Users:

An identification, analysis and evaluation of potential users will be undertaken to provide a set of user specifications as an input to the design of the system and the establishment of operating procedures. Additionally, a set of guidelines will be established to govern who can use the bank and what can be drawn from it.

    g.   Design, Physical Make-up and Location of the NESB:

Tasks b through e will provide the basic information upon which to establish the functional specifications of the system and will allow for the development of a system design.

The physical make-up will depend substantially upon the numbers and volumes of specimens, the methods of storage, the analytical instrumentation and laboratory requirements, and the numbers and kinds of people who will be provided access to the system.

The location will depend substantially upon the location of the users, the location of the sample sites, and, to an as yet undetermined degree, upon what now exists which may become a part of the system.

    h.   Design or Propose a Data Storage and Retrieval System:

The utility of the NESB will be expressed by the collection, maintenance, processing and dissemination of data. This data system, whether an existing off-the-shelf system, or a new set of system specifications will be based upon user requirements and specimen sample requirements. These requirements will be translated into more meaningful parameters for the design of the data storage and retrieval system. These considerations will include: data volume and compression for storage, frequency of user access to data, updating/amending data, data format, data processing, and data traceability. The NESB requirements may dictate a mix of data storage media and associated access systems to be most cost-effective. This mix could consist of:

        1.   Photographic storage media (microfilm and microfiche)
        2.   Hard copy volume
        3.   Digital storage media with interactive and non-interactive mode

    i.   Develop a Plan for Management and Operation of the Bank:

The management and operation plan for the NESB will consider the following: the maintenance requirements of the physical building(s) housing the bank, the storage facility and the data storage and retrieval system; the procedural requirements for the use of the bank, insuring the economic utilization by the users; outline of NESB support requirements; formulation of a management plan acknowledging the EPA as the lead agency with unambiguous authority for insuring that the NESB meets its objectives by satisfying the user's needs, and recognition of the need to update specimen and data base.

    j.   Budget Plan:

The budget plan will take into consideration the one-time set up costs at the inception of the NESB and then identify all of the cost elements and their contribution to the total maintenance costs.

At the present time, NBS is developing state-of-the-art methodology for sample collection, preparation, storage and analysis, thus satisfying the requirements of tasks d and e. In addition, NBS is preparing documentation addressing Tasks a, b, c and f. Tasks a, b, c and f are regarded as the statement of need, or feasibility study. The successful completion and acceptance of these tasks would warrant the completion of tasks g through j.

B.   Budget

The tasks required to develop the NESB have been designed to give the maximum amount of information in a step-wise fashion while remaining cost effective. Each series of tasks terminates at a GO-NO GO stage, with the exception of the methodology tasks. As a result of the urgent need for methodology protocols and the extended time required for the decision to develop the NESB, the methodology protocols will continue until the final GO-NO GO stage. It is my opinion that regardless of the outcome of the NESB, the methodology protocol development would provide the scientific community with state-of-the-art standardized protocols for sample collection, preparation, storage and analysis for a diversity of elements and chemicals in a variety of ecologically important materials. The cost benefit of this alone is astronomical.

The initial survey and evaluation task which provided us with the present knowledge on specimen collections and sampling, storage and analysis techniques cost approximately U.S. $100,000.00. Protocol development for sampling, specimen preparation, storage and analysis is currently costing about U.S. $200,000.00 per year. The preparation of the NESB need statement will cost about U.S. $50,000.00.

It is estimated that the remaining tasks g through j may cost about U.S. $300,000.00 to $400,000.00.   These tasks would provide detail descriptions for the physical design of banking system, a data storage and retrieval system, operation and management plan and an operation budget.

From our previous studies in the population studies program, the EPA has cost estimates for transportation, autopsy acquisition and analysis.   The cost for acquiring an autopsy set, consisting of twenty tissues per individual varied from U.S. $0.00 to $75.00.   The cost of shipping the tissues would vary depending upon the point of acquisition, storage, and analysis.   As an example, a container holding sixteen (16) autopsy sets and twenty-three (23) kg of dry ice cost approximately U.S. $30.00 to ship by air-express door to door from Los Angeles, California to Research Triangle Park, North Carolina; a distance of approximately 4830 km.

In these studies, the twenty tissues obtained from one autopsy set was analysed for twenty trace elements.   The cost of this analysis was approximately U.S. $ 1200.00.

BIBLIOGRAPHY

1. Banking the Environment.   National Bureau of Standards Dimensions.   **59**:147-149 (July 1975).
2. HAMMER, D.I.   A Community Health and Environmental Surveillance System – Overview, Progress and Perspectives.   Presentation at the Karolinska Institute, Stockholm, Sweden, September 14, 1971.
3. HAMMER, D.I. et al.   Environmental Epidemiology and Human Pollutant Burdens: Theoretical and Methodological Considerations.   Presented at the International Conference of the Permanent Commission and International Association of Occupational Health, Subcommittee on Toxicology of Metals, September 1971, Slanchev-Bryag, Bulgaria.
4. Report of a Meeting of Investigators on Trace Elements in Relation to Cardiovascular Disease.   (Joint WHO/IAEA Research Project) Geneva, February 1971.   Ecological Research Branch, WHO.

APPENDIX A
Ambient Air Monitoring

1. Total Suspended particulate (daily)
    a. Sulphate (daily)
    b. Nitrates (daily)
    c. Organic substances (monthly)
    d. Benz(α) pyrene(monthly)
    e. Trace metals (monthly)
2. Respirable particulate (daily)
3. Dustfall (monthly)
    a. Trace metals (monthly)
4. Sulphur Dioxide (daily)

APPENDIX B
Pollutant Burden Tissues

1. Maternal-Foetal tissue sets
    a. Placenta
    b. Maternal blood
    c. Foetal blood
    d. Maternal hair
2. Biopsy
3. Autopsy
4. Hair, urine, blood

APPENDIX C
Health Indicators and Covariates

1. Acute exposure (<24 hours)
    a. Reversible lung function changes
    b. Acute irritation symptoms
    c. Frequency and severity of asthma attacks
    d. Aggravation of Chronic Respiratory Disease (CRD) symptoms
    e. Aggravation of cardiac symptoms
    f. Daily mortality
2. Chronic exposure (>24 hours)
    a. Pollutant burdens (using man as an environmental dose indicator)
    b. Impairment of lung function
    c. Absenteeism
    d. Prevalence of CRD
    e. Frequency of Lower Respiratory Disease (LRD)
    f. Incidence of Acute Respiratory Disease (ARD)
    g. Mortality Studies

In designing these studies, the following covariates were taken into consideration:

1. Demographic — age, sex, ethnic group, socioeconomic status, bias.
2. Exposure — diet, water, smoking, occupation, migration, indoor-outdoor differences, daily movement
3. Susceptible populations

All the data that were integrated in this program were acquired from the following sources:

1. Exposure monitoring
2. Single-time questionnaire
3. Weekly diaries
4. Bi-weekly telephone contact
5. Spirometry in schools
6. Telephone contact during pollutant alerts
7. Tissue collection
8. Vital statistics

APPENDIX D
Subject Selection Criteria

1. Selection of Subjects
   Subjects will **include** the following:
   a. Age of subject will not be a restriction except as noted below under the exclusion heading.
   b. All subjects must be permanent residents of the county designated by the project officer.
   c. Subjects will include only those deceased persons whose bodies, if stored, have been maintained at decreased temperatures.
2. Subjects to be **excluded** are as follows:
   a. Newborns, if stillborn, or if less than term (premature).
   b. Any subjects over **one** year of age lacking at least **one** gram of collectable scalp hair
   c. Embalmed bodies.
   d. Subjects who are victims of homicides or suicides.
   e. Subjects who are victims of accidental poisonings or intoxication.
3. Collection of Tissue Sets.
The following tissues were collected and in the case of paired organs, the left organ was sampled.
   a. Scalp hair — at least 1 gram, however, 3 grams would be ideal, sampled from the occipital region.
   b. Axillary hair — all hair from both axillae.
   c. Pubic hair — (1 - 2 grams).
   d. Subcutaneous fat — abdominal in the navel area.
   e. Rib — T-10 or T-11 posteriorly.
   f. Muscle — left psoas muscle.
   g. Vertebra — the body of T-10.
   h. Femur — when possible, sample from the shaft.
   i. Thoracic aorta — from the arch at least $2cm^2$ in size, if possible, and as free from arteriosclerotic plaques as possible.
   j. Heart — left anterior ventricle, near the septal wall.
   k. Lung — lower lobe, left lung, anteriorly.
   l. Liver — cut approximately $5cm^3$ from the superior aspect of the right lobe.
   m. Pancreas — the tail.
   n. Renal cortex — lower left kidney.
   o. Adrenal — left.
   p. Ovary — left, or testis — left.
   q. Prostate — left lobe superior.
   r. Thyroid — left lobe, plus a section of the isthmus.
   s. Brain — cortex.
At least 10 grams of tissue from smaller organs and larger amounts from larger organs should be obtained. All specimens should be stored frozen as soon as possible after removal (within 1 hour after removal from the body). No special dissecting equipment is necessary. All that is necessary is that instruments coming in direct contact with the tissue be free from rust and cleaned before each case.

APPENDIX E
Additional Banking Efforts

1. The World Health Organization (WHO) is conducting a multinational program for collecting tissue specimens of the heart, brachial artery, aorta and diaphragm of autopsy tissue of persons that have lived in different geochemical environments and comparing this varying trace metal exposure to incidence of cardiovascular disease. Other tissues and disease states (hypertension, cancer) that may be related to environmental exposure are being planned or are underway [3]
2. The Center for Disease Control (CDC), Atlanta, Georgia, has been collecting human serum specimens from 1964. These specimens are being preserved for immunological testing. The collection contains over 30,000 specimens (1973).

3.   EPA's pesticide laboratory at Research Triangle Park, N.C. is in possession of a collection of human tissues chemically stabilized in formaldehyde. The collection was donated by the U.S. Naval Hospital, Bethesda, Md. in 1966. Some of the tissues predate the introduction of DDT.

4.   ERDA, Los Alamos Scientific Laboratory, New Mexico, has been collecting tissues from the New Mexico area since 1958. A portion of these tissues have been stored. Since 1970, this program has been expanded to include other parts of the U.S. A pathology report accompanies each specimen. Normally, both lungs and kidneys, a rib, sternum, thyroid, gonads, and lymph nodes are included. A gamma scan is taken on the fresh tissue. One half of a fat-free specimen of the large organs is vacuum dried and the other half is frozen at -20° C.

5.   EPA's Office of Pesticides Programs has been collecting and analysing human adipose tissue for chlorinated hydrocarbons, pesticides and PCBs since 1969. Tissues are being collected from 39 locations in the U.S. at the rate of 1,950 specimens annually. No systematic effort has been made however, to preserve, store and bank part of these tissues.

APPENDIX F
Tissue Preparation and Storage Techniques

1.   Low temperature ashing.

This is the method of choice for trace metal pollutants not subject to volatilization at the temperatures used.

2.   Freeze drying.

Lyophilized tissue can be maintained with a high degree of integrity for long periods of time at room temperature. It may be necessary to store some samples under a nitrogen atmosphere.

3.   Rapid Freezing of Tissue.

Storage of labile organic compounds and accessibility for microscopic pathology require freezing of whole tissue samples at temperatures of -40° C to -70° C. Initial and maintenance costs are factors to be considered.

4.   Chemical Preservation.

Traditionally, formaldehyde has been used to chemically preserve human tissue. In the past, impurities contained in the formaldehyde solutions drastically decreased the worth of the tissue for retrospective analysis. Reagent grade chemicals are now available that may circumvent this problem. Further development is desirable in this area because of its simplicity and low cost. Refrigeration is eliminated and the expertise for tissue sample preparation is readily available.

Other items of discussion that related to sample preparation included:

1.   Tissue Excising.

In order to prevent trace metal contamination of tissue samples, surgical instruments manufactured from titanium, beryllium, beryllium oxide ceramic and carborundum were suggested. The present availability of instruments fabricated from the above mentioned substances would prevent their widespread use.

This may change, however, if measurable contamination results from the commonly used stainless steel instruments. For the sampling of specific parts of tissue, a cork borer type instrument was suggested.

2.   Homogenation.

If tissue is to be used for retrospective analysis at different times by different laboratories and/or investigators, it may be necessary to preserve a sample of homogenous trace substance distribution. The inhomogenous distribution of trace substances in nearly all tissue would warrant homogenizing the tissue.

Studies requiring data on trace element tissue distribution would, of course, involve the preservation of the intact tissue.

3.   Supporting Samples.

In addition to tissue samples, a significant number of water, food and air (filters) samples may be useful in assessing pollutant levels in an area.

4. Containment of Preserved Specimens.

Pollutant levels in specimens must reach analysis in the same concentration that they were sampled.   One of the greatest sources of error in analytical work is sample contamination. A prime source of this contamination is the specimen container.   To reduce the possibility of contamination, the following container characteristics should be employed:

    a. Minimum interaction between specimen and container
    b. Minimum interaction between specimen and the external environment
    c. Capable of allowing partial specimen withdrawal without contaminating stored portion
    d. Container capable of withstanding possible temperature changes

5. Supportative Data

The usefulness of tissue analysis will be expanded by the inclusion of supportative data, including:

    a. Pathologist report
    b. Medication history
    c. Health history
    d. Occupational history
    e. Dietary habits

6. Data

The amount of data amassed by the specimen bank will be processed, stored, retrieved and disseminated through an 'Information Data Center'.

7. Legal Considerations.

The attaining of autopsy tissue is usually through authorized medical examiners and pathologists.   In the cases of accidental death, appropriate clearances can usually be attained. The importing or transporting of whole organs or cadavers are controlled by Local, State and Federal regulations.

8. Specimen Bank Advisory Board.

The potential multi Agency, Academic and Industrial involvement into the specimen bank would necessitate a management system for the Specimen Bank.   A Management Advisory Board should be established, with the following duties:

    a. Define the operational and management plans of the bank
    b. Review performance of various elements of the bank
    c. Approve utilization of samples and data

APPENDIX G
Collection Contents

	Number
Microorganisms	52
Viruses	14
Bacteria	45
Plants	272
Algae	21
Fungi	65
Lichens	38
Embryophytes	32
Bryophytes	46
Tracheophytes	72
Pteridophytes	90
Spermatophytes	154
Animals	361
Invertebrates	213
Vertebrates	235
Human Tissues	33
Fossils	19
Crustal Materials	168
Soils	76
Bedrock	52
Organic Detritus	16
Bottom Sediments	95

	Number
Water	115
Air	50
Gaseous	13
Particulates	41
Precipitation	17

Component of Interest in Specimens

	Number
Trace Elements	142
Pesticides	61
Microbiological	56
Mineralogical	76
Organic	61
Radionuclides	33
Medical	33
Other	408
Major Elements	34

Collection Types

	Number
Federal	143
State	103
Personal	14
Private Laboratory	31
Private Museum	13
University	345

MONITORING OF HUMAN SAMPLES
FOR ORGANOCHLORINE PESTICIDES AND RELATED COMPOUNDS

P.A. Greve
Laboratory for Toxicology
National Institute for Public Health
Bilthoven

1.   REVIEW OF CURRENT AND PAST PROGRAMMES

The occurrence of organochlorine pesticides and related compounds (O.C.'s) in human samples is still a matter of concern in many countries and many monitoring programmes are, or have been, in effect throughout the world.   This is the case not only in agricultural countries where spraying with organochlorine pesticides still is indispensable for obtaining satisfactory crop yields, but also in industrialized countries where the pesticides are manufactured or formulated and where - even if the use of the persistent organochlorine pesticides has been banned or largely reduced - the population is subjected to exposure to those pesticides through imported food stuffs.

Reviewing current and past human monitoring programmes is hampered by a number of difficulties :
--   aim, scope and presentation differ widely from one investigation to another, so that the figures can be compared with reserve only;
--   the analytical methods are not always standard ones, nor always clearly described;
--,   many of the programmes are published in not easily accessible journals so that the reviewer must rely upon Abstract Journals.

Nevertheless an attempt to summarize relevant data which have become available in the course of the last years has been made in the Tables I - III.   This summary is limited to the last four years as other reviews covering older data are available (Gatti, 1974; Wassermann, 1974[b]). Although many investigations are included in the tables no claim for completeness can be made. The samples investigated include fatty ('adipose') tissues (Table I), human milk (Table II) and blood samples (Table III).   Incidental investigations on organs (Kawanishi, 1973; Suzuki, 1973 and Vas'kovskaya, 1974) and excreta (Lee, 1973; Vas'kivs'ka, 1974 and Michail, 1974) are not included in the tables.

The figures mentioned in the tables refer to average (mean) concentrations when only one figure is given (sometimes however it was difficult to assess whether 'arithmetic mean',' geometric mean' or just 'median' was meant).   Ranges (minimum - maximum values) are given by two figures connected by a hyphen.   In some instances means values ± standard deviation could be given; maximum published values are denoted as such.

The concentrations in fatty samples (Table I) are always expressed on a fat basis in mg/kg, the concentrations in milk samples (Table II) are mostly expressed on a milk basis in mg/l (justified if Daily Intakes are to be calculated); unfortunately however some authors prefer calculating on a fat basis without giving the actual fat content of the samples investigated.   In Table II the figures on a fat basis are denoted by an asterisk.   The concentrations in blood (Table III) are expressed in µg/l; most figures are given on a whole-blood basis.   Some figures however, indicated as such, are given either on a plasma or on a serum basis.   There appears to be little or no difference between those three ways of presentation.

2.   COMMENTS ON THE FIGURES MENTIONED IN THE TABLES I - III

With due reserve, caused by restrictions mentioned above, the following general trends can be derived from the figures presented in the Tables I - III:
--   The highest residues of O.C.'s are reported for β-HCH (notably in Japan), p.p'-DDE and PCB's.   Surprisingly, only few authors mention HCB as a major residue; this compound must nevertheless be present in easily detectable amounts in most samples;
--   through the years a slow, but steady decrease for most O.C. residues, except for β-HCH and HCB, can be noted (Anonymous, 1974; Greve, 1976; Ramachandran, 1973, Suzuki, 1973; Sugaya, 1975; Brosnisz, 1973; Knoll, 1973; Yamada, 1973; Bojanowska, 1973);

-- residues in males tend to be higher than residues in females (Adamovic, 1973; Ritcey, 1973; Wassermann, 1974; Abe, 1974; Copplestone, 1973; Burns, 1975; Chase, 1973; Kaku, 1974);

-- urban (non-farming) individuals on the average seem to have higher O.C. residues than rural (farming) individuals (Vas'kovskaya, 1974; Hayashi, 1974; Inuyama, 1973; Matsuda, 1971; Miller, 1973; Yoshida, 1974);

-- only few systematic investigations on the correlation between the intake of O.C.'s and the residues in blood or body fat have been made, viz.: Anonymous (1974) for Σ DDT, and Shimizu (1974) for β-HCH;

-- little is still known about the correlation between O.C. levels in blood and in tissues, of Brown (1975) for Σ DDT, Inoue (1974) for -HCH and p.p.'-DDE, and Ware (1975) for Σ DDT in **cattle**;

-- human milk often contains more O.C. residues than cow's milk, and WHO/FAO practical residue limits for O.C.'s in product of animal origin are often exceeded; see Bauza (1975). Bronisz (1973), Luquet (1974), Miller (1973), Pesendorfer (1975), Rappel (1975) and Terplan (1973);

-- although food - and more especially food from animal origin - clearly is the major pathway for O.C.'s to man (Tokutsu, 1970; Acker, 1974 and 1974[a]) other incidental pathways have been found, viz.: HCB in chemical waste (Burns, 1975), DDT in house dust contaminated by spraying for insect control (Davies, 1972) and miscellaneous occupational exposures of workers (Burns, 1974; Kuwahara, 1974 and Siyali, 1973[a]);

-- the data on O.C. levels in samples from cancer patients are contradictory: Kawanishi (1975) reports higher levels, Mestres (1974) found no significant differences, Suzuki (1975[a]) found lower levels;

-- most authors who give an opinion on the subject state that no adverse effects of the O.C.'s levels found in human beings have been established; two authors however (Trebicka, 1974 and Yamada, 1974) correlate clinical symptoms ranging from premature birth and inadequate lactation to the delivery of dead or dystrophic foetuses to high levels of DDT-complex and β-HCH respectively. Two other authors (Siyali, 1974 and Stolfi, 1974) report that the O.C. levels in the mothers' blood are higher than those in the umbilical cord blood, thus suggesting a placental barrier;

-- fasting (Grosser, 1973) or administration of drugs (Sandifer, 1974; Davies, 1973) can diminish O.C. residues in man.

3.   MATERIALS

Traditionally, most investigations on human samples are being conducted with fatty tissues.   Autopsy samples of perirenal fat or biopsy samples of abdominal fat can, in the experience of the author, be obtained rather easily, provided a good personal contact is established between the clinic and the analytical laboratory, and guarantees are given with regard to the confidentiality of the patients' personal data.   Generally a 'depot fat' is preferred over 'recent fat' (cf Mestres, 1974).

Human milk samples generally are more difficult to obtain in an organized way, also because of the fact that breast-feeding is becoming less and less usual in many countries.   The urgence of such cumbersome investigations can be questioned, as they probably can, given the modern analytical possibilities, be replaced by investigations of blood samples.   If blood samples are to be investigated, analysis in the serum is easiest.   The partition of the O.C.'s over the blood components has, to the knowledge of the author, however, not yet been systematically investigated.   The precautions against deterioration during storage or transport include in the first place deep-freezing (at -20° C the samples can be stored for a few years without serious losses of the main O.C.'s).   The formation of TDE from p.p.'-DDT by anaerobic degradation is described by Mughal (1973).

For long-term collection for future reference storage in liquid nitrogen can be envisaged. If human milk samples are to be stored, they should be extracted first and the fat stored.   The fat content of the milk samples should always be stated in reporting O.C. levels in milk.   Preferably, the samples are stored in sealed glass ampoules; plastic containers are to be avoided. Sample size can generally be limited to appr. 2 g of fatty material.   The number of samples investigated is often too little in order to allow statistically valid conclusions.

For a survey, a number of 100 samples in one year can give a first impression about the general levels present and about the homogeneity of the group. If time-trends for the major contaminants in the order of 10 % a year are to be discerned with a certainty of 10 % , a study of 4 years comprising at least 65 samples a year (or 3 years comprising at least 155 samples a year) can be expected to give a reliable answer, provided the group is reasonably homogeneous (i.e. the concentrations are reasonably log-normally distributed) (calculations made by Mr. A.B. Leussink, National Institute of Public Health, The Netherlands, on the basis of data provided by the author). Minimally required background information on the donor of the samples includes: sex, age, eating habits, dwelling place(s) during at least five years, possible medication and professional or occasional exposure to pesticides. In reporting, the results obtained in "normal" samples should be separated from those "special" samples.

Investigations on organs, bone marrow, hair, excreta etc. are of less importance in monitoring work.

The sampling and rapportage can best be organized on a national basis, with frequent international exchange of experiences and rapid publication in an internationally accessible scientific journal.

4. ANALYTICAL METHODS

Many reliable methods for the determination of O.C.'s in fatty materials are available. If the analysis is carried out properly, the results obtained are equivalent, except for special cases, e.g. in the analysis for HCB when partition clean-up techniques are used (Greve, 1974[a]). However, there is a need for further standardization and harmonization of the methods, so as to make the results of the investigations better comparable. Exchange of samples between interested laboratories ('Round Robin samples') could be a first step in the desired direction.

The methods used should enable the analyst to determine at least : HCB, α-,β -, γ-HCH, heptachlor (seldom found), -epoxide, aldrin (idem), dieldrin, p.p'-DDE, o.p.'-DDT, TDE and p.p'DDT. Reporting values for 'ΣHCH' or 'ΣDDT'* is to be avoided as they do not give sufficient relevant information. PCB's should be analysed preferably either by capillary gas-chromatography (Schulte, 1974) or after perchlorination (Berg, 1972). Standardization of calculating methods is still lacking however for the first case. Litttle is still known about the occurrence of other O.C.'s than those listed above. Investigations in the authors' laboratory have revealed that roughly one half of the total organochlorine can be explained by the normal O.C.'s (cf. also Greve, 1974[b]).

Compounds mentioned in literature outside the normal ones include: δ-HCH (0.01 ppm in fat; Kawanishi, 1973), PCT (5 ppb in blood, Doguchi, , 1975), oxychlordane (0.14 ppm in fat; Biros, 1973), mirex (only qualitatively; Kutz, 1974[a]), DDA (4.6 - 33.7 ng/ml in urine; Lee, 1973; respectively 0.1 μ g/ml in urine; Vas'kivs'ka, 1974), 1,4-dichlorobenzene, 1,2,4,5,-tetrachlorobenzene and pentachlorobenzene (Morita, 1975[a]) and methylchlor (31.3 ppb in blood of occupationally exposed people, against 16.8 ppb in blood of a control group; Kontek, 1976).

The yearly costs of a normal O.C. monitoring programme in human fatty samples on a basis of 100 samples per year can be estimated as follows :

–	design and organization of the programme	Dfl.	2.000.-
–	collection and transport of the samples	"	500.-
--	storage of the samples	"	P.M.
–	analysis of the samples (incl. PCB's)	"	35.000.-
–	data processing and rapportage	"	4.500.-
		Total Dfl.	42.000.-

(price level August 1976)

---

* Moreover 'ΣDDT' sometimes includes o.p.'-DDT and /or TDE, sometimes p.p'-DDT and p.p'-DDE only.

REFERENCES

ABE, J. et al   (1974),   Nippon Eiseigaku Zasshi,   **29 (1)** , 93;   via Pest. Abstr.* 74 - 1573

ABE, J. and M. TAKAMATSU (1973), Nippon Noson Igakkai Zasshi, **22 (3)**, 280 - 1; via Pest. Abstr.. 74 - 0292,

ACKER, L. (1974), Deut. Lebensm. - Rundschau, **70 (1)**,   5 - 12

ACKER, L. and E. SCHULTE (1974[a]), Naturwiss., **61 (1)**, 32.

ADAMOVIC, A.M. and B. SOKIC (1973),   Arh. Hig. Rada Toksikol., **24**,   303 - 6 ; via Pest. Abstr, 75 - 0517.

ANONYMOUS (1974). Saga-Ken Kasei-Bu, Saga Prefectural Office, p. 464 - 80 ; via Pest. Abstr. 75 - 1856.

ANONYMOUS (1974[a]). Environ. Sci. Technol., **8 (13)**, 1065 - 8

BAUZA, C.A. (1975).   Arch. Pediat. Uruguay, **46 (1)**,   31 - 42 ; via Pest. Abstr. 75 - 2325.

BAUZA, C.A. (1975[a]).   Arch. Pediat. Uruguay, **46 (3)**, 139-148 ; via Pest. Abstr, 76 - 1615.

BERG, O.W. et al (1972). Bull. Environ. Contram. Toxicol., **7**, 338 - 47.

BIROS, F.J. and N.F. ENOS (1973). Bull. Environ. Contam. Toxicol., **10 (5)**, 257 - 60.

BOJANOWSKA, A. et al (1973). Pol. Tyg. Lek., **28 (51)**, 1999 - 2001 ; via Pest. Abstr. 75-0049.

BROSNISZ, H. and J. OCHYNSKI (1973), Pediat. Pol., **48 (4)**, 445-51; via Pest. Abstr. 75-1288.

BROWN, J.R. and L.Y. CHOW (1975). Bull. Environ. Contam. Toxicol., **13(4)**, 483 - 8 .

BURNS, J.E. (1974). Pest. Monit. J., **7 (3/4)**, 122 - 6 .

BURNS, J.E. et al (1974[a]). Arch. Environ. Health, **29 (4)**, 192 - 4.

BURNS, J.E. and F.M. MILLER (1975). **30 (1)**, 44 - 8.

CHASE, H.P. et al (1973), Rocky Mt. Med. J., **70 (11)**, 27 - 31 ; via Pest. Abstr. 74 - 0607.

COCISIU, M. et al (1975). Igiena, **24 (1)**, 31 - 5 ; via Pest. Abstr. 75 - 1845.

COPPLESTONE, J.F. et al. (1973), New Zealand J. Sci., **16 (1)**, 27 - 39 ; via Pest. Abstr. 74-0061.

DAVIES, J.E. (1972), West Indian Med. J., **21 (3)**, 172 ; via Pest. Abstr. 74 - 0820.

DAVIES, J.E. (1973). Environmental Pollution by Pesticides, Plenum Press, London, p. 313 - 33.

DOGUCHI, M. and S. FUKANO (1975), Bull. Environ. Contam. Toxicol., **13(1)**, 57 - 63.

ENGST, R. and R. KNOLL (1973), Ernährungsforsch., **18 (1)**, 1 - 8 ; via Pest.Abstr. 75 - 1827.

FISHER, I.L. et al (1975). Forensic Sci., **5 (2)**, 126 ; via Pest. Abstr. 76 - 0043.

---

* Pesticides Abstracts, Environmental Protection Agency, Washington - 8 - D.C. 20460.

GATTI, G.L. (1974). 'Problems raised by the contamination of man and his environment by persistent pesticides and organo-halogenated compounds', Luxembourg, Commission of the European Communities, Doc. EUR 5196, p. 383 - 424.

GRACA, I. et al. (1974). Pestic. Monit. J., 8 (3), 148 - 56.

GREVE, P.A. and R.C.C. WEGMAN (1974), Meded. Rijksfac. Landb. Wetensch. Gent, 39, 1301.

GREVE, P.A. et al (1974[a]). 'Problems raised by the contamination of man and his environment by persistent pesticides and organo-halogenated compounds', Luxembourg, Commission of the European Communities, Doc. EUR 5196, p. 187 - 217.

GREVE, P.A., (1974[b]), ibidem, p. 434.

GREVE, P.A. (1976). unpublished results.

GROSSER, V. and W. KNOLL (1973). Deut. Gesundheitsw., 28 (42), 1997 - 2000 via Pest. Abstr. 74 - 1039.

HALACKA, K. and F. VYMETAL (1973). Cesk. Hyg., 18 (8), 372 - 6 ; via Pest. Abstr. 75-1262.

HAYASHI, M. (1974).Shonika Shinryo, 37 (9), 1113 - 9 ; via Pest. Abstr. 74 - 2820.

HESSELBERG, R.J. and D.D. SCHERR (1974). Bull. Environ. Contam. Toxicol., 11(3), 202-5.

INOUE, Y. et al (1974). Nippon Eiseigaku Zasshi, 29 (1), 92 ; via Pest. Abstr. 74 - 1572.

INUYAMA, Y. and T. TAKASHITA (1973). Shimane-Ken Eisei Kogai Kenkyusho Nenpo, 15, 37 - 9 ; via Pest. Abstr. 75 - 1297.

ITO, K. and N. UMEMURA (1973). Nippon Koshu Eisei Zasshi, 20 (108), 406 ; via Pest. Abstr. 74 - 1073.

JONCZYK, H. et al (1974). Pol. Tyg. Lek., 29 (37), 1573 - 6 ; via Pest. Abstr. 75 - 1892.

JUSZKIEWICZ, T. et al (1975). Pol. Tyg. Lek., 30 (44), 1821 - 1824 ; via Pest. Abstr. 76-1640.

KAKU, T. (1974). Kurume Igakkai Zasshi, 36 (12), 1143 ; via Pest. Abstr. 75 - 2344.

KAWAI, Y. et al (1973). Shokuhin Eiseigaku Zasshi, 14 (3), 302 - 3 ; via Pest. Abstr. 74 - 0805.

KAWANISHI, A. et al (1973). Nippon Noson Igakkai Zasshi, 22 (3), 278 - 9 ; via Pest. Abstr. 74 - 0291.

KAWANISHI, A. et al (1975). Nippon Noson Igakkai Zasshi, 24 (3), 426 - 7 ; via Pest. Abstr. 76 - 0375.

KASAI, A. et al (1976). Jap. Soc. Rural. Med., 1 - 2, 48-55 ; via Pest. Abstr. 76 - 1648.

KNOLL, W. and S. JAYARAMAN (1973). Nahrung, 17 (5), 599 - 615.

KNOWLES, J.A. (1974). Clin. Toxicol., 7 (1), 69 - 82 ; via Pest. Abstr. 75 - 0527.

KONTEK, M. et al (1973). Pol. Tyg. Lek., 28, 860 - 2 ; via Pest. Abstr. 75 - 1290.

KONTEK, B. et al (1976). Pol. Tyg. Lek., 31 (7), 265-267 (1976); via Pest. Abstr. 76 - 1642.

KUTZ, F.W. et al (1974). Bull. Soc. Pharm. Envir. Path., 2 (3), no page-numbering.

KUTZ, F.W. et al (1974[a]). Environ. Entomol., **3 (5)**, 882 - 4; Via Pest. Abstr. 75 - 1825.

KUWAHARA, Y. (1974). Kurume Igakkai Zasshi, **37 (11)**, 639 - 53; via Pest. Abstr. 75 - 1283.

LEE, R.K. and S.A. PEOPLES (1973). Proc. West. Pharmacol. Soc., **16**, 240 - 3; via Pest. Abstr. 74 - 0067

LUQUET, F. et al (1974). Aliment. Vie, **62 (1)**, 40 - 69; via Pest. Abstr. 75 - 1814.

LUQUET, F. et al (1975). Pathol. Biol., **23 (1)**, 45 - 59; via Pest. Abstr. 75 - 1851   75-2346.

MATSUDA, H. et al   (1971). Ehime-Kenrit su Eisei Kenkyusho-ho, **33**, 43 - 8; via Pest. Abstr. 74 - 1042

MATSUNAGA, K. et al   (1975). Okayama-Ken Eisei Kenkyusho Nenpo, **22**, 35 - 8; via Pest. Abstr. 75 - 2931

MESTRES, R. et al (1974). Trav. Soc. Pharm. Montpellier, **34 (3)**, 267 - 74; via Pest. Abstr. 75 - 1580

MICHAIL, G. (1974). Nippon Noson Igakkai Zasshi, **22 (6)**, 773; via Pest. Abstr. 74 - 2595.

MILLER, G.J. and J.A. FOX (1973). Med. J. Aust., **2 (6)**, 261 - 4; via Pest. Abstr. 74 - 0060.

MORITA, M. et al (1975). Shokuhin Eiseigaku Zasshi, **16 (1)**, 53 - 4; via Pest. Abstr. 75 - 1574.

MORITA, M. et al (1975[a]). Environ. Pollut., **9 (3)**, 175 - 9; via Pest. Abstr. 76 - 0340.

MUGHAL, H.A. and M.A. RAHMAN (1973), Arch. Environ. Health, **27 (6)**, 396 - 8;

MUSIAL, C.J. et al (1974). Bull. Environ. Contam. Toxicol., **12 (3)**, 258 - 67.

OLSZYNA-MARZYS, A.E. et al (1973). Bol. Of. Sanit. Panamer., **74**, 93 - 107; via Pest. Abstr. 74 - 0020

PESENDORFER, H. (1975). Wien. Klin. Wochenschr., **87 (21)**, 732 - 6; via Pest. Abstr. 76-0660.

PESENDORFER, H. et al (1973). Wien. Klin. Wochenschr., **85 (14)**, 218 - 22; via Pest. Abstr. 74 - 0319

PFEILSTICKER, K. (1975). Monatschr. Kinderheilk., **121 (8)**, 551 - 3; via Pest. Abstr. 74-1065.

RAMACHANDRAN, M. et al (1973). Bull. WHO, **49 (6)**, 637 - 8.

RAPPEL, A. and W. WAIBLINGER (1975). Deut. Med. Wochenschr., **100 (6)**, 228 - 38; via Pest. Abstr. 75 - 1839.

RITCEY, W.R. et al (1973). Can. J. Public Health, **64 (4)**, 380 - 6; via Pest. Abstr. 74 - 0025.

SANDIFER, S.H. (1974). Pediatrics Supplement part II, **53 (5)**, 843-4 ; via Pest. Abstr. 75-0334.

SAVAGE, E.P. et al (1973). Pest. Monit. J., **7 (1)**, 1 - 5.

SCHULTE, E. and L. ACKER (1974). 'Problems raised by the contamination of man and his environment by persistent pesticides and organo-halogenated compounds', Luxembourg, Commission of the European Communities, Doc. EUR 5196, p. 435 - 46.

SHIMAMOTO, T. et al (1973). Ehime-Kenritsu Eisei Kenkyusho-ho, **35**, 71-3, via Pest. Abstr. 75 - 1544.

SHIMIZU, S. (1974). Nippon Koshu Eisei Zasshi, **21(4)**, 239 - 45; via Pest. Abstr. 74 - 1832.

SHIRAKAWA, M. (1974). Nippon Eiseigaku Zasshi, **29(1)**, 94; via Pest. Abstr. 74 - 1574.

SIYALI, D.S. (1973). Med. J. Austr., **2(17)**. 815 - 8; via Pest. Abstr. 74 - 1059.

SIYALI, D.S. and K.H. OUW (1973[a]). Med. J. Austr., **2(19)**, 908 - 9; via Pest. Abstr. 74 - 1062.

SIYALI, D.S. et al (1974). Med. J. Austr., **1(8)**, 285; via Pest. Abstr. 74 - 1829.

STACEY, C.I. and B.W. THOMAS (1975), Pestic. Monit. J., **9(2)**, 64 - 6.

STOLFI, E. et al. (1974). J. Eur. Toxicol., **7(5/6)**, 330 - 8; via Pest. Abstr. 75 - 2086.

SUGAYA, H. (1975). Nippon Noson Igakkai Zasshi, **24(3)**, 434 - 5; via Pest. Abstr. 76 - 0405.

SUGAYA, A. et al (1976). Jap. Soc. Rural. Med., **1-2**, 43 - 47; via Pest. Abstr. 76 - 1647.

SUZUKI, Y. et al (1973). Nippon Nosson Igakkai Zasshi, **22(3)**, 276 - 7; via Pest. Abstr. 74 - 0290.

SUZUKI, Y. et al (1975). Akita-Ken Noson Igakkai Zasshi, **22(1)**, 41 - 4; via Pest. Abstr. 76 - 0969.

SUZUKI, Y. et al (1975[a]). Akita-Ken Noson Igakkai Zasshi, **21(2)**, 1 - 4; via Pest. Abstr. 75 - 1837.

TAKAMIYA, T. and A. UCHIDA (1975), Nippon Noson Igakkai Zasshi, **24(3)**, 430 - 1; via Pest. Abstr. 76 - 0377.

TAKAMIYA, T. and A. UCHIDA (1976). Jap. Soc. Rural. Med., **1-2**, 57 - 59; via Pest. Abstr. 76 - 1649

TAKANO, H. (1972). Iwate-Ken Eisei Kenkyusho Hokoku, **15**, 88 - 91; via Pest. Abstr. 75-0015.

TERPLAN, G. (1973). Internist (Berlin), **14**, 230 - 5; via Pest. Abstr. 74 - 2066.

THIELEMAN, H. et al (1975). Z. Gesamte Hyg. und Ihre Grenzgeb., **21(9)**, 685 - 7; via Pest. Abstr. 76 - 0089.

TOKUTSU, K. et al (1970). Wakayama-Ken Eisei Kenkyusho Nenpo, **19**, 59 - 62; via Pest. Abstr. 74 - 0308.

TREBICKA-KWIATKOWSKA, B. et al. (1974), Pol. Tyg. Lek., **30(42)**, 1769 - 72; via Pest. Abstr. 75 - 1022.

VAS'KIVS'KA, L.F. (1974). Dopov. Akad. Nauk. Ukr. RSR, **Ser.B9**, 827 - 9; via Pest. Abstr. 75 - 0730.

VAS'KOVSKAYA, L.F. (1974). Vrach. Delo., **1**, 129 - 32, via Pest. Abstr. 74 - 1584.

WARE, G.W. et al (1975). Bull. Environ. Contam. Toxicol., **14(3)**, 285 - 8; via Pest Abstr. 75-2949.

WASSERMANN, M. (1974), Nippon Noson Igakkai Zasshi, **22(6)**, 772; via Pest. Abstr. 74-2558.

WASSERMANN, M. et al (1974[a]), Bull. Environ. Contam, Toxicol., **12(4)**, 501 - 8; via Pest. Abstr. 75 - 0521.

WASSERMANN, M. et al   (1974[b]). 3rd International IUPAC-Congress of Pesticide Chemistry, Helsinki.

YAMADA, A. (1974). Kurume Igakkai Zasshi, 37(11), 645 - 81; via Pest. Abstr. 75 - 1313.

YAMADA, A. and Y. SAKAMOTO (1973). Hiroshima-Ken Eisei Kenkyusho Fozoku Kogai Kenkyusho Gyomu Nenpo, 3, 57 - 8; via Pest. Abstr. 75 - 1562.

YAMAGISHI, T. et al (1972). Tokyo-To Eisei-Kyoku Gakkai-Shi, 50, 44 - 5; via Pest. Abstr. 74 - 0812.

YAMAGUCHI, S. et al (1972). Minzoku Eisei, 38(6), 309; via Pest. Abstr. 74 - 1064.

YOSHIDA, K. et al (1974). Nagasaki-Ken Eisei Kogai Kenkyusho-Ho, 13, 44 - 5; via Pest. Abstr. 75 - 1284.

ZARKOVIC, G. et al (1973). Arh. Hig. Rada Toksikol., 24, 381 - 91; via Pest. Abstr. 75-0763.

ZIMMERLI, B. and B. MAREK (1973). Mitt. Geb. Lebensmittelunters. Hyg., 64(4), 459 - 79.

TABLE I Fat samples   concentrations in ppm (milligram per kilogram) on a fat basis

Country	HCB	α-HCH	β-HCH	γ-HCH	ΣHCH	HEPO	p.p'-DDE	o.p'-DDT	TDE	p.p'-DDT	ΣDDT	dieldrin	PCB	first author (year)	remarks
FRG					6.8 10.9		2.9- 7.8			0.82- 2.0			2.9- 6.8	Acker (1974)	
FRG		0.01- 0.03	0.46- 1.3	0.06- 0.16	2.9- 8.2	0.06- 0.12	2.9- 6.2	0.03- 0.58	0.02- 0.03	0.88- 1.3		0.08- 0.23	6.8- 10	Acker (1974[a])	
Yugoslavia											12.8 10.2			Adamovic (1973)	males females
USA											7.6 6.0			Anonymous (1974[a])	1966 (calculated intake: 0.069 mg/day) 1970 (calculated intake: 0.025 mg/day)
Canada											5.83			Brown (1975)	significant correlation with levels in blood
USA			1.29				17.4				23.2	0.35		Burns (1974)	Mexican-Americans > Anglo-Americans
Rumania					4.76						12.4			Cocisiu (1975)	
Israel				0.18			10.8			1.48	11.7			Fisher (1975)	
Netherlands	0.7	<0.1	0.4	<0.1		0.1	2.8	0.1	0.6	1.4		0.2		Greve (1976)	samples from 1968/69 (median values given)
	1.2	<0.1	0.4	<0.1		0.2	2.8	0.1	0.1	0.8		0.2	2.2		samples from 1973/74 (median values given)
	1.2	<0.1	0.3	<0.1		0.1	2.7	<0.1	<0.1	0.5		0.1	1.8		samples from 1975 (median values given)
Czecho-Slovakia							2.2+ 1.6			3.2+ 1.8				Halacka (1973)	
Japan					3.43						6.28	0.16		Inuyama (1973)	
Japan					18.6						35.3	0.9		Kasai (1976)	
Japan		0.09	2.52	0.04			4.41	0.06	0.10	1.36		0.13		Kawanishi (1973)	σ-HCH: 0.01 ppm
Japan			2.96				8.64							Kawanishi (1975)	
Poland				0.15			7.62			5.72	14.3			Kontek (1973)	gastro-intestinal patients
USA		<0.1	0.3	<0.1		0.1					8.1	0.2		Kutz (1974)	
France											3.43- 4.55	0.20		Mestres (1974)	superficial fat
											4.0- 6.5	0.37			deep fat
Japan	0.21													Morita (1975)	
Austria				0.2	1.9		4.6			1.2		0.1	3.5	Pesendorfer (1973)	
FRG			0.26 0.32								0.94- 1.44			Pfeilsticker (1973)	6-7 month -old babies
			0.57								4.51 7.2				7 day - old baby fetuses
			0.45		6.3		2.10			1.10			4.5		mothers
India											21.8 (0.17- 176.5)			Ramachandra (1973)	1965: 24.3 ppm
Canada				0.02		0.04	3.43			1.02			0.12	Ritcey (1973)	males > females
Japan			0.76- 6.2				0.72- 4.1			0.07- 7.0				Sugaya (1976)	

TABLE I Fat samples   concentrations in ppm (milligram per kilogram) on a fat basis

Country	HCB	α-HCH	β-HCH	γ-HCH	∑HCH	HEPO	p.p'-DDE	o.p'-DDT	TDE	p.p'-DDT	∑DDT	dieldrin	PCB	first author (year)	remarks
Japan		0.10	2.30	0.02			3.24	0.10		0.76		0.16		Suzuki (1973)	samples from 1970
		0.03	2.96	0.02			1.27	0.06		0.60		0.21			samples from 1971
		0.04	3.92	0.02			2.82	0.06		0.80		0.43			samples from 1972
Soviet-Union											0.9–15.5			Vas'kovskaya (1974)	urban > rural
Israel											9.94	0.38	2.75	Wassermann (1974)	males > females
Uganda							1.4				2.3			Wassermann (1974[a])	samples from 0- 4 year - old
							1.9				3.8				samples from 5-24 year - old
							1.8				2.9				samples from 25-44 year - old
							1.3				2.4				samples from > 44 year - old
Yugoslavia											8.01			Zarkovic (1973)	samples from 0- 9 year - old
Switzerland	0.6–4.8		0.3–1.8				0.6–9.9			0.8–5.2	1.9–16.3	0.07–0.57	0.4–2.2	Zimmerli (1973)	

TABLE II   Milk samples   concentrations in ppm (milligram per liter), either on a milk basis or on a fat basis[x]

Country	HCB	α-HCH	β-HCH	γ-HCH	∑HCH	HEPO	p.p'-DDE	o.p'-DDT	TDE	p.p'-DDT	∑DDT	dieldrin	PCB	first author (year)	remarks
Japan			0.18 (0.02-0.46)								0.04 (<0.01-0.12)			Anonymous (1974)	
Uruguay			0.06		<0.01						0.23	0.03		Bauza (1975)	
Uruguay	0.01	0.02	0.04								0.07	<0.01		Bauza (1975[a])	
Poland											0.50 (0.15-1.73)			Bronisz (1973)	samples from 1968
											0.36 (0.15-0.67)				samples from 1970
DDR											8.2[x]			Engst (1973)	
Portugal							<0.01-0.70			<0.01-0.34	0.33	<0.01-0.03		Graca (1974)	∑ DDT 1.38 ppm in one case of occupational exposure
Netherlands	0.03	<0.01	0.01	<0.01	<0.01		0.06	<0.01	<0.01	0.03		<0.01		Greve (1974)	
Japan			"high"		0.10 (max. 0.88)	<0.01 (max. 0.02)					0.06 (max. 0.31)	<0.01 (max. 0.03)		Hayashi (1974)	non-farming mothers > farming mothers
Japan		<0.01	0.08	<0.01			0.08			0.02		<0.01		Inuyama (1973)	β-HCH and dieldrin: urban > rural
Poland													0.01-1.40[x]	Juszkiewicz (1975)	
Japan			0.03-0.05								0.08-0.13			Kawai (1973)	
DDR							0.14			0.07				Knoll (1973)	samples from 1969
							0.10			0.05					samples from 1970
			0.07				0.21			0.09			0.09		samples from 1973
USA											0.02-0.20			Knowles (1974)	
France	0.98[x]	0.04[x]	1.67[x]	0.06[x]	1.77[x]	0.28[x]	2.4[x]			0.84[x]	3.24[x]	0.23[x]		Luquet (1974 and 1975)	
Japan			0.07		0.07		<0.01			<0.01	<0.01	<0.01		Matsuda (1971)	farming mothers
			0.09		0.09		<0.01			<0.01	<0.01	<0.01			non-farming mothers
Japan					0.38						0.17	<0.01		Matsunaga (1975)	
Australia	2.20[x] 1.23[x]										8.6[x] 16.9[x]			Miller (1973)	rural urban
Canada										0.01	0.02-0.04			Musial (1974)	
Guatemala											0.34[x]-12.2[x]			Olszyna (1973)	
Austria			0.20[x]	0.05[x]	1.24[x]	3.38[x]				1.06[x]			1.54[x]	Pesendorfer (1975)	samples from Vienna
			0.28[x]	0.06[x]	3.67[x]	3.92[x]				1.76[x]			1.29[x]		samples from Mistelbach

TABLE II   Milk samples   concentrations in ppm (milligram per liter), either on a milk basis or on a fat basis[x]

Country	HCB	α-HCH	β-HCH	γ-HCH	∑HCH	HEPO	p.p'-DDE	o.p'-DDT	TDE	p.p'-DDT	∑DDT	dieldrin	PCB	first author (year)	remarks
FRG			0.02		0.15		0.08			0.03			0.10	Pfeilsticker (1973)	
USA		<0.01-0.04				<0.01	0.02-0.39		<0.01	<0.01-0.11		<0.01-0.01	0.04-0.10	Savage (1973)	rural district
Japan			0.11				0.05			0.02		<0.01		Shimamoto (1973)	
Japan			0.19 (max. 0.38)											Shimizu (1974)	3-4 µg β-HCH/day 0.17 ppm in milk
															67 µg β-HCH/day 0.60 ppm in milk
Australia	0.02									0.06		<0.01		Siyali (1973)	
Australia										<0.01-0.02				Stacey (1975)	
Japan			0.92-6.3				0.77-3.6[x]			<0.01-1.7[x]				Sugaya (1976)	
Japan		0.14[x]	0.65[x]	0.08[x]			2.20[x]	0.16[x]		1.17[x]		0.38[x]		Suzuki (1973)	samples from 1970
		0.06[x]	3.20[x]	<0.01[x]			2.48[x]	<0.01[x]		0.83[x]		0.21[x]			samples from 1971
		<0.01[x]	6.10[x]	<0.01[x]			2.77[x]	<0.01[x]		0.74[x]		0.29[x]			samples from 1972
Japan		<0.01	0.07	<0.01		<0.01	0.06			<0.01		<0.01		Takano (1972)	urban district
		<0.01	<0.01	<0.01		<0.01	0.06			0.02		<0.01			rural district
DDR											0.23[x] (<0.07-5)			Thielemann (1975)	TLC-technique
Japan			0.10								0.07 (0.04-0.13)			Tokutsu (1970)	urban > rural
Japan		<0.01	0.02-0.04	<0.01-0.10			0.01-0.03			<0.01-0.04				Yamada (1973)	residues were smaller than in 1972
Japan		<0.01	0.02	<0.01	0.02		0.02			<0.01	0.03	<0.01		Yamagishi (1972)	colostrum
		<0.01	0.03	<0.01	0.04		0.03			0.01	0.04	<0.01			milk
Japan		<0.01	0.09	<0.01			0.05		<0.01	0.01		<0.01		Yoshida (1974)	urban > rural

[x] The concentrations on a fat basis are denoted with an asterisk, the other concentrations are expressed on a milk basis.

TABLE III Blood samples concentrations in ppb (microgram per liter) on a whole-blood basis, unless indicated otherwise under "remarks"

Country	HCB	α-HCH	β-HCH	γ-HCH	∑HCH	HEPO	p.p'-DDE	o.p'-DDT	TDE	p.p'-DDT	∑DDT	dieldrin	PCB	first author (year)	remarks
Japan			2.3–17.9											Abe (1974)	males > females
			9.3–12.2											Abe (1973)	urban > rural (plasma)
Poland				84							30			Bojanowska (1973)	∑DDT 40 ppb in 1967
Canada											32			Brown (1975)	significant correlation with levels in fat
USA	40 (0-310)													Burns (1974[a])	occupational exposure (DCPA-spraymen)
	3.6+ 4.3−													Burns (1975)	males > females
											117			Davies (1972 and 1973)	unusual high exposure via dust (serum)
Japan							11.2						3.2	Doguchi (1975)	PCT: 5.0 ppb
USA							21							Hesselberg (1974)	cachectic patients
							3								controls
Japan			11.8+ 7.7−				18.9+ 11.3−			4.4+ 3.4−			4.9+ 1.9−	Inoue (1974)	significant correlation with levels in fat for β-HCH and DDE (plasma)
			57.7				20.4			8.4				Kaku (1974)	males > females; urban > rural (plasma)
Poland				11.0			59.9			18.6	84.1			Kontek (1976)	occupationally exposed people
				2.0			1.3			10.6	28.7				controls
Japan			40.0				19.6			14.2				Kuwahara (1974)	female farmers (maximum: 82 ppb β-HCH for pesticide factory personnel) (plasma)
USA											3-78			Sandifer (1974)	blacks > whites (neonates)
Australia	57.1										21.9			Siyali (1973[a])	workers in cotton-producing areas
	59.9										16.7				controls
Japan	11-34				11-48									Suzuki (1975)	farmers (pld > young)
			1.9– 7.7		1.8– 4.7									Takamiya (1975)	nursing mothers
			4.6		5.6										men from rural areas
			1.9		1.5									Takamiya (1976)	umbilical cord
			5.7		5.5										mother
			6.8		4.3										placenta
			13 (7-25)								11(5-20)			Tokutsu (1970)	nursing mothers (plasma)
Poland					2.7		44.6		1.7	17.2	63.4			Trebicka (1974)	mothers exposed to O.C.'s
							6.7			5.9	11.7				controls
Japan			282											Yamada (1974)	correlation of high β-HCH levels with gynaecological symptoms (plasma)
		4.4	10.5	4.2	19.1		8.2			1.1	9.3	3.0		Yamagishi (1972)	mothers'blood
		3.3	7.2	2.8	13.3		2.3			<0.1	2.3	<0.1			umbilical cord
Switzerland			3.4	0.4			14			5.3		1.1	11	Zimmerli (1973)	(serum)

<u>TABLE IV</u>   <u>Abbreviations used</u>

HCB = hexachlorobenzene

HCH = 1,2,3,4,5,6-hexachlorocyclohexane

HEPO = heptachlorepoxide

DDE = 1,1'-(dichloroethenylidene)bis[4-chlorobenzene]

DDT = 1,1'-(2,2,2-trichloroethylidene)bis[4-chlorobenzene]

TDE = 1,1'-(2,2-dichloroethylidene)bis[4-chlorobenzene]

PCB = polychlorinated biphenyls

SPECIFIC WORKING PAPER ON LEAD FOR BIOLOGICAL SPECIMEN COLLECTION

H. Grimes
Department of Clinical Biochemistry
Western Health Board
Regional Hospital, Galway

Summary

A study on the environmental exposure to lead of selected groups of the population of Ireland has been carried out.

No difficulties were encountered in collecting samples and a high response was obtained.

Specimens were analysed for lead by two laboratories in Ireland and 10% of these samples were also sent to two other laboratories outside Ireland.

A.   Review of past and current programmes :

A study was carried out in 1974 on selected groups of individuals to establish blood lead and Aminolevulinic Acid Dehydratase (ALAD) levels in adults and children living in the West of Ireland.   These included rural and urban dwellers, children of lead miners and children of agricultural workers.   In all, 1018 samples were analysed.

A further study was carried out in 1976 in which blood samples were taken from selected groups of individuals, i.e. pregnant women, recent army recruits and dock workers, from the four major population centres of Ireland.   375 samples were analysed for lead and ALAD enzyme activity levels.   The pregnant women and recent army recruits included both urban and rural dwellers.

It is hoped to carry out another study in 1977, again involving selected groups of individuals with emphasis on those who could be considered to be exposed to a higher lead burden or who are more susceptible to the effects of an increased lead burden.

TABLE 1

SUMMARY OF POPULATION STUDIED

	Selected Group	Number	
1974 Study	Office Workers	103	Male
		21	Female
	Blood Donors	55	Male
		46	Female
	Hospital inpatients	69	Male
		50	Female
	Voluntary Workers	29	Male
		14	Female
	School Children	144	Male
		342	Female
	Lead miners	145	Male
1976 Study	Pregnant women	155	
	Recent Army recruits	188	
	Dock Workers	32	

The first study established the range of blood lead and ALAD activity levels to be expected in a general population in the West of Ireland. It was used to study the Relationship between blood lead levels and ALAD activity.   It showed that the blood lead levels of children of Lead Miners did not exceed 35 μg/100 ml (1.7 μmol/l) as it was thought this group might have a higher exposure to lead through their fathers bringing it into the home environment. Some of the miners blood lead levels, as expected, were greater than 35 μg/100 ml (1.7 μmol/l) but did not exceed 80 μg/100 ml (4.0 μmol/l).

The 1976 study was undertaken to test guidelines which were developed for carrying out biological monitoring of populations for exposure to lead in the context of the E.E.C. Draft Directive on biological standards for lead (Doc. V/F/3373/3/74C). A small study was first planned to identify problems which might be encountered when carrying out a larger study. Quality control involving an intercomparison programme with a laboratory of the Federal Republic of Germany and one of the United Kingdom was incorporated into this programme. It showed that screening of preselected groups for exposure to lead could be easily carried out. It identified a group of workers with elevated blood lead levels who had previously not been considered to be industrially exposed to lead.

Both studies were limited by the finance available, and were carried out inexpensively by taking part of blood samples being taken from individuals for other purposes — such as pregnant women, blood donors and hospital patients, or from people who were easy to organize — such as army recruits, school children, office workers, or who were motivated to some degree such as dock workers. Personal contact may have influenced the high response from school children and office workers. The sampling team was assembled when required and was paid expenses and a fee only.

B.   **Rationale for interest or concern** :
'The European Community has an annual consumption of more than one million tons of lead, the most important uses of which include the following :
gasoline additives, electric batteries, paints, varnishes, enamels, plastics, ceramics, printing, pipes and certain insecticides. Some of these uses, by their very nature cause considerable quantities of lead to be spread through the environment.

The transfer of lead from the environment to man can occur in a variety of ways through inhalation, ingestion and cutaneous absorption.' (proposal for a Council Directive on biological standards for lead and on screening of the population for lead Doc. V/F/3373/3/74C).

To accurately assess current and projected levels of environmental exposure to lead, data is required on the following :
- Lead in air measurements ;
- Knowledge of industries involved with lead and their monitoring programmes ;
- Geological surveys as to the occurrence of lead ore ;
- Information as to the location of lead piping in the water supply ;
- Identification of food produced in a lead contaminated area ;
- Information as to the location of paints containing a high lead content.

In view of the difficulties in establishing the quantities of lead absorbed from any given exposure, the effects on the individual have to be assessed on the basis of the total body burden. The methods generally used to achieve this include measurements of the lead levels in blood and urine, and of red cell ALAD activity. The blood lead level indicates the individual's recent exposure to lead.

Lead selectively inhibits enzymes which require the participation of a sulphydryl group - one of these being Aminolevulinic Acid Dehydratase which is an enzyme involved in haem synthesis.

The incidence of lead poisoning has decreased remarkably since the beginning of this century. The main question now is the effect of subclinical lead poisoning particularly in relation to brain development in the child and possibly the effects of lead on the heart and kidney in the adult. Children are considered to be more sensitive to the toxic effects of lead, since it has been shown that they absorb greater quantities of lead from the diet. These effects may be further augmented in iron deficiency anaemia which is a common finding in the 1 - 5 year olds. Recent work suggests that the blood lead range 35 - 60 μg/100 ml (1.7 - 3.0 μmol/l) blood should no longer be accepted as harmless. (Alexander - Lead Symposium London 1974).

Ireland is a country with 3 million inhabitants and is not heavily industrialized — one third of the population resides in or around the capital city, Dublin. Environmental exposure to lead is thought not to be a problem and it is possible that even individuals industrially exposed to lead are not aware of its hazards to health or the risk to which they may be exposing their families to, by bringing it into the home environment by poor hygiene habits.

Factories known to use lead are monitored by a Government Department and are bound by certain regulations which require that their workers have periodic medical examinations. However, the extent and frequency of the medical examination and the monitoring of the worker's blood lead level is left to the discretion of the individual factory. There are some smaller groups such as mechanics, dock workers, plumbers, painters etc. who are not officially considered to be industrially exposed to lead and are therefore not under medical care. Monitoring of the general population's exposure to environmental lead had not previously been carried out in Ireland. It is desirable to establish to what extent environmental lead is a problem in a country which is becoming increasingly industrialized.

It is probable that the contribution of environmental lead from motor vehicle exhaust is negligible because of the country's low density population. Lead in air measurements are only available for Dublin and conform with the proposed air quality standards for lead (Doc. V/F/ 3373/3/74e).

The amount of lead which may be present in food and beverages in Ireland is controlled by legislation [Health (Arsenic and Lead in Food) Regulations 1972] . Samples are regularly collected by food sampling officers and analysed for compliance with these regulations. In general, the lead content in the Irish diet is low.

With regard to lead in water supplies, most piped supplies are from limestone areas and are not plumbsolvent. In addition, many of the houses, especially in rural Ireland, have been reconstructed or newly built in the past thirty years and do not contain lead piping. In Dublin city, lead piping is still present in many houses and approximately one third of the water supply for the city is plumbsolvent. In these houses, high lead values have been found especially in samples taken when taps are first opened in the morning. Residents in these areas are advised to allow the water to flow to waste before using it for human consumption.

Lead ore is mined, or about to be mined, in three centres in Ireland. The mining authorities appear to be very conscious of the hazards of lead and precautions are taken to prevent the development of lead poisoning.

Although paint, with a high lead content, does exist in many houses, lead poisoning in children as a result of licking such paint has not been reported. Two incidents of lead poisoning thought to be due to itinerant melting batteries have been reported, but not confirmed, in recent years. Subclinical lead poisoning may remain undetected in many children admitted to hospital.

C.   Consideration for human sample selection, collection, containment, shipment and storage

Selection

The Irish people do not have Social Security numbers or equivalent, so random selection was difficult for the surveys carried out to date. It was also felt that random selection of individuals could make the study difficult to manage and expensive to carry out. Therefore, in the first study the emphasis was on personal contact to motivate office workers to volunteer to participate in the study. School children were chosen because of their proximity to a lead mine. Selection was random in the sense that each location was visited on a day preselected by the sampling team and blood taken from any volunteers present on that day.

In the second study emphasis was placed on readily accessible population groups — pregnant women and recent army recruits. In the case of the pregnant women, clinics in the four major population counties were visited on a day preselected by the sampling team and samples were collected from volunteers attending the clinic on that day. It was subsequently found that the volunteers represented both rural and urban dwellers. Barracks with recent army recruits were similarly visited, except that the army authorities had been requested to provide recruits from the same geographical locations as the pregnant women. The third group in this study consisted of dock workers, working with lead concentrate, and once the purpose of the study was explained to them they agreed to participate. The methods of selection resulted in a high response rate.

Collection

Blood samples only were collected — and no difficulties were encountered. Once a group was chosen, a central place was arranged and the sampling team visited it on the preselected day. The sampling team was accustomed to working together and was familiar with collecting specimens for lead analysis.   The skin was carefully cleaned prior taking the sample and a venous sample of blood was collected into a syringe and the blood then subdivided into the appropriate blood tubes (EDTA tubes for Lead and Lithium Heparin tubes for ALAD activity analyses). The tubes were uncapped for a minimum length of time when the blood was being subdivided to reduce the exposure of the sample to the air.   All sampling equipment used was supplied by the sampling team, this included swabs, syringes, needles and blood tubes.   10 % of the sampling equipment was prechecked for lead contamination.

Shipment

In Ireland, because of the short distances involved, delivery of specimens to a central laboratory is not a problem.   In both surveys it was possible to have the bloods in the laboratory within six hours of being collected.   Samples were transported by car.

Storage

In both surveys, specimens were stored in a refrigerator initially, and then in a deep freeze at -20 °C.   The Lithium Heparin samples were stored in a refrigerator at 4° C until ALAD analyses were carried out.   ALAD activity was always measured within twenty-four hours of sampling. 10 % of these blood samples were also spotted onto filter papers and sent to a laboratory in the U.K. for lead analyses.   The same 10 % of the EDTA samples were further subdivided — a portion of these bloods being sent to a laboratory in the Federal Republic of Germany for lead analyses. These specimens were delayed for up to three weeks at Customs, despite labels identifying the contents.   The original EDTA samples were stored in their original containers deep frozen at -20 ^{o} C as there was usually a delay in carrying out lead analyses by the two Irish laboratories. This form of storage is simple but takes up a considerable amount of space. It was not intended to store the bloods after completion of the study.

Storing the specimens for future reference requires a very organized system — as retrieval is as important as storage.   The best system for large numbers is probably freezing blood samples in capillary tubes under liquid Nitrogen.   This enables the maximum of samples to be stored in the minimum of space. Such storage could be centralized.

Spotting of blood onto filter papers is another very convenient way of storing blood samples and is suited to both small and large surveys.   Contaminated filter papers may however give misleading results.

D.   Analytical procedures

ALAD

ALAD activity measurements were carried out on the Lithium Heparin samples using the European Standardized Technique (Doc. No 2318/2/73C).   Internal Quality Control was only possible due to the instability of the enzyme.   Each batch of samples included a blood specimen from at least one of four control individuals — whose ALAD levels had previously been established.

Despite the precautions taken to keep specimens for ALAD analysis cool, to avoid light when carrying out the analysis, and to analyse within 24 hours of the sampling, the ALAD activity of the controls in two batches was less than the established values by the same factor.   The excessive fall-off in enzyme activity was thought to be due to the high ambient temperature on these two days.

Lead

Lead analysis was carried out on all EDTA samples by two laboratories on the same campus, both using Atomic Absorption Spectrophotometry.   The EDTA samples which had been stored frozen at -20 °C were well mixed on a roller after thawing, and aliquoted for analysis. On completion of the analysis the specimens were again placed in a deep freeze. Each specimen was analysed in duplicate — if results were not in agreement repeat tests were carried out.

Pretreatment is minimal with both methods used — the Delves Cup Method simply involves predigestion with Hydrogen Peroxide and the Heated Graphite Atomizer requires dilution with a dilute solution of Triton - X - 100.

At each bleeding session blood was taken from at least one of the sampling team which served as a control blood to check precision in the lead analysis. Precision and accuracy were also monitored using a commercial control blood and specimens from the U.K. National Quality Control scheme for blood lead.

External Quality Control was monitored through participation in the U.K. National Quality Control scheme for lead and by exchanging 10 % of the samples with a German and a U.K. laboratory.

Sample contamination did not appear to be a problem. Some minor difficulties were experienced in analysis due to small clots, which were overcome by ultrasonification. Also difficulties were encountered in pipetting comparable microquantities of fresh blood for the Delves Cup Method, this was overcome by analysing specimens which had been frozen and rethawed.

E.   Programme design

The programme design for both surveys was simple. Questionnaires requested minimal information (see copy attached). The surveys were sufficiently small to be handled without computer analysis. The groups were chosen, in general, known to be easily accessible and the selection was random in the sense that it was not known in advance which individuals would be present on the day of sampling.

Both surveys were written up as a report and submitted to the Health and Safety Directorate in Luxembourg.

F.   Organizational aspects

The surveys were carried out under the auspices of the Irish Western Health Board. For the purpose of the Health Administration, Ireland is divided into eight Health Boards, each Health Board being under the direction of a Chief Executive Officer. The Board membership, i.e. the policy-making body, consists of elected representatives from the political, medical, nursing and paramedical fields. A committee of experts was convened by the Chief Executive Officer, and the survey planned with their help. Approaches were made by the Chief Executive Officer to his colleagues in the other Health Board Areas and in this way access was gained to the various population groups. In the case of children, the Chief Medical Officer of Health and School Managers were also approached.

In the two surveys conducted a centralized approach was used involving one sampling team for collection of specimens and two laboratories on the same campus for the analysis of the samples. This approach was possible because of the size of the country and the small number of samples involved. The advantage of one sampling team is that samples are collected in the same manner and the need for standardization of collection technique between different teams is avoided. This approach has worked very well in Ireland but might not be suited to countries with larger populations.

Sampling and analytical teams accustomed to working together were found to be extremely efficient. It was found preferable to have a member of the sampling team complete the questionnaire and by using standardized questionnaires this was carried out rapidly. Questionnaires filled in by volunteers were often found, on the first study, to be incomplete.

With regards to the determination of lead in blood, two laboratories from the same campus using different techniques were chosen to carry out the analyses on all samples because of the known difficulties with this measurement. In addition an Intercomparison Programme involving these two laboratories and two other laboratories, one in the United Kingdom and one in Germany was introduced. This approach was considered to be essential as it was the first time that such a monitoring of the general population for exposure to environmental lead was carried out in Ireland. It is hoped that the results obtained can thus be used for comparison with future studies in Ireland and in other countries. It did, however, involve additional work and expense.

At the present time, one of the major problems with blood lead measurements is the absence of stable reference standards containing known amounts of lead. The availability of such material would considerably reduce the amount of Intercomparison work which is now necessary to ensure comparability of results. The development of an International Quality Control Scheme is desirable. This would involve the distribution of blood specimens on a regular basis to laboratories engaged in surveys monitoring populations for exposure to environmental lead, and subsequent compilation of the results returned. Such a system would aid the comparison of results obtained in the various countries, and participation should be compulsory.

Experience has been gained through these surveys which can be used in planning future studies. This experience covered methods of approaching selected groups of individuals, the actual sampling, transportation and subsequent analysis of specimens.

G.   Ethical and Legal Considerations

It would appear that laws governing the carrying out of such surveys are not clear, but tend to follow the United Kingdom laws. However, a code of practice does exist. Blood specimens may not be taken from individuals under the age of eighteen years without written permission from, or verbal permission in the presence of, one of the parents or guardians. Blood may be taken from anyone over the age of 18 years who volunteers to participate in a survey. Usually medical personnel only are legally covered (insured) for any mishaps involved when taking blood specimens. Medical personnel prefer the results of such surveys to be given to the individual's doctor rather than to the individual himself. As a result of much discussion as to who was entitled to the result − it was decided to incorporate into future questionnaires a question regarding permission to send the individual's result to his doctor.

Although blood specimens only were collected in the surveys carried out, the system for using other tissues is as follows :
1.   Organ Transplant and Post Mortem Tissue :
Permission is obtained from the nearest relative to carry out the organ transplant or post mortem examination. Usually a general permission is given for the post mortem examination but on occasions may be limited.
2.   Placenta :
Placentas are usually disposed of or sent for Histological examination to the hospital laboratory. It is not customary to obtain permission if the placenta is to be used for research purposes.
3.   Foetuses :
Depending on the age of a foetus − it is disposed of or sent for post mortem examination. In the latter case permission is obtained from the mother.

H.   Cost estimates

The first study was not costed but an EEC Grant of £1,200 defrayed expenses incurred. Some analyses were incorporated into routine laboratory work and equipment was already available for the work within the laboratory.

The second survey involved the collection of 385 samples and involved a total of 1,675 hours. It was costed as follows :

1.   Time spent (man-hours)
2.   Cost of Equipment
3.   Cost of Consumable Materials

The personnel engaged on the survey were subdivided into three categories :

1.   Laboratory Technicians & Secretarial Staff
2.   Scientific and Junior Medical Staff
3.   Senior Administrative, Medical & Scientific Staff.

The time spent by each category was further subdivided into the following subgroups :

-    Travelling Time
-    Contact
-    Sampling
-    Laboratory (Analytical)
-    Administrative.

TIME IN MAN-HOURS (Total 1,675 hours)

Category	Travelling time	Contact	Sampling	Analytical	Administrative
1	-	-	-	276	80
2	360	-	75	135	-
3	274	20	30	-	100

A further 225 man-hours plus 100 man-hours transport time was spent by Category 3 personnel in five Meetings of a Steering Committee.

The capital cost of the laboratory equipment used was £18,000 at 1975 prices. The cost of consumable materials used was £627 at 1975 prices.

WESTERN HEALTH BOARD

Survey number

Questionnaire A   **Confidential**

Name: . . . .

Address: . . . .

Date of Birth: . . . .

Nationality: Irish ☐   If other please state which: . . . .

Husband's Occupation: . . . .

Number of Children: . . . .

Stage of Pregnancy (months): . . . .   L.M.P. . . . .

Period of Residence at present address (years): . . . .

If less than one year – previous addresses

during the last three years: . . . .

. . . .

. . . .

BEFORE PREGNANCY – No of Cigarettes approx. smoked per day less than 5 ☐ 5-10 ☐ 10-20 ☐ 20-30 ☐ actual number ☐

DURING PREGNANCY – No of Cigarettes approx. smoked per day less than 5 ☐ 5-10 ☐ 10-20 ☐ 20-30 ☐ actual number ☐

BEFORE PREGNANCY – No of Cigars/cigarellos smoked per day less than 5 ☐ 5-10 ☐ 10-20 ☐ more than 20

DURING PREGNANCY – No of Cigars/cigarellos smoked per day less than 5 ☐ 5-10 ☐ 10-20 ☐ more than 20

Have you smoked to-day ?   Yes ☐   No ☐

BEFORE PREGNANCY – No of glasses of BEER consumed per week/per one night out : less than 5 ☐ 5-10 ☐ more than 10 ☐

SPIRITS : " ☐ " ☐ " ☐

WINE : " ☐ " ☐ " ☐

DURING PREGNANCY – No of glasses of BEER consumed per week/per one night out : less than 5 ☐ 5-10 ☐ more than 10 ☐

SPIRITS : " " "

WINE : " " "

Have you consumed any alcohol to-day ?   Yes   No

Survey number

WESTERN HEALTH BOARD

Questionnaire B   **Confidential**

Name: ....

Home Address: ....

Date of Birth: ....

Length of time in Barracks: ....

Nationality: Irish   If other please state which ....

Previous Occupation: ....

Married or Single: ....

If less than one year in barracks -

previous addresses during the last

three years, if different to home address : ....

....

....

....

	less		greater
Number of Cigarettes approx. smoked per day :	than 10	10-20	than 20

	less		greater
Number of Cigars smoked per day:	than 5	5-10	than 10

Have your smoked to-day ?	Yes	No

	less		approx.
Number of Pints of BEER approx. consumed per week :	than 5	5-10	number
(glasses) SPIRITS :	less than 5	5-10	approx. number
(glasses) WINE :	less than 5	5-10	approx. number

Have you consumed any alcohol in the last 24 hours ?	Yes	No

Survey number

WESTERN HEALTH BOARD

Questionnaire C   **Confidential**

Name: ....

Home Address: ....

Date of Birth: ....

Married or Single: ....

Nationality: Irish ☐ If other please state which ....

Length of time at Docks: ....

Previous Occupation: ....

What cargo did you last handle ? ....   When ? ....

Do you agree to have the result of the test sent to your G.P. ?   Yes   No

If Yes, Name and address of General Practitioner: ....

....

If No, to whom: ....

....

	less		greater
Number of Cigarettes approx. smoked per day :	than 10	10-20	than 20
Number of Cigars smoked per day:	less than 5	5-10	greater than 10

Have your smoked to-day ?   Yes   No

	less		approx.
Number of Pints of BEER approx. consumed per week :	than 5	5-10	number
(glasses) SPIRITS :	less than 5	5-10	approx. number
(glasses) WINE :	less than 5	5-10	approx. number

Have you consumed any alcohol in the last 24 hours ?   Yes   No

BIOLOGICAL SPECIMEN COLLECTION FOR ANALYSIS OF RADIOACTIVITY

J. Harley
U.S. Energy Research and Development Administration, New York

Summary

Relatively high concentrations of radionuclides in the body have been shown to cause damage, and conservative reasoning would stipulate that any amount of any internal radionuclide would have a finite risk of producing an effect. Thus programs designed to document both natural and man-made radionuclide levels in the body are required.

Present programs have been limited in scope but are probably adequate for their prescribed purposes. In the environment, natural radionuclides and weapons test fallout contribute to body burdens and can be measured to estimate population effects if not individual doses. Occupational exposures also give useful information for high levels of exposure in a limited number of individuals.

Sampling requirements for present programs are generally limited to lung, bone, liver and kidney. Present programs have not included collection of reference samples, except for bone ash. Freeze-dried materials should be adequate for most purposes, if the organs can be selected. If not, it would seem desirable to retain a few cryogenically-preserved whole bodies for future reference.

Analytical procedures and equipment are adequate for sample analyses required, but improvements in in-vivo counting of x-ray emitters would be welcomed. Increased emphasis on quality control is needed so that valuable samples are not wasted.

Introduction

Radionuclides in tissue and excreta are examined principally to evaluate possible hazard to man. While the chemical characteristics of the elements involved control their intake and metabolism, the actual effects of radionuclides in the body are dependent on the radiation dose and thus the concentration and type of radiation emitter that is present.

Radiation dose is the common denominator in all problems of radioactive contamination of humans. In simplest terms, it represents the amount and distribution of energy transferred to an organ or tissue by the radiation. This is our best index of hazard, and is independent of the particular nuclide emitting the energy. Direct dose measurements in tissue, however, are not possible and it is necessary to determine radionuclide concentrations as a basis for dose calculation. These calculations are detailed in Spiers (1968) and ICRP (1968, 1971).

One special requirement for radioactivity measurement is that the usual levels of interest require large samples, up to several hundred grams of tissue or several days of excreta. The factor of radioactive decay means that short-lived radionuclides must be determined rapidly and that storage of samples is not possible for such cases.

The distribution of radionuclides within the body follows that of the corresponding stable elements. The major difference is that measurements soon after single acute exposures may not represent the equilibrium conditions existing for stable elements normally present in the body. This particularly appears as a non-uniformity of distribution, both organ-to-organ and within individual organs. It is most apparent for intake by inhalation. Here, the original deposit in the lung is usually redistributed over a period lasting days to years to other organs in the body while also being excreted. This affects the size of the tissue samples required, since in many cases only whole organs can be analysed if the organ burden is to be measured accurately.

There is a degree of simplification in radioactivity measurement in that sensitive apparatus exists for measuring the radiations emitted and that, in most cases, contamination of reagents and apparatus is not a problem. Also, unlike the organic contaminants, the elements concerned do not undergo changes during metabolism that alter their analytical behaviour. The most notable difference from other types of analysis is that many gamma-emitting radionuclides can be determined directly by in vivo counting of the individual in a whole-body counter.

In addition to the literature references that are part of the paper, a selected general bibliography is included to cover individual nuclides that may be of interest.

a.   Review of Past and Current Programs

Studies of radionuclides in human tissue and excreta have been chiefly concerned with six programs.

1.   Evaluating the possible hazard from fallout of radionuclides produced in nuclear weapons tests.
2.   Baseline studies for possible future contamination by radionuclides produced in the nuclear fuel cycle.
3.   Documentation of natural radioactivity with a view to comparing doses from natural and man-made sources.
4.   Evaluating the possible hazard to workers in the nuclear industry.
5.   The use of radionuclides as tracers in metabolic studies of interesting elements and direct metabolic studies of the radionuclides themselves.
6.   Medical applications.

While only the first three of these are actually related to radionuclides in the environment, the other three furnish basic data which are helpful in improving our understanding of radionuclide behaviour.   A number of these programs can be fitted together to develop an overall picture of element metabolism as well as its behaviour in the environment.   For example, fallout strontium-90 and cesium-137 have furnished significant data for understanding the behaviour of these elements in the biosphere while the natural radioisotopes of lead are furnishing comparable information for that element.

Fallout: The fallout programs in the United States included those at the Atomic Energy Commission and the Public Health Service, now the Environmental Protection Agency.   These covered analysis of bone samples for strontium-90 and plutonium, thyroid samples for iodine-131 and measurement of cesium-137 in the total body by in vivo counting.   Comparable measurements on strontium-90 were made in 23 countries, 11 of which produced sufficient data to obtain an age distribution.   (In all of the radionuclide programs, the age distribution is important because both the metabolism of the particular element and the expected dose response to the radiation may vary with age).   Sixteen countries carried out similar extensive measurements of cesium-137 by whole body counting.   These data are best summarized in the reports of the United Nations Scientific Committee on the Effects of Atomic Radiation (UNSCEAR, 1972).   A brief summary of the global dose commitment* for fallout is shown in Table 1, compared with other man-made sources and natural background radiation.   The commitment for the United States is broken down by radionuclide in Table 2.

Bioassay samples were not measured to any great extent for evaluating fallout.   Moghissi et al (1973) did follow the urinary excretion of a group of institutionalized children for ^{90}Sr and ^{137}Cs.

Baseline Studies: The data for baseline programs are chiefly available from fallout measurements.   The principal long-lived nuclides, ^{3}H, ^{14}C, ^{90}Sr, ^{137}Cs and plutonium are well documented and should provide adequate baseline data.   The short-lived radionuclides do not require baseline measurements.

Natural Activity: The global distributions of natural radionuclides are being documented at a few institutions.   In the United States, a large effort is being expended on the radioactive daughter products of radon, both for the occupational exposure of uranium miners and for the environmental levels in certain specific areas, such as the uranium mill tailings piles in the western states and in the phosphate rock mining areas of Florida.   Most of the work is on exposure to airborne dust, but increasing interest is being shown in the tissue content of ^{210}Pb as an index of past exposure.   Dose estimates broken down by radionuclide are shown in Table 3.

---

*   The dose commitment concept has been adopted for environmental contamination where the dose from the radionuclides will be delivered over a period of years.   It is the cumulative dose to infinity to a population group from a specific practice, e.g. a series of nuclear explosions, and is thus not directly comparable to annual doses from natural background and other sources.

TABLE 1

Estimates of World-Wide Average Dose Commitments from Man-Made Environmental Radiation and Annual Doses from Natural Background
(Adapted from UNSCEAR, 1972)

	Atmospheric Tests[a]	Cratering Experiments[b]	Electrical Power Production[c]	Annual Doses From Natural Background (mrad y^{-1})
	(mrad)	(mrad)	(mrad)	
Gonads				
External	84	1.7×10^{-2}	4.5×10^{-4}	72
Internal	35	0.6×10^{-2}	4.7×10^{-4}	21
Rounded Total	120	2×10^{-2}	9×10^{-4}	93
Bone-lining cells				
External	84	1.7×10^{-2}	4.5×10^{-4}	72
Internal	95	0.6×10^{-2}	4.7×10^{-4}	20
Rounded Total	180	2×10^{-2}	9×10^{-4}	92
Bone Marrow				
External	84	1.7×10^{-2}	4.5×10^{-4}	72
Internal	76	0.6×10^{-2}	4.7×10^{-4}	17
Rounded Total	160	2×10^{-2}	9×10^{-4}	89

a   Dose commitments resulting from atmospheric tests carried out before 1971. For ^{14}C, only the doses accumulated up to the year 2000 were taken into account. The total dose commitment to the gonads and bone marrow due to ^{14}C is about 140 millirads, and that to cells lining bone surfaces is about 170 millirads.

b   Dose commitments resulting from peaceful nuclear explosions conducted before 1972.

c   Dose commitments per year of generation of electricity (1970).

TABLE 2

Mean Dose Commitments (mrad) in the United States from Nuclear Testing Through 1970
(Adapted from NCRP, 1975)

	Mean Dose Commitment
External	80
Internal	
^{90}Sr, Bone marrow	45
endosteal cells	65
^{137}Cs, gonads	15
^{239}Pu, lung	2
bone	0.2
^{131}I, thyroid	unknown
^{85}Kr, skin	0.02
^{3}H, gonads	2
^{14}C, gonads	12*
^{55}Fe, gonads	<1
red blood cells	3

*   This is the dose commitment to the year 2000. The total dose commitment, to be delivered over many lifetimes is 140 mrad.

TABLE 3

Summary of Dose Equivalent Rates (mrem/y) from Various Radionuclides Composing the
Natural Background Radioactivity in the United States for External (E), Airborne (A) and
Internal (I) Exposures
(Adapted from NCRP, 1975)

Radionuclide	Mode of Exposure	Gonads	Lung	Bone Surfaces
^{14}C	I	0.7	0.7	0.8
^{40}K	E	8	8	8
	I	19	19	15
^{87}Rb	I	0.3	0.3	0.6
Uranium Series	E	6	6	6
^{238}U (^{234}U)	I	0.8	0.8	4.8
	A	-	0.2	-
^{226}Ra	I	0.2	0.2	6.6
	A	-	0.2	-
^{222}Rn	I	0.4	0.4	0.4
^{218}Po (^{214}Po)	A	-	90	-
^{210}Pb (^{210}Po)	I	6	3	24
	A	-	11	-
Th Series	E	12	12	12
^{232}Th	I	0.0	0.0	0.7
^{228}Ra	I	0.3	0.3	8.0
^{212}Pb (^{212}Bi)	A	-	3	-
^{220}Rn	I	0.0	0.0	0.2

Occupational Exposure: Another source of information on radionuclides is the occupational experience, where about one individual in 1000 is receiving radiation exposure (UNSC EAR, 1972).   The earliest work was on the dial painters who ingested radium when painting luminous numbers on watch, clock and instrument faces.   The largest numbers of individuals affected were in the United States and in Switzerland and this work is well referenced (Martland, 1927; Aub et al 1952; Wenger and Soucas, 1965).   The U.S. cases are being followed at the Center for Human Radiobiology, part of the Argonne National Laboratory.   A second group has been the uranium miners exposed to inhalation of radon daughter products and many of whom have showed a distinctive form of lung cancer.   The greatest number of lung cancers have appeared in the United States (Saccomano, 1964; Lundin et al, 1971) but significant data were also obtained from Sweden (Renard et al, 1972) and are expected from other countries where miners are exposed to radon daughters.   Tissue and excreta analyses have been used to develop the information required to evaluate past exposures for comparison with effects.

Other occupational studies are largely limited to bioassay where excreta are used to estimate the burden of a particular nuclide that is retained by the individual worker.   This routine type of measurement is expanded sharply in cases of accidental high exposures where it is necessary to evaluate significant amounts taken in by the worker.   These cases, if properly handled, can also furnish useful scientific information on the metabolism of the particular element. Some bioassay programs are really designed to supplement engineering control of occupational exposure but the data obtained should still be useful.

Bioassay programs are required by the regulations of many countries even though the interpretation of bioassay data in terms of body burden is extremely dubious (Dolphin and Jackson, 1964; Dolphin, 1972; Harley, 1962, 1964).   It is noteworthy that publications on this topic have been few during the period 1970–75 as compared with earlier periods when numerous predictive models were being developed (e.g. Beach and Dolphin, 1964; Jackson, 1964; Lawrence, 1960).

A number of workers who received a relatively high exposure during the early days of the atomic energy program in the United States have signed agreements with the Plutonium Registry, now called the Transuranic Registry (Norwood and Newton, 1975). This means that the person has agreed that at his death suitable autopsy specimens may be taken for measurement of radionuclides involved. The individual also carries an identification card so that, if death occurs away from his own physician, suitable arrangements can be made for obtaining specimens.

The transuranium program is intended to measure both the total body burden and the distribution of transuranics among the various organs. The sampling protocol therefore requests whole organs, including lung, liver, spleen, thyroid, kidney, gonads and brain as well as samples of certain tissues, including lymph nodes, bone, blood, muscle, fat, skin and teeth. These are generally preserved in formalin by the pathologist before shipment to the central analytical laboratory. Where possible, samples are preserved and shipped in the frozen state. At the laboratory, radioactive tracer is added and the sample is first dried and then dry ashed. The ash is dissolved in acid, made up to a known volume and an aliquot taken for analysis. The remainder of the solution is stored in case of loss during analysis and for future reference.

Metabolic Studies: The metabolic studies on humans must rely on intake and excretion data, rather than tissue samples. A number of short-lived gamma emitters have also been tested by in vivo counting of human volunteers (e.g. Harrison, 1967). Typical metabolic balance studies using fallout ^{90}Sr and tracer ^{85}Sr have been described by Spencer et al (1967, 1972). These rely on analysis of weekly diet and excreta samples from individuals maintained on hospital metabolic wards. More general discussions may be found in Spiers (1968).

Medical Applications: The present medical applications of radionuclides do not require either tissue analysis or bioassay. On the other hand, a number of past applications, such as treatment with radium-bearing water (Gettler and Norris, 1933) and use of Thorotrast (ThO$_2$) as an x-ray contrast medium (Risø Symposium, 1973) have required analysis of autopsy specimens in evaluating exposures.

Summary: The current major programs for monitoring human tissue for radionuclides are the fallout program and the Transuranium Registry program. There are numerous samples being analysed in various laboratories to evaluate specific occupational exposures or to take advantage of the availability of samples but these cannot be called programs.

The past programs have largely been additional fallout measurements carried out at a number of laboratories around the world. The number of samples collected and analysed has decreased steadily along with the general public interest in fallout.

In most cases the amount of sample that became available was used in its entirety. In our own laboratory, excess bone ash was reserved for future reference. Some of this material was used for the determination of other radionuclides such as radium-226, lead-210 and plutonium. Unfortunately, such ashed samples did not receive specific handling to avoid contamination with trace metals or loss of volatile materials so they may not be useful for additional programs.

The current fallout and Registry programs would appear to be adequate for the very specific and limited goals that they were designed to meet. There was no real effort to collect specimens for future reference.

b.   **Rationale for Interest or Concern**

Interest in the body content of radionuclides arises from the health effects shown to result in dial painters and uranium miners. The concept that any dose, no matter how small, has a finite chance of producing health effects has extended our interest to lower levels of radioactivity in the body. This concept of a linear, non-threshold response to a pollutant is the basis of all current standards for radiation protection (NCRP, 1971) and for risk estimation (NAS, 1972).

The radionuclides of concern are a very small fraction of the total number that exist naturally or are produced by nuclear explosions, nuclear reactors or by activation. The ones of interest have been selected on the basis of their characteristics for potential radiation hazard. These characteristics include the amount produced, the expected chemical and environmental behaviour, the metabolic fate of the radionuclide and the sensitivity of the human organ to the particular radiation produced. There is only one case where the toxicological properties are most siginificant, that is the intake of soluble uranium compounds, where chemical kidney damage is more significant than radiation. Table 4 indicates the characteristics of the radionuclides which are currently considered to be of most interest.

TABLE 4

Characteristics of Radionuclides, Including Maximum Permissible Body Burdens

Radionuclide	Source	$T_{1/2}$	Radiation Emitted	Maximum Permissible Body Burden**	Critical Organ
				(μCi)	
^{3}H	Natural, Weapons	12.6 y	.02 MeV β	300	Total Body
^{14}C	Natural, Weapons	5700 y	.16 MeV β	300	Fat
^{55}Fe	Activation	2.6 y	x-rays	1000	Spleen
^{90}Sr	Fission	28 y	.55 MeV β	2	Bone
		64 h	2.3 MeV β		
^{129}I	Fission	1.7×10^{10} y	.15 MeV β	3	Thyroid
^{131}I	Fission	8 d	.61 MeV β	0.7	Thyroid
			.36 MeV γ		
^{137}Cs	Fission	30 y	.51 MeV β	30	Total Body
			.66 MeV γ		
^{210}Pb	Natural	22 y	.06 MeV β	0.4	Kidney
^{210}Po		138 d	5.3 MeV α	0.03	Spleen
Natural U	Natural	4.5×10^9 y	4.2 MeVα*	0.005	Kidney
Natural Th	Natural	1.4×10^{10} y	4.0 MeVα*	0.01	Bone
^{239}Pu	Activation	2.4×10^4 y	5.2 MeV α	0.4	Bone
^{241}Am	Activation	460 y	5.5 MeV α	0.05	Bone

*   The half-life and radiation listed are for the parent of the series. Several radionuclides with various half-lives and emissions form the series.

**   ICRP, 1959.

The best assessment of current and projected levels of environmental exposure are given in the reports of the U.N. Scientific Committee (UNSCEAR, 1972). They include data on radionuclides from natural sources, weapons testing and the present and projected use of nuclear power. Data for medical use of radioisotopes are also included although they are not pertinent to the present discussion. Table 1 in the previous section compares the radiation doses to be expected from the various environmental sources mentioned.

The major pathways for human exposure depend on the chemical characteristics of the particular element involved. The chief difference from considerations of other toxic elements is that insoluble particulates which are inhaled and retained by the lung can produce damage in the lung itself. More soluble compounds may be transported to other organs such as bone or liver where they are retained. Some radionuclides are more critical when taken into the body by ingestion. This explains the emphasis on following dietary levels of several radionuclides produced in nuclear explosions and nuclear power production as well as a few naturally present in the environment. The ingestion hazard in most cases is from foods but in a limited number of local situations the intake of drinking water may outweigh other constituents of the diet.

c. **Consideration for Human Sample Selection, Collection, Containment, Shipment and Storage.**

The specific tissues most useful for evaluating exposure to a radionuclide depend on the particular element and to some extent on the route of intake. In most cases the critical organ would be the desired sample since the concentration in that organ is of greatest significance. Many times, of course, a number of organs will be collected to confirm the distribution of the element in the body. In all cases where inhalation is the route of intake, lung would be a desired tissue with bronchial or lymphatic tissue often being an additional requirement. In the case of excreta, the route of intake is frequently as significant as the chemical form of the radionuclide. Those substances that are readily metabolized or transported from the lung will be found in the urine. Insoluble substances which are ingested or transported from the upper respiratory tract will be found in the faeces. In two cases, exhaled breath is of possible interest. In one case, radon-222 is measured as an indication of radon-226 contained in the body and, in the other case, exhaled carbon dioxide will contain carbon-14 in proportion to the body content.

The precautions or special techniques for obtaining specimens for radionuclide analysis are perhaps less stringent than those for many other pollutants. Contamination is rather rare in normal laboratory operations. The greatest difficulty is that of obtaining a true fresh weight of the tissue samples. Experience with the Transuranium Registry shows that autopsy weights are generally valueless. This is required since radiation dosimetry is based on the mass of an organ as it exists in the living person.

In general it has been found that the standard wide-mouthed polyethylene bottles are the most satisfactory containers. For tissue samples a small amount of formalin is normally used as a preservative, largely to make later sample handling less unpleasant. Urine samples may be preserved by adding 1 percent hydrochloric or nitric acid or a small amount of merthiolate, while faeces samples are preserved the same as tissue.

Storage conditions do not affect the analysis except in the case of tritium. This nuclide, particularly when it is in the form of tritiated water, is subject to exchange with atmospheric water vapor. This exchange is reduced but not eliminated by freezing, so sealed glass containers must be used. For all other nuclides low temperature storage is used only to reduce spoilage.

Long-term storage of samples requires pre-treatment. One simple approach is freeze drying followed by storage in sealed plastic containers. This will maintain material in useable form without loss of any radionuclides except tritium as tritiated water. Freeze dryers with capacities of several kilograms are available and the product lends itself both to storage and to blending in preparation for taking sub-samples. If such equipment is not available, ashing is a possible alternative. Wet ashing results in the least loss of volatile constituents but of course offers the greatest opportunity for contamination by radionuclides in reagents. Dry ashing offers the opposite conditions. Preservation of the original material in formalin or alcohol offers no advantages and frequently complicates later procedures of aliquoting or analysis.

d. **Analytical Procedures.**

In many cases the sample as received must be analysed in its entirety to give the required sensitivity. If this is not true, considerable precautions are necessary in taking aliquots since many radionuclides, particularly those that are recently taken in, are not uniformly distributed in the particular organ. In such cases the sample must be homogenized before attempting to take a representative aliquot. As mentioned above, freeze-dried material can be readily homogenized in a blender and a sub-sample taken. The same is true for a sample that has been dry ashed. Wet ashed samples are usually not aliquoted, since the effort spent in wet ashing is directly proportional to sample size and it is preferable to take the aliquot first.

In the case of the Transuranium Registry, whole organs are dry ashed and then dissolved in acid before taking the necessary aliquot. This does simplify the homogenization if a clear solution can be obtained.

Radiochemical analysis involved separation of the desired radionuclide both from the bulk matrix constituents of the sample and from the other radionuclides with comparable emissions. In some cases the sample can be measured directly by gamma spectrometry without any separation but this is only true for relatively high concentrations of radioactivity. In the more usual sample, separations are necessary to prepare the sample in a form suitable for counting and to eliminate other radionuclides which would interfere with the measurement.

None of the normal substances present in tissue need interfere with a proper radiochemical analysis for a desired constituent.

The available analytical methods comprise an extensive literature since analysts have a considerable reluctance to use procedures developed by others. A few manuals of collections of tested procedures exist (Harley, 1972; PHS, 1967; Holmes, 1967) and these are recommended as the primary source for seeking out useful techniques. A few other procedures are given in the General Bibliography. The methods selected should specify their applicability to different sample types and indicate their other characteristics, particularly sensitivity and freedom from interference. For reference, a list of nuclides determined by various procedures is given in Table 5.

TABLE 5

Measurement Characteristics of Selected Radionuclides

Radionuclide	Major Radiation Emitted	Method of Measurement	Sensitivity*
^{3}H	.02 MeV β	Combustion Liquid Scintillation Counting	1
^{14}C	.16 MeV β	Combustion Liquid Scintillation Counting	1
^{55}Fe	x-rays	Chemical Separation x-ray Counting	1
^{90}Sr ^{90}Y	.55 MeV β 2.3 MeV β	Chemical Separation β Counting of ^{90}Y	0.4 0.4
^{129}I	.15 MeV β	Chemical Separation β or x-ray Counting Neutron Activation	0.4 1 10^{-5}
^{131}I	.61 MeV β .36 MeV γ	Chemical Separation β Counting Direct Gamma Spectrometry	0.7 4
^{137}Cs	.51 MeV β .66 MeV γ	Chemical Separation β Counting Direct Gamma Separation	0.6 4
^{210}Pb ^{210}Po	.06 MeV β 5.3 MeV α	Chemical Separation, β Counting Chemical Separation α Spectrometry	0.4 0.4
Natural U	4.2 MeV α	Chemical Separation Fluorimetry	10^{-8}g
Natural Th	4.0 MeV α	Chemical Separation α Spectrometry	0.1
^{239}Pu	5.2 MeV α	Chemical Separation α Spectrometry	0.1
^{241}Am	5.5 MeV α	Chemical Separation α Spectrometry	0.1

*   As defined in Harley (1972) in dpm per sample and 400 minute count for radioactivity.

Solution standards are generally available for the radionuclides most commonly determined. Others must be standardized by the individual laboratory or obtained by interlaboratory exchange. The best sources for standards are the various national standardizing bodies for individual countries or in the case of Britain and France the Atomic Energy Authorities. Standards from commercial suppliers have not always been satisfactory and some assurance of their quality should be obtained before they are purchased.

The most useful standards, of course, are those where the radionuclide of interest is contained in the sample matrix to be analysed. Such materials are seldom available and it is necessary for each laboratory to gradually generate a large set of 'standard' samples for its own use. Here, the 'standard' value is obtained by repetitive analyses or interlaboratory comparison. The only continuing source of these standards is the IAEA (International Atomic Energy Agency).

Quality control is one of the most important features of radiochemical analysis of tissues since the samples are usually not replaceable and broad replication is not possible. A program as described in the HASL Procedures Manual is desirable*.

One favorable feature of radiochemical analysis is that it is usually possible to check the chemical recovery of the separation procedures either gravimetrically, by adding stable carrier, or radiometrically with an isotopic tracer. This feature, however, as well as other features relating to quality and accuracy do not extend back into the sample collection stage or even the early stages of preparation. Testing these steps is part of the method development and need not be done on every sample if this would multiply the required effort.

e. Program Design.

The present programs of tissue analysis for radionuclides have involved either general populations (as for weapons test fallout) or very limited populations of workers in the occupational programs. Descriptions of some of these are referenced in the General Bibliography.

The largest number of individuals measured was in the cesium-137 whole body counter programs. In theory it was relatively easy to obtain the desired population distribution since this is an in vivo process. In reality, of course, the good whole body counters were operated at large research institutions which were not necessarily well located in population centers. Thus the group measured frequently tended to be laboratory personnel and thus to be limited in many characteristics such as age, sex, economic status and dietary habit. This was the largest program but only a few thousand individuals were measured during the period of highest fallout. These were mostly limited to inhabitants of western countries.

The next largest program was the strontium-90 bone program and almost as many total samples were measured. After about 1960, the various groups all required that specimens were only acceptable from accidental or other sudden deaths where there was no evidence of metabolic disease. In several programs the geographical region included was limited so that correlation with dietary intake might be attempted. Complete information on life history was not always available but at least the individuals were known to be residents of the locality at the time of death. The only other information absolutely required in this program was age at death.

While there were certain differences in the information collected in various fallout programs the minimum required data always seemed to be included. Age, sex, date of death, cause of death and geographical area were most often requested and would probably not be added to in any future comparable program.

The occupational programs, particularly the Transuranium Registry require considerably more information since they are intended to correlate body burden with past exposure. The actual individual exposure, however, was not well known at the time when the highest exposures were taking place, therefore the most interesting cases tend to be the most poorly documented. Present exposures are better known, but considerably lower.

The total mass of data collected in the programs described was small and did not require formal procedures for storage and retrieval. The occupational programs have tended to become computer oriented, since information on individual exposures is more detailed than in the case of general populations.

---

*   An excerpt is appended to this report.

The method of interpretation has been a matter of choice for the individual scientist preparing the report. The only guidelines that have been developed have been those for units of concentration, pCi/g Ca for ^{90}Sr, pCi/gK for ^{137}Cs and pCi/kg tissue for most other radionuclides.

f.   Organizational Aspects

The existing programs for tissue collection are very limited and are directed toward specific goals. This means that any attempt to utilize these for other purposes may receive only secondary attention, since the primary project will not collect samples and handle them in a way that they are suitable for broader use.

The only advantage to a centralized approach is that cost can sometimes be reduced. This is possible through more efficient use of expensive counting equipment and greater efficiency in having a single quality control program. This approach leaves the program at the mercy of a single group — not always desirable.

A coordinated international program would be most valuable in the field of sampling if there is a need for broad geographical coverage. Coordination of laboratory analyses, standardization and the like are essentially no different than coordination of laboratories of the same country.

The requirement for quality control programs is recognized but not always observed. It certainly is a prime requirement for any system producing data from which scientific conclusions are to be drawn. Both this topic and the requirement for reference standards have been discussed in earlier sections. There are no specific needs for training, etc. since the total effort of measurement and data interpretation is so limited in scope.

g.   Ethical and Legal Considerations.

In covering this topic, I must limit my remarks to the United States, since comparable information is not available to me for other countries. The laws and regulations affecting sample collection and storage vary from state to state within the United States. In the simplest case, the medical examiner or other medical officer has the legal right to take tissue samples for any purpose during any autopsy required by law. In other cases the permission of next of kin is required and in still others, there are no rights whatsoever granted to the medical officer and autopsy samples are not directly available. Where consent is required, religious beliefs may often be the controlling factor.

The Transuranium Registry system is based entirely on a signed document of consent executed by the individual that will permit an autopsy and sample collection after his death. The individual also receives a small sum to help defray the funeral expenses. This is not a system which could be broadly applied to the general population.

In considering the financial aspects of tissue sampling programs it is certainly necessary to contribute towards the expenses of the medical officer and his assistants. Such payments do cause difficulty however and they have become the center of heated arguments which have cut off sources of many tissue samples in most large metropolitan areas.

Our laboratory has had no problems with transportation of specimens across state or national borders, however care must be exercised to insure protection of samples during shipment.

h.   Cost Estimates.

The only cost data available to the writer are those from the Health and Safety Laboratory and these are largely limited to collection of a few hundred vertebrae specimens in large metropolitan areas and to measurement of only a few radionuclides. The total cost of the HASL bone program is approximately $150,000 per year. As a continuing program, the design costs were incurred many years ago and cannot be developed here. They were certainly not greater than $10,000. The collection and transport of samples is around 10percent of the total. Storage costs for the limited number of samples are negligible. Analytical costs run about 60percent of the total and the costs of scientific supervision,data handling, and interpretation are about 30percent.

The other available cost data are our operating costs for radiochemical analyses. Strontium-90 and cesium-137 run about $75 while plutonium runs about $700. These costs include everything except equipment, since it is not possible for us to estimate the equipment cost which would be applied to this particular project.

Another general guideline is that the Laboratory considers that analytical services cost $50,000 per man-year including salary and benefits, administrative needs, materials and supplies and overhead.

REFERENCES

AUB, J.C. et al (1952). The Late Effects of Internally-Deposited Radioactive Materials in Man. Medicine **31**, 221-329.

BEACH, S.A. and G.W. DOLPHIN (1964). Determination of Plutonium Body Burdens from Measurements of Daily Urine Excretion. Proceedings of Symposium on Assessment of Radioactive Body Burdens in Man, IAEA, Vienna.

DOLPHIN, G.W. and S. JACKSON (1964). Interpretation of Bioassay Data. Proceedings of Symposium on the Assessment of Radioactive Body Burdens in Man, IAEA, Vienna.

DOLPHIN, G.W. (1972). Some Problems in Interpretation of Bioassay Data. Proceedings of Symposium on Assessment of Radioactive Organ and Body Burdens, IAEA, Vienna.

GETTLER, A.O. and C. NORRIS (1933). Poisoning from Drinking Radium Water, JAMA **100**, 400.

HARLEY, J.H. (1962). Indirect Methods of Estimating Radionuclide Body Burden or Exposure. Proceedings of Symposium on Radioactive Contamination of Workers. EURATOM Report EUR 2210, Munich.

HARLEY, J.H. (1964). Sampling and Analysis for Assessment of Body Burdens. Proceedings of Symposium on the Assessment of Radioactive Body Burdens in Man. IAEA, Vienna.

HARLEY, J.H. (1972). HASL Procedures Manual. US ERDA Report HASL-300. This manual is updated annually.

HARRISON, G.E. et al (1967). Distribution of Radioactive Ca, Sr, Ba and Ra Following Intravenous Injection into a Healthy Man. Int. J. Radiation Biol. **13**, 235-247.

HOLMES, A. (1967). Determination of Radionuclides in Materials of Biological Origin. Proceedings of a Symposium. U.K. Atomic Energy Authority Report AERE-R 5474.

ICRP PUBLICATION 2 (1959). Permissible Dose for Internal Radiation. Report of the International Commission on Radiological Protection. Pergamon Press, Oxford.

ICRP PUBLICATION 10 (1968). Evaluation of Radiation Doses to Body Tissues from Internal Contamination due to Occupational Exposure. Report of the International Commission on Radiological Protection. Pergamon Press, Oxford.

ICRP PUBLICATION 10A (1971). Assessment of Internal Contamination Resulting from Recurrent or Prolonged Uptakes. Report of the International Commission on Radiological Protection. Pergamon Press, Oxford.

JACKSON, S. (1964). Estimation of Internal Contamination with Uranium from Urine Analysis Results. Proceedings of Symposium on Assessment of Radioactive Body Burdens in Man. IAEA, Vienna.

LAWRENCE, J.N.P. (1960). PUQFUA: An IBM-704 FORTRAN Code for Determining Plutonium Body Burden from Urine Assays. US AEC Report LA-2329.

MARTLAND, H.S. (1927). Occupational Poisoning in Manufacture of Luminous Watch Dials. JAMA **92**, 466.

MOGHISSI, A.A. et al (1973). Radiobioassay Program of the Institutional Total Diet Sampling Network. Rad. Health Data and Reports **14**, 129-144.

NCRP (1975). Natural Background Radiation in the United States. Report of the National Council on Radiation Protection and Measurements, Washington.

NORWOOD, W.D. and C.E. NEWTON, Jr. (1975). U.S. Transuranium Registry Study of Thirty Autopsies. Health Physics **28**, 669-675.

PHS (1967). Radioassay Procedures for Environmental Samples. U.S. Public Health Service Report PHS-999-RH-27.

RENARD, K.G. et al (1972). Lung Cancer Among Miners in Sweden. Gruv forskningen serie B No. 167. Svenska Gruv föreningen, Stockholm.

RISØ SYMPOSIUM (1973). Proceedings of the Third International Meeting on the Toxicity of Thorotrast. Danish Atomic Energy Commission – Risø Report No. 294.

SACCOMANNO, G. et al (1964). Lung Cancer of Uranium Miners on the Colorado Plateau. Health Physics **10**, 1195-1201.

SPENCER, H. et al (1967). Effect of Low and High Calcium Intake on ^{90}Sr Metabolism in Man. Int. J. Applied Radiation and Isotopes **18**, 605-614.

SPENCER, H. et al (1972). Effect of Orally and Intravenously Administered Stable Strontium on ^{90}Sr Metabolism in Man. Radiation Research **51**, 190-203.

SPIERS, F.W. (1968). Radioisotopes in the Human Body. Academic Press, New York.

UNSCEAR (1972). Ionizing Radiation: Levels and Effects. Report of the United Nations Scientific Committee on the Effects of Atomic Radiation. United Nations, New York.
WENGER, P. and K. SOUCAS (1965). La contamination et l'accumulation du radium et du radiostrontium chez les horlogers suisses. Radiol. clin. biol. **34**, 67-71.

ADDED REFERENCES:
LUNDIN, F.E., J.K. WAGONER and V.E. ARCHER (1971). Radon Daughter Exposure and Respiratory Cancer: Quantitative and Temporal Aspects. NIOSH and NIEHS Joint Monograph No. 1, National Technical Information Service, Springfield, Va.
NCRP (1971). Basic Radiation Protection Criteria. National Council on Radiation Protection and Measurements, Report 39, Washington.
NAS (1972). The Effects on Populations of Exposure to Low Levels of Ionizing Radiation (BEIR Report). National Academy of Sciences — National Research Council, Washington.

GENERAL BIBLIOGRAPHY

Analytical Procedures
Tritium Measurement Techniques. Report No. 47 of the National Council on Radiation Protection and Measurements. NCRP, Washington (1976).
B. SANSONI and W. KRACKE. Rapid Determination of Low-Level Alpha and Beta Activities. IAEA Symposium — Rapid Methods for Measuring Radioactivity in the Environment. STI/PUB-289 CONF 710705.

Tritium
A.G. EVANS (DuPont). New Dose Estimates from Chronic Tritium Exposures. Health Physics **16**, 57-63 (1969).
A.A. MOGHISSI and R. LIEBERMAN. Tritium Body Burdens of Children — 1967 to 1968. Rad. Health Data and Reports **11**, 227-231 (1970).

Carbon-14
W.S. BROECKER et al. Bomb ^{14}C in Human Beings. Science **130**, 331-332 (1959).
R. NYDAL et al. Bomb ^{14}C in the Human Population. Nature **232**, 418-421 (1971).
Carbon-14 in Total Diet and Milk 1969-70. Rad. Health Data & Reports **12**, 42-44 (1971).

Iodine-129
J.K. SOLDAT et al. Radioecology of Iodine-129. USAEC Report BNWL-1783 (1973).
F.P. BRAUER et al. Natural Iodine and Iodine-129 in Mammalian Thyroids and Environmental Samples in the United States. USAEC Report BNWL–SA–4694 (1973).

Lead and Polonium-210
E.J. BARATTA and E.S. FERRI. Po-210 and Pb-210 Concentrations in Human Tissues. Am.Ind.Hyg. Assoc.J. **27**, 438 (1966).
R.L. BLANCHARD. Body Burden, Distribution and Internal Dose of ^{210}Pb and ^{210}Po in a Uranium Miner Population. Health Physics **21**, 499-518 (1971).
R.L. BLANCHARD. Concentrations of ^{210}Pb and ^{210}Po on Human Soft Tissues. Health Physics **13**, 625-632 (1967).
R.L. BLANCHARD et al. Blood and Skeletal Levels of ^{210}Pb – ^{210}Po as a Measure of Exposure to Inhaled Radon Daughter Products. Health Physics **16**, 585-596 (1969).

Radium
J.B. HURSH and A. LOVAAS. Radium-226 in Bone and Soft Tissues of Man. Nature **198**, 265-268 (1963).
H. SPENCER et al. Intake and Excretion Patterns of Naturally Occurring Radium-226 in Humans. Radiation Research **56** 354-369 (1973).

Thorium
A.S. GOLDIN et al. Radionuclides in Autopsy Samples from Thorotrast Patients. Health Physics **22**, 471-482 (1972).
A. KAUL. Distribution and Excretion of Thorium and its Daughters in Thorotrast Patients. Proceedings of Symposium on Assessment of Radioactive Body Burdens in Man. IAEA, Vienna (1964).
H.F. LUCAS et al. Natural Thorium in Human Bone. Health Physics **19**, 739-742 (1970).

Uranium

E.I. HAMILTON.   Concentration of Uranium in Man and His Diet.   Health Physics **22**, 149-53 (1972).
G.A. WELFORD and R. BAIRD.   Uranium Levels in Human Diet and Biological Materials.   Health Physics **13**, 1321-24 (1967).

Plutonium

E.E. CAMPBELL and J.F. McINROY.   Plutonium and Environmental Metals in Man.   CONF$-$730577$-$1 (Nov. 1973).
E.E. CAMPBELL et al.   Plutonium in Autopsy Tissue.   USAEC Report LA$-$4875 (1973).   See also LA$-$5633$-$PR (1974) for errata.
Metabolism of Compounds of Plutonium and Other Actinides.   Report of the International Commission on Radiological Protection.   ICRP Publication No. 19.   Pergamon Press, Oxford (1972).
B.G: BENNETT.   Transuranic Element Pathways to Man.   Proceedings of IAEA Symposium on Transuranium Nuclides in the Environment.   IAEA, Vienna (1976).
C.R. RICHMOND.   Current Status of Information Obtained from Plutonium Contaminated People.   Proceedings of the Fifth International Congress of Radiation Research.

BIOLOGICAL MONITORING OF TOXIC METALS IN HUMAN POPULATIONS USING HAIR AND NAILS

D. Jenkins
Pan American Health Organization, Mexico

Summary

Biological monitoring of human biological materials can be used to determine the presence, amounts, changes, trends, and the biological effects of physical, chemical, and biological pollutants in human populations.

Direct measurement of the amounts of toxic metals accumulated or concentrated in human hair and nails is effective for monitoring the levels of certain toxic metals including antimony, arsenic, cadmium, chromium, cobalt, lead, mercury, nickel, selenium, tin and vanadium. Human hair has been proven to be valuable for measuring environmental exposure gradients for antimony, arsenic, cadmium, lead, mercury, selenium and vanadium, and for children only for chromium, nickel and tin, but not for cobalt, copper and zinc. Levels of toxic metals in hair have been used in showing occupational exposure, poisoning, and correlating with certain diseases.

Advantages and disadvantages of hair for use in human biological monitoring and need for the international standardization of collecting methods, washing procedures, analysis and storage are discussed. Program design requires statistical consideration of human target populations at risk, baseline control measurements, and optimal descriptive information for individual samples. Hair and nail samples are relatively easy to collect, have small volume and require no special containers or refrigeration for storage.

Many existing laboratories in the world obtain good accuracy and precision in measurement of hair samples and use international standards. These and additional required laboratories could be combined into an international biological network system. No legal or ethical restrictions were noted on use of hair or nails, and they do not appear to have the same implications involved in post mortem specimens, or blood and urine from living persons. It is difficult at present to make cost estimates on a biological monitoring system using hair and nails.

Introduction

Biological monitoring of human tissues, organs, secreta and excreta can be used to determine the presence, amounts, changes, trends, and the biological effects of physical, chemical, and biological pollutants in human populations. It is important to determine past and recent exposures to determine baseline values and trends, dose-effect relationships, and to be able to define standards and control measures to protect humans from the health hazards of present and emerging environmental pollutants.

Biological organisms such as man continuously integrate their responses through time and react to all synergistic and antagonistic effects of combined pollutants and stresses. They give actual responses instead of predicting biological effects from chemical and physical measurements of the environment by instruments. Biological monitoring then resolves the extremely difficult task of extrapolating from these measurements to determine biological responses.

Biological monitoring can be conducted in two ways:

1. Direct physical or chemical measurement of the amounts of pollutants (residues) accumulated or bio-concentrated in the human body and its products. This is especially effective, particularly for toxic pollutants that occur in low levels in the environment at the threshold of measurement capability. (This will be discussed in further detail).

2. Monitor the impact or effects of pollutants on man, rather than the presence of the pollutant itself. This is important but very difficult. It involves detailed epidemiological studies of human health with complex variables, and/or laboratory experiments on animals and limited studies on man. In field studies, the combined effects of many other components of the environment, including nutrition, disease organisms, and social effects, often outweigh the effects of a single pollutant unless it occurs at very high levels and is extremely toxic. (This will not be discussed further except the correlation of threshold and toxic levels to accumulation or concentration levels in the human body and its products).

In this report only toxic metals and metalloids will be considered in biological monitoring of human populations. These include antimony, arsenic, beryllium, boron, cadmium, chromium, cobalt, copper, lead, mercury, nickel, selenium, tin, and vanadium.

In biological monitoring of human populations, the selection of the optimal tissues, secreta or excreta and organs is of critical importance, particularly in living subjects, without causing harm or damage. It is important to determine which parts of the body and products accumulate or concentrate the toxic metals and retain them for periods of time. The biological materials from living humans, which have been collected, include blood, urine, faeces, hair, nails, sweat, placentae and foetuses. Blood and urine have been used extensively for determining levels and exposures of toxic metals in man. For very recent exposures, blood and urine are excellent biological indicators for certain metals. However, for most metals, the levels in blood and urine decrease rapidly following cessation of exposure. Placentae and foetuses are also of value for certain metals but only in restricted segments of the population. They are unsuitable for measuring levels in children and men who are often in the most exposed target populations. Sweat is difficult to obtain and measure and the levels are transient.

For measurement of levels of toxic metals for long continuing periods, or especially for measuring exposure to high levels during past periods, hair and nails appear to be superior to blood and urine for certain toxic metals which are highly concentrated in the hair and nails.

Sequestering tissue such as hair and nails immobilize elements and take them out of equilibrium with the rest of the organism. These tissues, as well as lung and kidney, can be used as indices of chronic over-exposures, and for diagnosing disease conditions or deficiencies related to toxic trace metals. Hair is being studied for use of trace element concentrations for hair individualization and identification in a manner similar to identification by fingerprint analysis. Hair and nails are also used in forensic science to determine poisoning and evidence of ingestion of abnormal amounts of toxic metals.

The Global Environmental Monitoring System (GEMS) of the United Nations Environmental Program has selected human hair as one of the important monitoring materials for the biological monitoring program.

a.   **Review of Past and Current Programs**

There is an extensive literature on the use of human hair and nails for biological monitoring of human populations. About 300 references have been consulted and the data have been compiled and evaluated for use for biological monitoring systems and networks (Jenkins, 1977). The concentration levels of toxic metals in hair and nails have been determined in all regions of the world, but none on a continuing basis, or as a network over a wide geographical area. The levels of toxic metals in hair have been correlated with various factors (see Table including a) environmental exposure gradients (from smelters, mines, highways, and other sources), b) occupational exposure levels, c) geographic area or region, d) historical trends, and e) disease and physiological or pathologic effects associated with nutritional excesses or deficiencies. Sample collection factors have been studied including effects of a) sex, b) age, c) hair color, d) comparison of scalp, pubic, axillary, chest, and facial hair, and e) concentration variation in relation to distance from scalp.

Human hair is a representative and meaningful tissue for monitoring levels of antimony, arsenic, cadmium, chromium, cobalt, copper, lead, mercury, nickel, selenium, tin and vanadium. There are not enough data for beryllium and boron in hair to state whether they are accumulated or concentrated in hair.

Hair levels of toxic metals have been clearly correlated with environmental gradients as follows: **antimony** − for a refinery; **arsenic** −for copper, lead and zinc smelters, zinc-copper mines, thermal power plant, and high levels in drinking water; **beryllium** − no data; **boron** − no correlation with environmental gradients; **cadmium** − for lead, zinc, and copper smelters, use of cadmium on golf courses, (but no correlation with epidemic and non-epidemic areas of itai-itai disease); **chromium** − environmental exposure gradient reflected in children's hair only; **cobalt** − no correlation with environmental gradients; **copper** − no correlation with environmental gradients; **lead** − for lead, zinc, and copper smelters, petrochemical industry, highways and high vehicle density or use, and lead processing plants; **mercury** − mercury smelters, urban to rural gradient, and from areas with high levels in food; **nickel** − urban to rural gradient - children only; **selenium** − for geographic areas with high Se levels; **tin** − for urban to rural gradient only in children; **vanadium** − urban to rural gradient exposures in adults and children. Zinc in hair was not correlated with environmental gradients.

TABLE 1
POSSIBLE CLINICAL USE OF HAIR AND NAILS FOR HELPING DIAGNOSE OR INDICATE DISEASE OR DEFICIENCY STATES*

Antimony	—	Toxic to humans and animals.
Arsenic	—	Arsenite is toxic; arsenical polyneuritis.
Beryllium	—	Toxic; causes cancer of lung.
Boron	—	Low toxicity to mammals.
Cadmium	—	Toxic; causes arterial hypertension, pregnancy toxaemia, itai-itai disease; is most insidious and widespread health hazard, causes congenital abnormalities.
Chromium	—	Causes diabetes mellitus; cancer of lung; deficiency causes atherosclerosis, hypercholesteremia, hyperglycemia; accumulates in lung.
Cobalt	—	High Co implicated in myocardial insufficiency; may play a role in immune reactions.
Copper	—	Absence of gene for Cu homeostasis causes hepatolenticular degeneration; high Cu implicated in various collagen diseases, rheumatoid arthritis; and infections.
Lead	—	Toxic; lead poisoning, subclinical states from moderate level, with ill-defined asthenia, neurosis; mental retardation in children.
Mercury	—	Methyl Hg is highly toxic; mercury poisoning, Minamata disease, causes congenital abnormalities.
Nickel	—	Causes cancer of lung; in myocardial infarction Ni increases in blood; causes congenital abnormalities.
Selenium	—	Essential element; excess causes alopecia; causes tumours.
Tin	—	Toxic; accumulates in lung.
Vanadium	—	May have a role in cholesterol and fatty acid metabolism; accumulates in lung.

* Modified after Schroeder and Nason (1971).

The use of hair for measuring environmental exposure gradients is therefore of value for measuring antimony, arsenic, cadmium, lead, mercury, selenium, and vanadium, and for children only for chromium, nickel and tin. Hair was not useful for measuring environment gradients for cobalt, copper, and zinc, and unknown for boron and beryllium.

Hair levels of toxic metals have been used to show occupational exposures to antimony, arsenic, cadmium, lead, mercury and nickel. Hair has proved to be valuable for determining the exposure experience, and for certain metals, using sensitive techniques, for dating the exact time or period of high exposure.

Hair and nails may be valuable for diagnosing or correlating with disease states. The various diseases or deficiency states caused by or correlated with the fourteen toxic metals are shown in Table 2.

Fingernails and toe nails have been studied for toxic metal levels for arsenic, chromium, copper, lead, mercury, selenium, and vanadium. They have been found of value in arsenic for correlating with exposure to high arsenic water levels and arsenic poisoning; in chromium in correlating with disease states, in mercury with high exposure to Hg in food, in selenium with exposure of people to areas with high Se levels; and in vanadium with occupational exposure in the oil industry and vanadium ore workers. Nails have not been used as extensively as hair. A rather extensive correlation study has been conducted by Masironi (1975) using levels of toxic metals in toe nails correlated with cardiovascular disease.

There are certain advantages and disadvantages of using hair as a tissue for biological monitoring. These are compared below:

A. Advantages of Hair as a Biological Monitoring Tissue

1. Certain toxic metals accumulate or concentrate in hair.
2. Metals are retained and provide a linear historic record over time, of the time and period of exposure (do not decrease rapidly as in blood and urine after cessation of exposure). Hair is stable and samples several hundred years old have been analysed.
3. Samples are easily obtained from clipping hair from subjects, from barber shops, and using historic hair samples and other sources, with minimum legal problems.

4.   Require only plastic sacks or simple containers for storage.
5.   Do not require dry ice or refrigeration for storage and transport.
6.   Hair is easily transported and has little weight or volume.
7.   Standardized methods are available for collecting hair samples.
8.   Standardized methods are available for washing and preparation of samples.
9.   Standardized methods are available for analysis and use of standards.
10. Storage of aliquots is simple for re-analysis and study of historic trends (no decomposition or changes reported).
11. For certain metals there is excellent correlation with environmental exposure gradients, e.g. distancefrom smelters, mines, and other sources.
12. For certain metals there is good correlation with natural geographic occurrence as with Se or As.
13. For certain metals there is good correlation with excess or deficiency disease states.
14. For certain metals there is good correlation with occupational exposure.

B.   Disadvantages of Hair as a Biological Monitoring Tissue.

1.   External contamination of hair can be a source of error. This can come from hair dyes, shampoos, soaps, cosmetics, free oils, hair sprays and lacquers, as well as dust and dirt from hands and the atmosphere.
2.   In cases where external contamination of scalp hair is suspected it may be necessary to compare scalp hair with axillary, pubic, chest, or face hair. Hair at the base of the scalp in the rear of the head has been recommended as the area least contaminated from external sources.
3.   Washing procedures before analysis may affect the results for some metals depending on the procedure used. Detergents, organic solvents, and especially chelating agents remove various amounts of exogenous surface contamination. Standardized sample preparation procedures must be used.
4.   There is variation in the level of metals with distance from the scalp, depending on the exposure history. The distance of hair from the scalp must be measured and reported.

TABLE 2
MONITORING OF TOXIC METALS IN HUMAN HAIR AND NAILS IN VARIOUS REGIONS OF THE WORLD*

	Sb	As	Cd	Cr	Co	Cu	Pb	Hg	Ni	Se	Sn	V
Canada	G	O		S	S	O	G,O,W	S,O,W		S		
United States	S,H	G,O,H	G,O,S	G,S,H	S,H	G,S,H	G,O,W H,N	G,O,F H,N	G,O,H	G,S,H	G	G,S,H N
Central America		W					G,S,O	G,S,O		G		
South America		W						S		G		N
Great Britain		G,O,S				G,S,N	G,O	G,S				
Europe		G,O,H	O			S	G,O,W	G,S,F O	O			
Middle East						G	O,F	F,S				
Africa	O						O					
S.E. Asia							S	F,S				
Australia and N.Z.	S	S				S	O,S	S		S		
Japan		G	F,W				G,O	G,S,F O				
New Guinea, Samoa					N			F				N

Monitoring Objectives		
G	— Environmental **gradient**	
O	-- Occupational exposure	
S	— Sampling Base Line	
F	— Food	
W	— Water	
H	— Historical	
N	— (Nails)	

*   From Jenkins (1977).

b.   **Program Design**

Statistical considerations of biological monitoring should clearly include the human target populations at risk, for example, around sources such as smelters, mines, local high concentrations in soil and water supply, urban areas including metal processing industry, manufacturing areas, and populations at risk from occupational exposure, and eating contaminated foods. It is also necessary to monitor unexposed human control population groups in rural and isolated areas including islands to determine background baseline levels. For many of these metals there are now regional baseline data or control data to compare with exposed populations at risk. These data should be subjected to statistical evaluations to determine the validity of the data and to determine what additional data are required. Until this is accomplished, the magnitude of a proposed monitoring program is still subject to the outcome of the evaluation.

The optimal descriptive information required for each individual sample includes the following:

1.   Age, sex, race, skin and hair colour.
2.   Occupation, length of time in occupation, other occupational history.
3.   Exposure to toxic metals
    a)   Urban or rural;
    b)   Occupational special exposure;
    c)   Hobbies, vacations, special foods, water, use of pottery, smoking habits;
    d)   Cosmetics, hair care, washing frequencies, dyes;
    e)   Environment — live near smelters, mines, traffic, metal industries, etc.;
4.   Hair sample — location on scalp or elsewhere, distance from scalp, how collected, date, amount ;
5.   Special remarks — disease, alopecia, skin or other disorders, illness, hospital or medical history if applicable. Living or dead, cause of death if applicable;
6.   Special remarks — e.g. socioeconomic group, education .

Procedures to standardize information collected. — It is necessary to agree on an international standardization on the size of hair sample, location on scalp, distance from scalp, and length of hair.

Sample preparation requires international agreement and standardization of washing procedures including use of detergents, organic solvents, and chelating agents. Also included is the method of drying and reporting the basis of measurement, e.g. wet, air dry, oven dry (temp.), and ash. The accurate and optimal methods of analysis should be agreed upon, and standardized analytical samples should be used. The results should be reported as ppm (preferably oven dry weight) and precision of analysis should be reported. The number of samples, range, arithmetic and geometric means, median, standard deviation, or standard error and other statistical data and tests of significance should be reported.

Data storage should be accomplished by national centers or regional centers of certain United Nations agencies such as WHO and UNEP. The retrieval of data should be included in the storage system. Interpretation of the data should be the responsibility of competent and responsible authorities in countries and in international agencies.

c.   **Organizational Aspects**

Existing programs should be used to the maximum extent possible. There are existing laboratories in many of the countries which already use international standards and obtain good accuracy and precision of measurement. Many of these laboratories require information on international standardization of sample collecting methods, sample preparation, measurement methodology and supply and use of standardized samples, reporting of measurements, and storage of aliquot samples. These laboratories and additional ones as required could be combined into an international human biological monitoring network with internationally standardized methodology, data storage, and tissue bank collections for future reference.

d.   **Ethical and Legal Considerations**

In reviewing 400 references on use of human hair and nails from a large number of countries of the world, no reference was made to laws, regulations, or restrictions on collection and storage of specimens from living persons, or restriction of the data from open publication. Use of hair and nails does not appear to have the same implications involved in post mortem specimens, or even of blood and urine from living persons. However, this should be looked into further since it is possible that some data have not been published due to restrictions. There has been no reference made to difficulties in the international transportation of hair samples across state or national borders. For example, duplicate hair samples collected in Mexico were sent to Mexico City and to the United States for confirmatory analyses.

e.   Cost Estimates

It is not currently possible to estimate the numbers of baseline sample sites and the number of samples required for determining dangerous exposures, using hair for biological monitoring. This should be determined in the context of a larger human biological monitoring program using blood, urine, and other human biological materials.

It is currently unknown how many existing laboratories at present have the capability to make accurate analyses of samples of human biological materials. A more important unknown is the number of new or additional laboratories required to give suitable world network coverage.

For biological monitoring of historic trends of the levels of toxic materials in human beings, stored hair samples could be used extensively in the world in existing laboratories.

Without estimates of the number of samples and sites required, it can only be said that since no heavy containers and refrigeration are required, the cost of collection, transport of samples, and storage of samples is much less than the equivalent number of blood and urine samples. However, analysis and data processing costs would be comparable.

TABLE 3

REPORTED LEVELS OF TOXIC METALS IN HUMAN HAIR WITH TENTATIVE 'NORMAL' AND TOXIC* LEVELS (ppm)**

	Reported Range	'Normal' Range	Threshold Effects	Acute or Chronic Effects	Death
Antimony	0.03–47.0	0.03–24.0 [a]	unknown		
Arsenic	0.0–1,585.0	0.0–2.0	3.0	12.0	
Cadmium	0.1–9.3	0.1–3.0 [b]	levels not correlated with toxicity		
Chromium	0.0–6.43	0.0–4.0	unknown		
Cobalt	0.0–3.11	0.0–1.0	unknown		
Copper	7.8–486.0	7.8–120.0	unknown		
Lead	0.0–1,880.0	0.0–70.0	12.5 infant 70.0 in children [c]		94.7–124.0
Mercury	0.01–2436.0	0.01–30.0	50.0-200.0	200.0-800.0	500.0+
Nickel	0.0–15.6	0.0–11.0	unknown		
Selenium	0.3–30.0	0.3–13.0	8.0–30.0	8.0–30.0	
Vanadium	0.006–271	0.006–2.71	unknown		

*   Levels are tentative estimates from visual inspection of data only. Data are incomplete on toxic effects, and experts vary in interpretation.
a)   most below 9.0.
b)   one Cd worker with 1,000.0.
c)   exposed adults frequently over 100.0 with no symptoms.
**   From Jenkins (1977).

LITERATURE CITED

JENKINS, D.W., 1977. Toxic Metals in Human and other Mammalian Hair and Nails. EPA. Report of Contract No. 68-03-0443. Las Vegas, Nevada. pp. 174 (submitted for publication).
LISK, D.J., 1974. Recent Developments in the Analysis of Toxic Elements. Science 184:1137.
MASIRONI, R., 1974. Trace Elements in Relation to Cardiovascular Di sease.WHO Pub. No.5, p. 45.
SCHROEDER, H.A. and A.P. NASON, 1971. Trace Element Analysis in Clinical Chemistry. Clin. Chem. 17:461.

TRACE ELEMENTS IN HUMAN TISSUE

T. Kneip, M. Kleinman and D. Bernstein
University Medical Center, New York
and
R. Riddick
Office of the Medical Examiner, Washington D.C.

Summary

Past and current design of human biological sampling programs for the analyses of trace metals in human tissues are described. The requirements of a clear definition of the purposes of these collections are set forth in terms of statistical considerations, the populations and tissues of interest, as well as descriptive information that would be pertinent to the study. Protocolsfor sampling and methods of analyses are discussed that will fulfil the goals of the program and obtain the overall accuracy and precision required to interpret the results.

The design and preliminary results of the New York University study of 'Trace Metals in Human Tissues' are presented. Included is an intercomparison of different methods of analyses, procedures employed to reduce variance in the data, costs and some of the conclusions drawn from the results.

Review of Past and Current Programs

The distribution of trace metals in human tissues has received increasing attention in recent times. The current efforts owe much to the basic work done some years ago. Early investigators such as Tipton (1963, 1963a, 1964) and Perry (1962) initially concentrated on the overall distribution of many trace elements in various tissues in an attempt to establish 'normal' levels. With few exceptions, studies performed since that time are limited to the analyses of either a specific element in one or more tissues or multielement analyses of a single tissue.

One of the first and most comprehensive studies of trace metals in human tissues was that performed by Tipton et al (1963). The main objectives of that work were 'to determine the concentration of as many tissue and organs (sic) from as many normal individuals from as many locations in the United States in as short a time as possible and thus to throw light on the elemental composition of 'standard man'.' The study was successful in establishing ranges for the concentrations of trace metals in human tissues. However, the design of the program was such that the sampling protocol and analytical techniques contributed significantly to the overall variance of the data.

The autopsies were performed by many different prosectors in cities throughout the country resulting in possible sampling variability and difficulty in maintaining strict quality control during sample collection. In addition, the limit of detection for the spectrographic method of analysis for the tissues was such that many of the analyses were below the limit of detection and precision was poor for the many positive values which were near the limits of detection.

One of the major conclusions resulting from Tipton's program was that trace metal concentrations in many tissues varied as a function of age and geographical location as expected. These factors account for much of the overall variability found in trace metal concentrations as determined in the Tipton study.

Many of the limitations in Tipton's work were overcome in varying degrees in later studies (Molokhia, 1967; Barry and Mossman, 1970; Barry, 1975; Rancitelli et al, 1969; Friberg, 1974; Morgan, 1969; Curry and Knott, 1970; and Livingston, 1971). However, all of these studies involve determination of single elements in several tissues, several elements in one tissue, or one element in one tissue.

Small samples were taken for analysis in many cases, even though the distribution of many trace elements is known to be non-uniform within organs. Though the analytical instrumentation has been greatly improved and the precision of measurements increased, most studies have compromised on the analytical procedures in order to obtain results more expediently. Tipton (1963) used dry ashing for speed and control of contamination, but lost volatile materials during ashing (Gorsuch, 1970).

Recent studies by NIOSH (Sweet and Crable, 1975; Brown and Taylor, 1975a; and Filby, 1975b) have focused on multielement methods for the analysis of lung and lymph nodes. Both spark source mass spectrometry and neutron activation methods were used in studying the trace metal concentrations of coal miners' lungs, and other lungs obtained at autopsy. The latter included tissues from a number of elderly and severely or chronically ill patients. The results of both studies indicate wide variations in trace element concentrations to exist in these populations as measured by the techniques used. The lack of 'normal' tissues has complicated interpretation of this data.

The findings of NIOSH confirmed the earlier findings of Molokhia (1967) that sampling of small sections of lung would contribute to large variations in the results, and a homogenizing technique was developed for sample preparation.   The problem of non-uniform distribution of trace elements in tissues must be recognized whenever extremely sensitive analytical techniques are used for measurement, permitting analysis of small tissue samples.

Our program has been in progress at New York University Medical Center by cooperation between the Departments of Forensic Medicine and Environmental Medicine, with goals of accurate and precise measurement of several trace elements in five tissues.   The data was intended and has been used for studies of relationships between tissue concentrations and environmental sources of exposure as well as in seeking correlations to microhistological findings.   We have emphasized the use of whole organ or maximum available fractions (>1/2) thereof and painstaking sample preparation and analysis.

Program Design
Statistical Consideration
Most experiments in which health aspects of human trace element burdens have been evaluated were retrospective studies.   From among the total population sampled, one group of cases was selected possessing a characteristic of etiological interest and a second group selected which did not have the characteristic.   For example, an important characteristic might be whether or not a subject smoked.

One can then statistically determine whether higher body or organ trace element burdens are found in smokers than in non-smokers.   A retrospective study is an economical way of drawing inferences about a population; however, great care must be taken to ensure that the cases are representative of the population at large and that biases are not injected by the way in which samples are obtained.   For example, if tissues are drawn from all persons who died in a hospital, one might expect many inferences drawn to be unrepresentative of a healthy population.   Matching of test and control samples may also be very difficult.

There have been a few prospective studies in which subjects received controlled doses of specific trace elements and the uptake and distribution of these elements were followed by monitoring the metabolic balance (Kehoe, 1971; Spencer, 1974).   In general, prospective studies are expensive and require extremely involved methodologies and facilities (i.e. a metabolic hospital ward).

The design of a retrospective study should begin with determination of the overall purpose.   In our study, we were interested in determining whether changes in concentration of trace elements in airborne particulates significantly influenced the trace metal burdens of tissues of residents of New York City; secondly, whether such changes had a health impact, as indicated by histological differences in respiratory organs (lungs and lymph nodes) of the subjects studied;   and thirdly, whether relationships between element concentrations in specific tissues could be indicative of a given source of pollutants.

Population Groups: Factors in the design of the study are:

a)   Cause of death: A study of trace element distributions in normal subjects must avoid subjects with histories of extensive medication, abuse of drugs, chronic disease, disease related mortality and mortality due to old age.   Cases of accidental or other rapid causes of death should be selected.

b)   Age: in examining a normal adult population, subjects should be between 20 and 40 years of age.

c)   Sex: One would anticipate that differences exist between men and women with respect to trace element metabolism for certain elements, therefore, balance should be sought in the overall selection.

Choice of Specimens: The specimens selected should meet two major criteria.

a)   They should include tissue from those organs which are of interest with respect to the goals of the study.   For example, for our study we chose tracheo-bronchial tissues (including the first bifurcation), lungs and respiratory lymph nodes since they would be the first targets of an inhalation insult from air pollutants.   We chose liver and kidney because these organs are involved in detoxification mechanisms and bone (vertebra) as representative of calcareous tissues for which several toxic elements have shown an affinity.

b)   The specimens obtained must be representative of the whole organs from which they are obtained.

Magnitude of Program: The size of a program is proportional to the number of questions to be answered and the level of confidence required in the final results. We have found, however, by reducing sampling and analytical variation through analysis of whole organs with precise techniques, and restricting the population with respect to age and cause of death, that we can observe statistically significant differences between lung concentrations of Pb and Cd in smokers and non-smokers with only 15 cases in each category.

With as few as 50 cases we observed significant trends in lung and lymph nodePb concentrations over a 4-year period with correlation ($p \leq 0.05$) to a decrease in ambient atmospheric Pb in New York City.

Optimal Descriptive Information Required

The minimum information required for evaluating data obtained in this type of study include age, cause of death, height, weight, medical history, smoking and occupational history, and sex. Information about the person's place of residence and economic and ethnic background is also necessary.

Certain jobs may directly expose a subject to emissions from a given source. Histories of exposure from occupations should be obtained on subjects whenever possible; and, in fact, the availability of such information is a prime requirement before accepting a case for study.

Finally, information about the specimen itself is required:

1) Autopsy protocol
2) Organ
3) Total organ weight (wet)
4) Sample taken (if not whole organ)
5) Method of storage
6) Condition of sample
7) Length of storage time
8) Method of analysis
9) Analytical results

Procedures to standardize information collected

All results should be reported as concentrations in the MKS system, for example, micrograms per gram organ weight. All information necessary to define what is meant by 'wet' weight, and all factors needed to convert from wet weight to dry weight or to ash weight should be given.

Recommended procedures for data storage, interpretation and retrieval

While the most universal data storage format (other than the printed page) is the computer card, large data bases stored on this medium often become unwieldy. We, therefore, recommend as an alternative that data be stored in card image form (80 column records) on IBM compatible tapes which can later be used as entries to data management and analysis programs. Raw data tapes should be saved as backups for the data in case of losses of information on the analysis tape or disc files.

There are several good computer program packages available which provide for storage and retrieval, management of the data base, and flexible analysis and interpretive capabilities. We have had excellent success with a program system supplied and supported by the University of Michigan called Osiris. Other packages such as the UCLA Biomedical Data programs (BMD) and the SPSS (Nie et al. 1975) programs are also useful.

Organizational Aspects

All programs must provide samples to fulfil the immediate goals, but should also take into consideration other goals. The most important factors are the integration of the data with that of other programs and provision of reserve samples. When samples are obtained for specific purposes, the usefulness of such samples in additional programs is of considerable importance. Where the sample size permits as large a portion as possible should be held as a tissue bank. Obviously, storage is a consideration in this situation. Samples should be placed in sealed plastic containers and held frozen as whole tissues or tissue sections to minimize any potential contamination. (If protection for possible analysis of organic compounds is desired, the sample should first be wrapped in two layers of aluminum foil before placing in a glass container).

Any steps of sample preparation may reduce the usefulness of the reserve samples through contamination or loss of materials later considered of importance for analysis. Where sample preparation must be done, adequate blanks must be run and preserved with prepared sample reserves to provide assurance as to blank concentrations (or definition of contamination). A detailed record of the procedural steps will permit determination of recovery factors for elements not originally measured.

Ethical and Legal Considerations

We will address only the considerations for post mortem samples. Confidentiality is maintained through coding of the samples by the pathologist. The information, whether historical, pathological, or analytical, is stored under the code assigned and publication of data undertaken only with identification by arbitrarily assigned sample numbers. The published data can then be followed back to a specific case only by access to both laboratory notebooks and the pathologist's files. This effectively prevents loss of confidentiality.

Samples may be obtained only by determination by the pathologist that the analytical data may be useful in the autopsy system and as part of a program approved by review boards of both the United States National Institute of Health and the New York University Medical Center. Both the review of the overall program and the case by case evaluations prevent an indiscriminate approach to obtaining tissue samples. Transport is restricted to within the State of New York. It would be expected that both interstate and international transport would require knowledge of and conformance to additional rules and regulations.

New York University Study

It is essential that the pathologist be a member of the study team and have adequate time to do the primary sampling in an extremely careful manner. Handling and cutting of the tissues must be minimized to avoid contamination; however, organs such as lymph nodes must be separated at the time of the autopsy. A written autopsy protocol must be prepared by the pathologist and analyst in advance. The NYU protocol is available on request.

We have examined various types of equipment used for homogenization of tissues. These have included the 2-quart stainless steel Waring Blender, and a Virtis Ultrasonic homogenizer. Neither will homogenize the fibrous connective tissues present in human lungs. A mass of clumped, mingled fibrous material must be removed from blades if short homogenizing times are used. The ultrasonic unit produced a stratified slurry after several hours with a residue of connective tissue fragments in one layer. These methods are not particularly convenient and fail to produce completely uniform homogenates. Uniform subsampling remains difficult.

Contamination is of course of constant concern. Materials of construction may contribute contaminants unless special tantatum or titanium parts are obtained (Sweet and Crable, 1975), and water used for production of slurries must be of the highest purity possible. Tissues are handled with rubber or plastic gloves and plastic covered tongs or forceps only.

Analytical Procedures

The organs sampled are the tracheo-bronchial tubes, lung, respiratory lymph nodes, liver, kidney, and bone. The samples are taken from the freezer and allowed to slowly defrost in a refrigerator for at least 24 hours. Each sample is removed from the plastic shipping bag and is placed in an individual glass tray. Any fluid or blood present in the sample is allowed to drain. The wet weight of the sample is then obtained. Using surgical scissors and scalpel the samples are cut into 1-inch cubes.

The cubes are then placed in hot nitric acid on a magnetic stirring hotplate one at a time, each cube being allowed to dissolve before the next one is placed into the acid. Approximately 1 litre of acid is used for the large samples such as lung, liver and kidney, and approximately 100 ml of acid are used for the smaller samples. The samples are allowed to boil to incipient dryness. Heating is continued and small increments of HNO_3 are added until a clear straw-colored solution is obtained. This solution is filtered, the insoluble residue is ashed at 550°C in a muffle furnace, and re-extracted with 50 ml HNO_3. The extract is combined with the solution obtained from wet ashing and diluted to a known volume. Each sample is analysed by Atomic Absorption Spectrophotometry for cadmium, chromium, copper, iron, lead, manganese, nickel, and zinc.

As part of our ongoing quality control program, samples containing known trace element concentrations are analysed with each batch of samples processed. Although this adds substantially to our analytical load (10-20 percent), the increased confidence in the accuracy of our results is well worth this level of effort.

During the past three years, standard reference materials prepared by the National Bureau of Standards (NBS Bovine Liver, NBS Orchard Leaves) and the International Atomic Energy Agency (IAEA Fish Solubles and IAEA Diced Mashed Potatoes), have been analysed. The results of our analyses are in good agreement with the reported values and the precision of the determinations measured by the 95 percent confidence limits about the mean, are generally as good as those reported by either NBS or IAEA.

Results

The most often neglected factor in reporting data is the definition of the base for calculations. Much of the data in the literature is reported on a wet tissue weight basis. However, data is frequently reported on a dry or ash (or calcium) basis. In these latter cases, care should be taken to determine and report loss on drying or loss on ignition values to provide for full intercomparison with other data.

We have obtained data for average weight losses for whole lungs by freeze drying, low temperature ashing, and muffle furnace ashing at a final temperature of 450°C. These are shown in Table I, with literature values for comparison. Correction factors should be supplied with all data reported allowing conversion to and/or from wet weight to dry or ash weight bases.

TABLE I

Weight Losses from Whole Human Lung Samples including Bronchi
After Freeze Drying, Low Temperature Ashing (LTA) and Muffle Furnace Ashing (MFA)

		Losses, percent by Weight	
Sample	Freeze Dried (a)	LTA Total (b)	MFA Total (c)
1	83.8	98.7	99.1
2	81.7	98.5	98.8
3	80.6	98.6	99.1
4	74.2	97.9	98.6
5	78.9	98.3	99.0
6	82.0	98.3	98.8
7	82.8	98.6	98.8
8	81.2	98.5	99.0
Average loss, percent	80.6 (± 1.1)(d)	98.4 (± 0.09)	98.9 (± 0.06)
Average residue, percent	19.4 22.5 (e) 20.0 (f) 18.0 (g)	1.6	1.1 1.1(e)

(a)   Whole lung frozen with liquid nitrogen crushed, homogenized in a Waring Blender, and 300 to 500 g freeze dried.

(b)   Five 2 g samples of dried homogenate were ashed 22-24 hours at 160-200 watts power in a five compartment Tracerlab LTA (Model 600).

(c)   One 10 g sample of dried homogenate was ashed at 250° C for 16 hours and at 450°C for an additional 24 hours in a muffle furnace.

(d)   All errors given as 1 standard deviation of the mean value (standard error).

(e)   Tipton et al, 1963a; Dried at 100°C – 24 hours and ashed at 450°C for 24-48 hours, Tipton et al. 1963.

(f)   Molokhia, M.M. and Smith, 1967 – Vacuum dried.

(g)   McKenzie, J.M., 1974.

Analyses of standard samples are given in Table II. Determinations were carried out by the same methods used for the tissue samples. In addition, two series of interlaboratory comparisons were carried out with the New York Health and Safety Laboratory of the Energy Research and Development Administration.

Twenty-four air filters were divided and analysed for lead with no significant difference found by use of a paired t test ($\alpha \leq 0.01$). Values ranged from 800 to 2000 μg Pb/m^3 air. Fourteen duplicate dustfall samples were also analysed for lead, cadmium, nickel and vanadium. No statistically significant differences were found; however, the NYU results were about 30 percent higher for Ni at 200 μg/cm^2 and Cd at 25 μg/cm^2.

Ranges are given in Table III for our data to that reported by Tipton (1963a). All the elements for soft tissues as well as bone, as measured by NYU, are compared to the corresponding tissues and elements reported by Tipton.

TABLE II
Results of Analyses of Standard Samples

National Bureau of Standards Bovine Liver Samples (1g aliquots)

Element	Number of Analyses	Mean & 95 percent Confidence Limit (μg/g)	N.B.S. Values (μg/g)
Iron	29	279 ± 58	270 ± 20
Copper	30	187 ± 10	193 ± 10
Zinc	30	131 ± 5.8	130 ± 10
Manganese	29	9.8 ± 0.4	10.3 ± 1.0
Cadmium	36	0.26 ± 0.10	0.27 ± 0.04
Lead	30	≤ 0.5	0.34 ± 0.08

International Atomic Energy Agency Fish Solubles (1g aliquots)

Element	Number of Analyses	Mean & 95 percent Confidence Limit (μg/g)	N.B.S. Values (μg/g)
Zinc	6	21.5 ± 1.8	18.9 ± 1.3
Copper	6	5.0 ± 0.4	5.3 ± 0.6
Manganese	5	4.8 ± 0.2	4.7 ± 0.6
Nickel	6	2.1 ± 0.4	–
Lead	6	2.3 ± 0.6	--

International Atomic Energy Agency Dried Mashed Potatoes (10g samples)

Element	Number of Analyses	Mean & 95 percent Confidence Limit (μg/g)	N.B.S. Values (μg/g)
Iron	6	18.8 ± 1.1	18.6 ± 1.1
Copper	6	3.7 ± 0.1	4.2 ± 0.3
Manganese	6	2.3 ± 0.02	2.4 ± 0.1
Zinc	6	12.3 ± 0.3	11.9 ± 0.3
Cadmium	5	0.18 ± 0.01	0.23 ± 0.02
Chromium	6	0.39 ± 0.02	Not reported
Lead	6	< 0.5	Not reported
Nickel	6	0.52 ± 0.08	Not reported

While the acid dissolution is a destructive method, a major fraction of the solution remains and is useful for further studies. We have already obtained data on vanadium, manganese and aluminum by instrumental neutron activation analysis (INAA) and have in progress radiochemical analyses for Pu-239. The latter were preplanned and a Pu-241 tracer was added during dissolution to facilitate recovery factor calculations.

The efforts to reduce variance by selection of cases, limiting the age range, analysis of whole organs, minimal handling, and use of more precise analytical techniques has resulted in data of greater precision in the NYU studies than that reported by others. As a result, correlations have been obtained between tissue concentrations and airborne metal concentrations (Bernstein et al, 1974; Bernstein, 1975).

TABLE III
Tissue Concentrations From Studies of Tipton and NYU
Mean and Standard Error — μg/g wet weight

LUNG	Tipton (a)				NYU	
	n Max. 141	$\bar{X}$	S.E.	n Max. 54	$\bar{X}$	S.E.
Essential						
Fe	120	290	15	53	128	12
Cr	139	0.20	± 0.02	36	0.052	0.005
Cu	141	1.30	0.03	51	1.04	0.04
Mn	141	0.24	0.020	52	0.080	0.008
Zn	141	14.0	0.4	53	0.9	0.4
Adventitious						
Cd	71	-0.5 to 0.5 (b)		52		0.04
Pb	141	0.67	0.06	50		0.009
Ni	70	-0.05 to 0.05 (b)		44		0.02

TABLE III (Continued)

	Tipton (a)			NYU		

TRACHEA (b)   **TRACHEA and R.M.S. BRONCHUS**

	n Max. 60	$\bar{X}$	S.E.	n Max. 29	$\bar{X}$	S.E.
Essential						
Fe	56	31	3	29	70	9
Cr	53	0.012 to 0.045 (b)		21	0.08	0.01
Cu	60	0.65	0.08	28	1.4	0.1
Mn	54	0.14	0.01	29	0.21	0.02
Zn	60	9.8	0.6	26	12	2
Adventitious						
Cd	7	- 0.5 to 0.5		28	0.25	0.04
Pb	60	0.58	0.06	27	0.28	0.03
Ni	31	- 0.05 to 0.06		26	0.23	0.04

LYMPH NODES

	n Max. 29			n Max. 29		
Essential						
Fe				49	96	8
Cr				33	0.29	0.06
Cu				47	1.05	0.08
Mn				45	0.14	0.01
Zn				48	7.8	0.5
Adventitious						
Cd				42	0.15	0.02
Pb				41	0.39	0.05
Ni				33	0.5	0.1

LIVER

	n Max. 150	$\bar{X}$	S.E.	n Max. 55	$\bar{X}$	S.E.
Essential						
Fe	127	150	8	54	52	6
Cr	115	0.003 to 0.013 (b)		26	0.033	0.006
Cu	148	6.8	0.5	51	5.2	0.6
Mn	148	1.3	0.07	54	0.53	0.06
Zn	150	38.0	1.1	54	40	3
Adventitious						
Cd	146	1.6 to 1.9 (b)		52	0.9	0.1
Pb	150	1.50	0.09	53	0.60	0.05
Ni	27	- 0.05 to 0.05 (b)		48	0.14	0.02

KIDNEY

	n Max. 145	$\bar{X}$	S.E.	n Max. 50	$\bar{X}$	S.E.
Essential						
Fe	123	69	2	48	73	10
Cr	117	0.007 to 0.016 (b)		27	0.07	0.02
Cu	143	2.7	0.06	48	2.3	0.1
Mn	143	0.91	0.04	50	0.68	0.03
Zn	145	49	1.4	49	35	2
Adventitious						
Cd	145	32	1.2	49	16.5	1
Pb	145	1.20	0.072	48	0.47	0.03
Ni	30	- 0.05 to 0.05		42	1.0	0.3

TABLE III (Continued)

	Tipton (a)		NYU	
		$\dfrac{n}{\text{Max. } 52}$	$\overline{X}$	S.E.
BONE (c)				
Essential				
Fe		49	90.6	9.1
Cr		29	0.46	0.05
Cu		51	0.49	0.03
Mn		37	0.049	0.007
Zn		52	27	2
Adventitious				
Cd		44	0.06	0.01
Pb		51	2.8	0.3
Ni		48	0.9	0.1

(a) Tipton and Cook, 1963; Reported values divided by 100 to adjust from ash to wet weight basis.
(b) 95 percent Confidence interval for the median reported when a normal distribution was not observed.
(c) One-half of the body of three thoracic vertebrae.

Intertissue and interelement burden correlations, correlations of metal concentrations to microhistological findings and differentiation between tissue burden patterns for smokers and non-smokers have also been obtained in ongoing computer evaluations. These results are only possible due to the precision in the analytical data obtained.

Costs

	Direct	Overhead (at 75 percent of salaries)
Design of Program		
Literature search, 1 man week	$250	$188
Draft proposals, statistics, protocols, 2 man weeks	500	373
Total		$1,313
Collection and Transport		
100 cases, 5 organs each case		
SAMPLING, HISTORIES, INTERPRETATION:		
Pathologist, 1/3 man day/case = 330 man days	$45,000	$34,000
Sampling Total (Min.)		($79,000)
HISTOLOGY: Sectioning, preparation, staining, records, history, reading		
Technician clerk, 1/2 man day/case = 500 man days	$20,000	$15,000
Pathologist, 1/6 man day/case = 190 man days	22,000	17,000
Equipment, technicon instrument (slide preparation)	5,000	
Microscope	2,500	
Sampling Total (Max.) (includes minimum total)		$161,000
TRANSPORT: Dependent on program		
Storage of Samples		
Containers per case, 100 cases at 4.00/each	400	
Freezers (2), 0.3m³ each (max. capacity about 40 cases each)	800	
Total		$1,200
Analysis of Samples		
100 cases, 5 tissues each case, 1 man week per case = 100 man weeks ∿ 2 man years	$20,000	$15,000
Subtotal		$35,000

	Direct	Overhead
SUPPLIES: per case at 5 tissues per case		
Reagents $50 x 100 cases	5,000	
Glassware	5,000	
Miscellaneous	2,000	
EQUIPMENT:		
Atomic absorption Spectrophotometer	15,000	
Hotplates	1,000	
Fume hood with acid gas scrubbing system	7,500	
Laminar flow hood	2,500	
Miscellaneous	2,000	
Subtotal		$28,000
TOTAL		$75,000

Data Processing

100 cases, 5 tissues for 8 metals plus histology and histories resulting in approx. 130 variables.

	Direct	Overhead
Supervision, evaluation, data handling, computer operation = 1 man year	12,500	9,375
Subtotal		$21,875
Central Processor Time	5,000	
Terminal costs	1,000	
Peripheral hardware	500	
Miscellaneous supplies	1,000	
Subtotal		$7,500
TOTAL		$29,375

Grand Total Costs (100 cases)

Including Histology	$267,888
Without Histology	$185,888

Summary and Conclusions

Human biological sampling programs require clear definition of the purpose for these collections.   Sampling, storage and sample preparation methods cannot be thoroughly defined unless the goals of the program are well defined.

The overall accuracy and precision required in the final measured values should be explicitly stated as a part of the goals.   Failure to consider these factors during the planning stage or reliance on understanding through implicit expressions may result in a failure to obtain useful data.

In an effort to maximize both accuracy and precision, our program has been designed following several principles:

1. The pathologist is a participating member of the study team.
2. Cases are selected to conform to criteria in terms of overall health, age, etc.
3. A serious effort is made to obtain a complete case history.
4. Whole organs are obtained, packaged and frozen by the pathologist.
5. Handling and sectioning is minimized during the autopsy.
6. Whole organs are prepared for analysis with minimal handling and subdivision, using the simplest procedure possible.
7. Rigid protocols are followed in the autopsy, sample handling and analytical stages.
8. Quality control is maintained by carrying blanks and standards through the procedure at ratios of from 1:5 to 1:10 to the samples run.
9. Data evaluation includes screening by medical, biological, physical and mathematical specialists, computer correlation analysis, and re-examination of significant correlations to differentiate logical relationships from artifacts often encountered in such studies.

The efforts based on these principles have resulted in correlation of airborne trace metal measurements to lung and lymph node burdens, interelement tissue burden correlations, and correlations of trace element concentrations to histological findings and smoking histories. Preliminary results of these studies have been reported and an overall final evaluation is in progress for future publication.

REFERENCES

TIPTON, I.H., M.J. COOK, R.L. STEINER, C.A. BOYLE, H.M. PERRY, Jr. and H.A. SCHROEDER, 'Trace Elements in Human Tissue, Part I. Methods'. Health Physics, 9:89-101 (1963).

TIPTON, I.H. and M.J. COOK, 'Trace Elements in Human Tissue, Part II. Adult Subjects from the United States'. Health Physics 9:103-145 (1963a).

TIPTON, I.H. and J.J. SHAFER, 'Statistical Analysis of Lung Trace Element Levels'. Archives of Environmental Health 8:58-67.

PERRY, M.M., Jr., I.H. TIPTON, H.A. SCHROEDER and M.J. COOK, 'Variability in the metal content of human organs'. Journal Laboratory and Clinical Medicine 60:245-253 (1962).

MOLOKHIA, M.M and H. SMITH, 'Trace Elements in the Lung'. Archives of Environmental Health 15:745-750 (1967).

BARRY, P.S.I. and D.B. MOSSMAN, 'Lead concentrations in human tissues'. British Journal of Industrial Medicine 27:339-351 (1970).

BARRY, P.S.I., 'A comparison of concentration of lead in human tissues'. British Journal of Industrial Medicine 32: 119-139 (1975).

RANCITELLI, L.A., R.W. PERKINS, and A.D. RENZETTI, Jr., 'The Multielement Analysis of Human Lung Tissue'. Report BNWL-1051 Part 2 (1969).

FRIBERG, L., M. PISCATOR, G.F. NORDBERG and T. KJELLSTROM, Cadmium in the Environment .CRC Press (1974).

MORGAN, J.M., 'Tissue Cadmium Concentration in Man'. Archives of Internal Medicine 123: 405-408 (1969).

CURRY, A.S. and A.R. KNOTT, ''Normal' Levels of Cadmium in Human Liver and Kidney in England'. Clin. Chim. Acta 30:115-118 (1970).

LIVINGSTON, H.D., 'Measurement and Distribution of Zinc, Cadmium, and Mercury in Human Kidney Tissue'. Clinical Chemistry 18:67-72 (1972).

GORSUCH, T.T.., 'The Destruction of Organic Matter'. Pergamon Press, New York (1970).

SWEET, D. and J. CRABLE , Robert A. Taft Laboratories NIOSH, 4676 Columbia Parkway, Cincinnati, Ohio 45226 USA. Personal co mmunication (1975).

BROWN, R. and H. TAYLOR, 'Trace Metal Analysis of Normal Lung Tissue and Hilar Lymph Nodes by Spark Source Mass Spectrometry'. HEW Publication No. (NIOSH) 75-129 (1975a).

FILBY, R.H., 'Elemental Analysis of Human Lung Tissue and Other Selected Samples Utilizing Neutron Activation Analysis, HEW Publication No. (NIOSH) 75-187 (1975b).

KEHOE, R.A., 'The Metabolism of Lead in Man in Health and Disease'. In: The Harbin Lectures 1960, London. McCarquodole and Co. Ltd. (1961).

SPENCER, H., D. OSIS, E. WIATROWSKI, C. NORRIS and P. RITZMAN, 'Plasma Levels and Excretions in Fluoride in Relation to Fluoride Intake in Man'. In: Trace Substances in Environmental Health VIII, D.D. Hemphill, ed., University of Missouri, Columbia (1974).

NIE, N.H., C.H. NULL, J.G. JENKINS, K. STEINBRENNER and D.H. BENT, 'Statistical Package for Social Research'(SPSS), McGraw Hill, New York (1975).

BERNSTEIN, D., T.J. KNEIP, M.T. KLEINMAN, R. RIDDICK and M. EISENBUD, 'Uptake and Distribution of Airborne Trace Metals in Man'. In: Trace Substances in Environmental Health VIII. D.D. Hemphill, ed. University of Missouri, Columbia (1974).

BERNSTEIN, D., 'Trace Metals in Human Tissue'. In: Trace Metals in Urban Aerosols, Report to EPRI. M. Eisenbud, T. Kneip, eds. (1975).

McKENZIE, J.M., 'Tissue Concentration of Cadmium, Zinc and Copper from Autopsy Samples'. New Zealand Medical Journal 79:1016-1019 (1974).

PESTICIDES AND PERSISTENT SUBSTANCES – BIOLOGICAL SPECIMEN COLLECTION

F. Kaloyanova, I. Benchev, G. Georgiev, N. Izmirova and N. Risov
Institute of Hygiene and Occupational Diseases, Sofia, Bulgaria

I. ORGANOCHLORINE PESTICIDES AND PERSISTENT CHEMICALS

I. REVIEW OF PAST AND PRESENT PROGRAMS

Surveys of organochlorine pesticides (OCP) and in recent years of PCB, in human tissues have been mainly limited in time and magnitude to selected populations in many countries. In most of them no effort has been made at adequate sampling plans and the earlier surveys (up to 1965) suffer from poor analytical methodology. Their main objectives have been to study age, sex, race differences in storage and exposure, to establish regional patterns, study the effect on populations with high occupational exposure and to come up with average national levels for comparison with results from other nations (4, 5, 6, 11, 17, 21, 24, 28, 30). Even values from a small number of samples have been useful in giving an approximate estimate of the degree of exposure for countries with varying geographical, social, ethnical and racial backgrounds. The validity of making further conclusions from an inadequately planned survey of organochlorine pesticides (OCP) in human tissues is highly questionable.

The only effort at a more systematic monitoring of pesticide residues in humans is the National Human Monitoring Program for Pesticides as a part of the National Pesticide Monitoring Program of the U.S.A. (16) started in 1967 and revised in 1971. The earlier Program for Community Pesticide Studies (12) has been recently revised. Sampling for PCB has been introduced in 1969 and regular analysis for these compounds is made since 1971 (16, 19, 29).

The utility of this program has been proved in the exhaustive review of the pesticide situation in the Mrak report (21) and it is being continued along the same lines. On the basis of the data available Deichmann (30) has been able to suggest average levels for the whole of the U.S.A. for comparison with other nations.

Through periodic evaluation of the results from the monitoring definite trends toward decreasing levels have been revealed (5, 21, 30). A more modest monitoring program is in operation in the United Kingdom (1, 24) and the results have also shown a downward trend for the past 5-7 years.

II. BASIS FOR INTEREST OR CONCERN

The persistent OCP and the PCB have been the primary cause of concern for well over 15 years mainly because of their resistance to biodegradation in the environment and the ability for bioaccumulation in the biological chains. Human beings store DDT and other OCP for long periods in their fat tissues and latest assessment does not rule out DDT as a potential carcinogen in man (5) although epidemiological data are inconclusive. Dramatic restrictions and total ban on agricultural application of DDT have been introduced in recent years in most developed countries with the corresponding fall of contamination levels in the environment. In many samples, however, a leveling off of the concentration is observed and taking into consideration the slow rate of elimination of the main metabolite of DDT - DDE from humans (15) its residues in humans are expected to remain for a long period. In addition some developing countries still use sizeable quantities of DDT and there are still no adequate substitutes for DDT in public health programs. Thus further inputs of DDT in the environment should be expected for at least some time to come.

PCB are widely used in electrical capacitors and transformers, plasticizers for waxes, heath transfer liquids and hydraulic liquids for mining equipment. Although voluntary restrictive action has been undertaken by some producers existing legal arrangements in the main producing and consuming countries are unable to impose further restrictions or a ban on their production or to stimulate the search for adequate new substitutes. Further pollution by PCB can be expected and exposure of humans by the routes already established.

Food is the main resort for the general population for both types of compounds but there is accumulating evidence that other routes of exposure can be substantial and are worth further investigation.

III   CONSIDERATIONS FOR SAMPLING AND SAMPLE PREPARATION

Fat

The most suitable and indicative tissue for monitoring the levels of OCP and PCB in humans is fat.   Data are available showing remarkably uniform distribution of OCP in the fat from different sites of the body.   This simplifies the removal of the necessary portion of fat in any case of surgical intervention.   By far the most common case is the adipose tissue from the abdominal region avoiding the site of the waist belt.   A piece of about 2.5g is removed, freed of skin or other non-fatty material, dried with a paper towel, and weighed to the nearest 0.01g.   Biopsy samples can easily be taken by (a) a small incision in the abdomen; (b) a suitable syringe introduced in a previously warmed site of the abdominal region.   For **biomonitoring** the sample is put in a small non-plastic container and (a) analysed immediately when possible; (b) frozen and stored for short periods of up to one week; (c) preserved in 10% formalin for longer periods.   Exact data are scarce regarding the behaviour of the various OCP compounds and the PCB under such storage conditions, but there is evidence which suggests that even under deep freeze transformation of DDT into DDE takes place.   The fate of these compounds in **specimens for future reference** is not known.   The biological importance of the different metabolites of the OCP and PCB is great enough to warrant the initiation of studies in this respect.

Blood

Blood is a much more easily available tissue and has been used extensively to assess exposure to and body burden of OCP and PCB.   Several studies have established varying but generally high degrees of correlation between blood and fat levels of OCP and particularly of total DDT which obviates the need for taking fat samples.   There is, however, some difference in the interpretation of the results.   Davis (3) finds blood DDT levels indicative of only very recent exposure in contrast to DDE which reflects chronicity of DDT exposure.   He also finds enough consistency in DDE levels of individuals from the general population to consider blood as a tissue with a high potential for measuring long-term exposure to DDT.   Apple (2) also established that DDE in blood is an indicator of only chronic exposure and that high increases in oral DDT intake do not affect its level.   Schafer (26) however questions the suitability of relating blood levels to the total body burden of the general population.   He suggested future studies with a more general sampling plan and stresses that mathematical models used to observe correlations in most studies are empirical curve fits and that additional data may reveal a more reliable mathematical form.   In a recent study Ware (27) concludes that analysis of blood samples of beef animals could provide an accurate estimate of total DDT residues in the carcass.

The advantages of blood for large scale biomonitoring for OCP and PCB are such that they justify a further discussion and study of this point.

Meanwhile blood sampling for biomonitoring is done by venipuncture.   Heparin, ETDA, or sodium or potassium citrate are equally good anticoagulant agents when analysis on whole blood is carried out.   For gas liquid chromatography determination 1 - 1.5ml are enough.   In most earlier studies serum was separated by centrifugation.   Analyses on whole blood have lately almost completely replaced serum (cf. IV.4).

The samples should be analysed as soon as possible since changes in DDT components occur even at deep freeze temperatures.

Storing of blood specimens for future reference should pose a serious problem.   Freeze drying is a possibility, but losses in volatile compounds such as BHC could be considerable, and codistillation of other compounds cannot be ruled out.

IV   ANALYTICAL PROCEDURES

1.   Organochlorine pesticides

A high quality of the results to be assured and maintained throughout the program by means of adequate methodologies is of prime importance for any successful monitoring activity.

An excellent review of the requirements and guidelines for pesticide monitoring methodology is given in ref. (8) which should be largely consulted.

The basic steps in the analysis of OCP in biological samples, and fat in particular, are well developed and are firmly established in research, control and monitoring.   Progress in standardization and unification of methodologies however has been slow even for national programs, and individual workers prefer their own modifications of the same sequence of procedures. The most widely used procedure is the FDA multiresidue method for organochlorine insecticides (14, 18). The Mills, Onley, Gaither procedure has undergone extensive validation and is regularly scrutinized for further improvements and additions (14). This is a good procedure to start with. A possible direction for further development is its miniaturization for fat samples as has already been done for other human tissues (14). This should not involve taking smaller fat sample but rather taking a smaller aliquot of the hexane extract from a 2.5 - 5g fat sample.

Clean-up is carried out in two steps: a liquid-liquid partition with acetonitrile and separation on a Florisil column. A possible time-saving modification which might well be part of a miniaturized procedure is by avoiding the liquid partition and pipetting an appropriate aliquot directly on the column, or using acetonitrile instead of hexane as extraction solvent.

The parameters of chromatographic mobility are poor evidence for identification purposes. This serious drawback of the multiresidue methodology based entirely on chromatographic techniques has been well recognized for the past ten years and alternate methods and confirmatory tests are now obligatory. This is especially so when a non-specific detector such as the electron capture detector is used which is the case of the OCP and the PCBs. A wide variety of interfering substances go through the whole procedure and can cause grave misinterpretation of the chromatogram.

Combined gas liquid chromatography - mass spectrometry equipment has proved invaluable for the identification of pesticide residues and PCBs. It is now almost a standard equipment in advanced pesticide monitoring laboratories but its price is prohibitive for its wide inclusion in monitoring network. It will most appropriately be used in a centralized laboratory for particular cases which failed to be resolved by other means.

A wide battery of techniques for identity confirmation should be mastered by the monitoring chemist. Currently the most valuable are the following:

1) Microcoulometric detection systems provide a high degree of specificity for halogen compounds and give a solid identification evidence.

2) The thin layer chromatography is a chromatographic system different from the gas phase chromatography and is a good qualitative tool. Sensitivity is the main limiting factor and pooling of samples may be necessary to provide sufficient material. Thin layer chromatography provides strong negative confirmation but care should be exercised in interpreting positive identification since often the chromatographic behaviour of substances even in different chromatographic systems is correlated (24).

3) Extraction p-values have proved useful for identification at the residue level. Good clean-up is essential for reliable results.

4) Suitable chemical reactions can be carried out with the OCP to obtain derivatives changed retention parameters in different chromatographic systems or enhanced detector response. This is a widely used approach which offers many possibilities.

5) Infra-red spectroscopy is the classical technique for unambiguous identification of organic compounds and has been used successfully in pesticide residue analysis. Low sensitivity is the main obstacle and means are sought to overcome it. Very thorough clean-up is an absolute condition for the application of this technique.

2.   Polychlorinated biphenyls

The PCBs go through all steps of the analysis of OCP and interfere in the final identification and quantitation by gas liquid chromatography with electron capture detector. It is now common practice of various techniques to be used to deal with this situation and the most widely used is to separate the PCBs from the cleaned extract on a silicic acid column (9, 14, 18). The PCBs fraction is then injected into a gas chromatograph. Now the main difficulties lie in the interpretation of the chromatogram and the quantitation owing to the great variety in PCB composition, the possibility of metabolic changes, degradation products, selective storage and different behaviour of the various PCB fractions in the chromatographic systems used to isolate, clean up and determine the compounds. Various approaches have been employed such as using the DDE response as a reference, perchlorination of the mixture to obtain a single peak, using synthetic mixtures of PCBs. There is no generally accepted method, but the quantitation by comparison of the peaks with those of a standard formulation most closely resembling the PCBs pattern of the biological sample seems to be the most promising at present (9, 14, 19). Further elaboration of this approach is recommended through the development of a series of reference Arochlors based on the data of R.C. Webb and A.C. McCall (J.Chromay Sci. 11, 366-73, 1973).

These complexities add up to the problems already outlined for OCP and the need of unified methodologies for PCBs cannot be too strongly emphasized if any valid comparisons are to be made in a monitoring system.   The development of adequate procedures for the analysis of PCBs in human samples should receive a high priority.   Since this task is likely to take some time an interim agreement should be reached for at least guidelines (if not standards) for PCBs methodology.   For preliminary studies designed to identify potential areas of monitoring for PCBs in humans, simplified procedures, even thin layer chromatography, may be useful (14, 16, 29).

3)   Expression of results for fat tissues

When taking specimens from the body non-fat tissues are usually removed and their proportion in the samples is not controllable.   This dilution by non-fatty material may cause considerable error so it is recommended that results should be expressed on a 'hexane extractable lipids basis'.   In so far as extraction procedure is standardized and adhered to reproducibility of the 'hexane extractable lipids' values should be reproducible enough to eliminate the need for more exhaustive and time- and reagent-consuming extraction procedure for the lipid content of the sample.   For sample for future reference, however, long storage in refrigeration (or in preserving media) might affect the amount of lipids available for a simple hexane extraction.   This is a point that should be considered in some detail.

It is advisable that the results be given together with data allowing recalculation to a 'wet weight' basis should the need arise, or for future reference.

4)   Blood samples

The most widely used method for OCP in blood has been the Dale method in which a simple extraction with hexane is performed on the serum (14, 18).   Protein bonding of DDT and other OCP has been established both **in vitro** and **in vivo** which leads to low recoveries of hexane extractable OCP.   In subsequent modification the author himself introduces treatment of the serum with formic acid to release bound DDT and its metabolites without degradation (JAOAC 53, 1287, 1970).   Several other methods also envisage treatment of whole blood with mineral acids to liberate the OCP from the blood structures and good recoveries have been reported.

Methods for whole blood have obvious advantages for large-scale monitoring, because serum separation is avoided and smaller samples are needed.   Variations have been demonstrated in the concentration of OCP among whole blood, serum and red cells so that the analysis of whole blood gives the most meaningful results.   A validation study on an agreed procedure for OCP in whole blood should prove useful.

5)   Standards, quality control

Chromatographic techniques form the backbone of present-day multiresidue methods for OCP and PCBs.   Since chromatographic evidence is presumptive in nature, i.e. retention of the sample and reference material are compared and identity is presumed established when these are equal, the supply of high-quality and reliable standards and reference material becomes of paramount importance.   Centralized supply of certified reference standards of OCP and their metabolites and isomers and of mixtures of PCBs should be an integral part of the implementation of any monitoring program.

A thorough system of checking for and maintaining a high quality of analytical performance should be in constant operation in the monitoring network. This system should envisage:

A)   Intralaboratory controls which involve scrupulous maintenance of cleanness in the laboratory, purity of reagents and reliability of standard solutions, strict adherence to methods, and a systematic check on the performance of individual analysis by means of **internal check** samples;

B)   **Interlaboratory checks** for all participating laboratories.   These are best carried out by a central laboratory which takes overall responsibility for the analytical performance of the monitoring program through (a) determining the precision of the analytical methodology; (b) checking the precision and accuracy of analytical results of the individual laboratories; (c) keeping a constant watch over methodology and detecting weaknesses; (d) organizing an **interlaboratory check samples** program to gauge and correct the performance of the laboratories.

In evaluating the accuracy of analytical results agreement should be reached for levels of accuracy in the determination of OCP and PCBs in fat and blood samples at various concentrations. On the basis of realistic assessment of the factors involved in the analysis of microconcentrations of OCP in environmental samples Gunther has suggested some guidelines shown in the table. The second column in the table consists of the values officially accepted in the Federal Republic of Germany for the analysis of OCP in foodstuffs of animal origin.

Level of pesticides mg/kg	Limits of Gunther *	Accuracy ± % F.R.G. **
10	10	12.5
1	10	25
0.1	25	50
0.01	50	100
0.001	100	200

*   Gunther F.A., Pure Appl. Chem. 21, 355-76, 1970.

**   Bundesgesundheitsblatt No. 18, 6 Sept. 1974, 269-75.

The impressive volume of pesticide residue analyses performed in various forms of monitoring programs does not seem to be matched by corresponding quality control programs comparable to the ones instituted in clinical chemistry laboratories. The experience of EPA in this respect is valuable (14) but more exchange of information and experience is needed and recommended.

V   PROGRAM DESIGN

The **objectives** of the monitoring should be clearly defined as they determine the design of the program.

1.   The selection of population groups

A.   For sampling representative for the whole country healthy adults of both sexes aged between 20-45 years should be randomly selected (4, 24, 28). Cases of accidental (trauma) surgery or illness of short duration should be used. Chronically ill or very old persons should be excluded. When arrangements have been made biopsy on volunteers should be performed as described in III. Efforts should be made for adequate geographical representation. Useful general directions for pesticide sampling are given in ref. (7) and the guidelines for pesticide monitoring in humans adopted by the National Pesticide Monitoring Program of the U.S.A. are given in ref. (16).

B.   If stratification by age, socioeconomic status, race, health condition, degree of exposure or any other factors is sought then appropriate statistical tests should be applied to determine the number of samples and levels of confidence for the varying groups keeping in mind the considerations developed further and in V.2.

There is a vast body of data showing that concentration distribution of DDT and OCP in human fat (1, 10, 11, 13, 22) and blood (23, 24) and of PCB in fat and blood (13) and in wildlife specimens (31) show a definite departure from normal Gaussian distribution and have a positive skew. In such cases the geometric mean is the more appropriate parameter than the arithmetic mean (22, 23) and indeed the values calculated by the two methods differ significantly (1, 13). Increased number of samples may be necessary in order to reveal significant trends or differences in a population with non-Gaussian distribution (Holben, 31). The importance of this finding has failed to receive the necessary recognition and should be firmly established in future programs for sampling plans, the treatment and the interpretation of the results.

2. The magnitude and scope of the program

The scope of a biomonitoring program based on purely statistical sampling considerations is not feasible, because laboratory facilities and cost/benefit considerations are limiting factors. Rather the total capacity of the available laboratories should be determined and the sample size thus obtained should then be distributed by randomization in space and time and the proper statistical techniques applied, due consideration being given to the factors outlined in V.1. Earlier formulae suggested by Quinby (20) for the number of samples cannot be considered adequate now.

3. Descriptive information

Individual samples should be accompanied by descriptive information, which again depends on the aims of the program.

Basic information should include name, age, sex, race, occupation, general health status, date and place of sampling, weight of sample. **Additional information** may include more detailed health status and illness record, eating habits, and other specific data.

All information should be uniform and standardized. Prepared forms for ticking off entries with minimum of writing are more acceptable.

Reporting and presentation of analytical results should also be standardized. Results for fat should be expressed on a 'hexane extractable lipids' basis and geometrical means and corresponding ranges ($p = 95\%$) should be given together with other pertinent information which has been agreed upon. Modern methods for data storage, interpretation and retrieval should be used.

VI ORGANIZATIONAL ASPECTS

1. **Assessment of programs.** A very thorough assessment should be made of existing and planned monitoring programs. For this purpose it would be advisable to have an agreement on some guidelines on how to do the assessment itself. Monitoring per se, on a 'just-to-know' basis is a wasteful activity.

Monitoring has immediate value for identifying areas that need attention, in assessing trends in human exposure, establishing regional patterns, etc. In planning future programs attention should be paid to **long-range uses** and benefits of human monitoring for OCP and PCBs, such as evaluating long-term effects on population health, for forecasting and directing future development of plant protection and industrial development strategies, use of the data in models for study and prediction of behaviour of chemicals in the environment.

The program should be made flexible to accommodate future changes in pollution patterns and human exposure. An example is the inclusion of PCBs and other non-pesticidal persistent chemicals in pesticide monitoring programs. Wide-ranging coordination should be sought between biological monitoring and other programs such as community studies, health histories, nutritional surveys and other epidemiological surveys (25).

2. **Centralization vs. decentralization of laboratory services.** The degree of centralization or otherwise is determined by several factors: objectives and magnitude of the monitoring program, availability of laboratory facilities and trained personnel, cost considerations. Modern residue methodology makes use of highly sophisticated and costly equipment which cannot be supplied to smaller regional laboratories. On the other hand automation of the analytical procedures for the determination of OCP and PCBs in human samples has not reached (and is not likely to reach in the foreseeable future) such a stage as to allow the centralized handling of a large volume of samples collected from a network of widespread laboratories.

A carefully balanced regionalization seems to be the best answer for the time being. In some cases a two-level structure can be introduced in which a number of smaller laboratories do the sampling and prepare the samples up to a point and send it to a better equipped centralized regional or national laboratory for analysis. The smaller laboratory can also perform some analyses.

3. **Coordination of programs.** Substantial benefits can result from pooling efforts, and resources in coordinated monitoring programs. Lack of coordination at national level should not be tolerated and quick measures should be undertaken to remedy existing situations. Bilateral coordination and coordination between groups of countries in various fields of moni-

toring have a long history and in various fields of monitoring activities have been practiced for some time with varying degrees of success. Coordination in pesticide monitoring has been achieved for wildlife among several European countries.

Attempts at a coordination on a global scale are illustrated by programs such as Worldwatch, GEMS. There is little experience in international monitoring of humans and the subject is open to wide and detailed discussions, due consideration being given to all problems of logistics, international arrangements, political, ethical and legal aspects.

4. Field and laboratory training. Provisions for field and laboratory training should be made in the monitoring program and should receive great encouragement. Well-planned and carefully prepared training courses offer considerable savings in time and human effort for mastering different techniques and methods at the various stages of the monitoring activity. Periodic checks, examinations, and seminars should be carried out to maintain and update knowledge, methodology and analytical skills.

VII ETHICAL AND LEGAL CONSIDERATIONS

Monitoring of humans inevitably touches upon sensitive ethical issues and complex legal arrangements. These are serious enough on a national level and should be clearly stated in a code of practice to be part of the program structure. The issues become still more complex when some kind of across-the-frontiers coordination is contemplated. These problems, however, are not insoluble and a compilation of existing ethical aspects and legal arrangements in the participating countries is a useful start. Agreement can be sought after within a working group.

VIII COST ESTIMATES

Cost estimates are essential for any existing or planned program. Unfortunately very little data are available for pesticide monitoring for various reasons: most of the calculations whenever they exist at all are reserved for internal use and are released for general reference only with reluctance, much of the information is locked in internal reports, which although not confidential in character also reach a very restricted number of officials, most of the programs have not been evaluated at all. It is impossible even to review in brief this point without the help and cooperation of competent and responsible experts.

A re-examination of existing programs for cost estimates is strongly urged.

REFERENCES

1. ABBOTT D.C., G.B. COLLINS, R. GOULDING. Organochlorine pesticide residues in human fat in the United Kingdom 1969-71. Brit. Med. J. 1972, 2, 553-556.
2. APPLE G., D.P. MORGAN, C.C. ROAN. Determination of serum DDT and DDE concentrations. Bull. Env. Contam. Toxicol. 5, 16-23, 1970.
3. DAVIS J.E. et al. An epidemiological application of the study of DDE levels in whole blood. Am. J. Publ. Hlth. 59, 435-41, 1969.
4. DAVIS J.E. Pesticide residues in man. In Environmental pollution by pesticides, Ed. C. Edwards, Plenum Press, London, 1973; pp. 313-333.
5. DDT — A review of scientific and economic aspects of the decision to ban its use as a pesticide. U.S. EPA, Washington, July 1975; EPA 540/1-75-002.
6. DURHAM W.F. Body burden of pesticides in man. In Ann. N.Y.Acad.Sci., 160 (Art. 1) 183-195, 1969.

7. Guidelines on sampling and statistical methodologies for ambient pesticide monitoring. FWGPM, Washington, 1974.

8. Guidelines on analytical methodology for pesticide residue monitoring. FWGPM, Washington, 1975.

9. Hazards to health and ecological effects of persistent substances in the environment - PCBs. Report of a working group. WHO, Regional Office for Europe, 1975.

10. KALOYANOVA-SIMEONOVA F., Z. MICHAILOVA, G.K. GHEORGHIEV, et al. Organochlorine pesticides in the fat tissue of the general population in Bulgaria. 17th Intern. Congress Occup. Med. Buenos Aires, Sept. 1972.

11. KALOYANOVA-SIMEONOVA F., E. FOURNIER. Les pesticides et l'homme, Masson, Paris, 1971.

12. KLEMMER H.W. Human health and pesticides – Community pesticide studies. Res. Rev. **41**, 55-63, 1972.

13. KRAUL I., and O. KARLOG. Persistent organochlorinated compounds in human organs collected in Denmark 1972-1973. Acta Pharm. Toxicol. **38**, 38-48, 1976.

14. Manual of analytical methods. Analysis of pesticide residues in human and environmental samples. Ed. J.F. Thompson, EPA, Washington, 1972.

15. MORGAN D.P., C.C. ROAN. Loss of DDT from storage in human body fat. Nature, **238** (5361) 221-223, 1972.

16. National Pesticide Monitoring Programme (Revised). Pestic. Monitor. J. **5**, (1) 35-71, 1971.

17. PCB – Environmental Impact. Environ. Res. **5**, (3) 249-362, 1972.

18. Pesticide Analytical Manual, 3 vol. FDA Washington, 1968.

19. PRICE H.A., R.L. WELCH. Occurrence of PCB in humans, Environ. Hlth. Perspect. **1**, April, 1972; 73-78.

20. QUINBY G.E., W.J. HAYES Jr., J.F. ARMSTRONG, W.F. DURHAM. DDT storage in the U.S. population. JAMA, **191**, 175-79; 1965.

21. Report of the Secretary's Commission on pesticides and their Relationship to Environmental Health, U.S. DHEW, Washington,1969.

22. ROBINSON J., A. RICHARDSON, C.G. HUNTER, A.N. CRABTREE, H.J. REES. Organochlorine insecticide content of human adipose tissue in South-Eastern England. Brit. J. Ind. Med. **22**, 220-29, 1965.

23. ROBINSON J., C.G. HUNTER. Organochlorine insecticides: Concentrations in human blood and adipose tissue. Arch. Env. Hlth. **13**, 558-563, 1966.

24. ROBINSON J. Persistent pesticides. Ann. Rev. Pharmacol. **10**, 353-78, 1970.

25. Safe use of pesticides, WHO Techn. Rep. Ser. 1973; No. 513.

26. SCHAFER M. Pesticides in blood. Res. Rev. **24**, 19-39, 1968.

27. WARE G.W., W.P. CAHILL, B.J. ESTESEN, J.A. MARCHELLO. Using blood DDT residues to predict fat residue in beef animals. Bul.Env.Contam.Toxicol. **14**, 285-88, 1975.

28. WASSERMANN M., L. TOMATIS, D. WASSERMANN. Organochlorine compounds in the general population in the seventies and some of their biological effects. Pure Appl. Chem. **42**, (1-2) 189-208, 1975.

29. YOBS A.R. Levels of PCB in adipose tissue of the general population of the nation. Env. Hlth. Perspect. **1**, (1) April 1972, 279-281.

30. DEICHMANN W.B. The chronic toxicity of organochlorine pesticides in man. In Pesticides and the Environment. A continuing controversy. Intercontinental Med. Book Corp. N.Y. 1973, pp. 347-420.

31. HOLDEN A.V. International Cooperative Study of Organochlorine Residues in Terrestrial and Aquatic Wildlife 1967/68. Pestic. Monitoring J. **6**, (3) 117-35 (1970).

II.   ORGANOPHOSPHATE PESTICIDES

II.   BASIS FOR INTEREST OR CONCERN

The investigation of cholinesterase activity (ChEA) is a very important test in the preliminary examination of persons exposed to occupational risks of pesticides.   An inhibition of ChEA is often established which could be explained   by a chronic exposure of these workers for a long period of time or may be due to an individual peculiarity.

Changes in ChEA are observed in steatosis, grave forms of infectious and toxic hepatitis, cirrhosis, carcinomes, liver coma, etc. and the level of ChEA correlates with the degree of parenchymatous lesion.

People engaged in production and application of pesticides in Bulgaria are under constant medical supervision.   It is carried out by the district physicians under the management and with the assistance of the district Hygiene and Epidemiologic Inspection and its Toxicological laboratory, which carries out the testing, and in the district hospitals.

A system of ChEA testing is known to prevent manifest intoxications and to detect incipient ones.   The level of ChEA is the basic criterion for the exposure of workers handling organophosphate and carbamate pesticides.

Blood contains two types of enzymes which hydrolize the choline esters: acetylcholine esterase (true or erythrocyte cholinesterase) present in erythrocytes and brain, and cholinesterase (pseudocholinesterase or serum cholinesterase) which is predominantly synthesized in the liver.

Most of the organophosphate and carbamate pesticides inhibit the plasma cholinesterase more readily than the erythrocyte enzyme but there are important exceptions (Groff, 1966). In addition to the cholinesterase other esterases are present in the serum.

According to their electrophoretic behaviour they are classified as A-, B- and C-esterases (Augustinsson 1958; Uriel 1963).

'A-esterases' known also as arylesterases hydrolize more readily phenyl acetate than phenyl butyrate and are almost inactive towards aliphatic esters.   They are resistant to organophosphorous compounds.   These enzymes possess a high electrophoretic mobility and usually move along the albumin components.

The 'B-esterases' hydrolize both aliphatic and aromatic esters, but not the choline esters. They are susceptible to organophosphate compounds.   After electrophoresis they move close to the alpha-globuline fraction.

The 'C-esterases' (the cholinesterases) hydrolize to a greater extent the cholinesters rather than the aliphatic and aromatic esters.   They are susceptible to the organophosphate compounds.   On electrophoresis they are located between the alpha- and beta-globulines.

We have been recently carrying out studies on the effect of organophosphates on the activity of 'B-esterases' (aliesterases).   The results so far obtained do not support a view that this type of esterase is more sensitive to organophosphates than the cholinesterases (Izmirova, Izmirov, 1976) (3).

III   CONSIDERATIONS FOR HUMAN SAMPLE SELECTION

Each year at the start of the plant protection activities a preliminary examination of the workers is carried out including tests on the cholinesterase activity and some liver function tests.

In the course of the season tests for ChEA are performed to evaluate the exposure of the workers and to identify possible light intoxications.   Another thorough examination is carried out at the end of the season.

Because of unfavourable working conditions prevailing in glass houses tests for ChEA in serum or plasma are carried out as exposure tests 2-3 times during the period of intensive spraying with organophosphates and carbamates.

In our studies for ChEA in serum or plasma blood is drawn from the finger tips of the workers.

Serum — No special cooling equipment is necessary at ambient temperature up to 20° C when samples have to be transported to the laboratory.   After a period of 1 to 24 hours the samples are centrifuged at 6,000 rpm for 5 min., the serum is decanted and kept in a refrigerator until analysed.

Plasma — The analysis is carried out on the spot.   Blood is drawn from the finger tip or the ear lobe with the help of a sterile lancet and a heparinized calibrated capillary tube.

At higher temperatures the samples are transported by special cooling equipment, but no freezing of the blood samples is permitted before the separation and decantation of the serum (plasma).

IV   ANALYTICAL PROCEDURES

An extensive review of the methodologies for ChEA determination covering the literature up to 1975 has been prepared by Vandekar (14).   The methods of Hestrin (9) and Weber (15) have been adopted as standard in Bulgaria.

For large-scale examination of workers in contact with organophosphate and carbamate pesticides a quick paper test has been developed for ChEA in serum or plasma and a test kit for ChEA in plasma has been suggested (Izmirova et al, 1971 (2); Benchev et al 1976 (1)).

The sensitivity of the paper test is better than that of the Merck paper test and the precision and the accuracy of the test are of the same order as those of the Hestrin method (Izmirova, Benchev 1969) (4), (Table 1).

The test kit does not require any equipment, can be carried out by a person without special training and is applicable under field conditions.

TABLE 1

Comparative evaluation of the paper test for cholinesterase activity and
the hydroxamic colorimetric method of Hestrin, 1961

Results obtained with the Hestrin method IU/ml		Results obtained with the paper test IU/ml
X		Y
1,55		1,40
1,60		1,50
1,40		1,50
1,50		1,50
1,50		1,40
1,72		1,80
1,80		1,80
1,85	a = 0,0470	1,80
1,75	b = 1,00986	1,70
1,80	γ = 0,9539	1,70
1,94	Sx = 0,3693	1,90
2,05	F = 1,06	1,90
2,10	Sy = 0,3928	2,00
1,90	Vx = 17,9	2,00
2,00	Vy = 19,3	2,00
2,00		2,00
2,18		2,25
2,20		2,00
2,25		2,00
2,10		2,25
2,25		2,25
2,40		2,50
2,45		2,50
2,25		2,25
2,50		2,50
2,50		2,50
2,60		2,75
2,66		2,50
2,55		2,25
2,60		2,75

V   PROGRAM DESIGN

Threshold limits of Inhibition of ChE activity.   Different values are reported in the literature.   As a result of studies performed on agricultural workers (Kaloyanova-Simeonova, 1959) (5) we assume an inhibition of 30% below the pre-exposure level as an index for absorption of organophosphate compounds.   Those working with inhibition of ChEA higher than this percent are removed from work to avoid poisoning.   Gage (1967) (7) proposed as a safe threshold the same percent for ChEA both for plasma and erythrocytes.   Strict control and safety measures should be taken with values of inhibition between 25 and 30% without interrupting the work process.   A 30% drop in ChEA requires interruption of the exposure.   Teizinger (1969) (13) is of the same opinion.   According to Michaux et al (1970) (11), Podolak (1971) (12) a drop of 25% in serum ChEA and of 20% in erythrocyte ChEA should be a signal for removing the worker from the working place.   Zavon (1965) (16) reports that the normal fluctuations of ChEA vary with 25% in separate individuals, therefore the initial level should be known.   As a general guide levels below 50% of the mean values for the general population are taken as indicative of significant depression by Mastromateo (1971) (10) and at levels below 25% it is recommended that workers should be removed from further exposure and the test repeated.

After the introduction of the quick paper test for ChEA in serum or plasma Izmirova et al (1971) suggest as normal values 2,3 - 3,0 IU/ml.   At levels below 2 IU/ml the person should be removed from further exposure to organophosphates.

REFERENCES

1.   BENCHEV I., KALOYANOVA F., IZMIROVA N.   Raboten komplekt za opredeljane na holinesterazna aktivnost v plazma Ref. No. 265 MNZ, 1976.
2.   IZMIROVA N., BENCHEV I., KALOYANOVA F.   Reaktivni hartii za opredeljane na holinesterzna aktivnost v serum.   Pat. Reg. No. 15148 INRA (1971).
3.   IZMIROVA N., IZMIROV I.   (Unpublished data, 1976).
4.   IZMIROVA N., BENCHEV I.   Sravnitelna otsenka na Barz method s reaktivni hartiiiki i metoda na Hestrin za opredeljane na holinesterazna aktivnost v serum.   Letopisi na HEI godina III, 1969, XIV.
5.   KALOYANOVA F.   Effects of certain organophosphorous insecticides upon cholinesterase activity in persons in conditions of agricultural labour.   Sb. Trudove na HIOTPZ 6, 1959, 105-114.
6.   KALOYANOVA F.   Cholinesterase activity as a biochemical indicator for monitoring exposure to certain pesticides.   International Conference on Env. Sensing and Assessment Vol. 1, Nevada 1975, 13-2, 1-3.
7.   GAGE J.C.   The significance of blood cholinesterase activity measurements.   Residue Reviews 18, 1967, 159-173.
8.   GROFF W.A., L.A. MOUNTEK, Van M. SIM.   A multichannel analytical system for continuous monitoring of blood cholinesterase.   Technical Symposium New York Oct. 19 (1966).

9.   HESTRIN S.   The reaction of acetylcholine and other carboxylic acid derivatives with hydroxylamine and its analytical application.   J.Biol.Chem. **180** (1949), 249.

10.   MASTROMATEO K.   Cholinesterase testing program in persons exposed to organic phosphorous insecticides.   Int. Workshop Pest. Com. Amsterdam 1971.

11.   MICHAUX P., H.L. BOITEAU, F. TOLOT.   Valeur et limites du dépistage clinique et biologique en pathologie professionnelle.Arch. Mal. Prof. Med. Trav. Sec. Soc. **32**, (1971) 1-2 Jan-Fév. 1-124.

12.   PODOLAK M., B. SUZKI.   Human exposure to phosphororganic insecticides taking into account the action of these compounds on particular phenitypes of cholinesterase.   Int. Workshop Pest. Com. Amsterdam 1971.

13.   TEISINGER I.   Les tests biologiques d'exposition.   Cahiers de Notes Documentaires. Note No 766, 65-71, d'après Pr. Lekarstvi v. **21** No 9 (1969).

14.   VANDEKAR M.   Monitoring of cholinesterase activity in people exposed to insecticides during WHO trials.   WHO (VBC) 75.603.

15.   WEBER H. Rasche und einfacheUltramikromethode zur Bestimmung der Serumcholinesterase.   Dtsch. Med. Wochenschrift **91**, 1961, 1927-32.

16.   ZAVON M.R.   Blood cholinesterase levels in organic phosphate intoxication.   J. Amer. Med. Ass. 192 (1), 1965, 137.

17.   AUGUSTINSSON K.B.   Electrophonetic separation and classification of blood plasma esterases.   Nature, vol. 181 pp. 1786-89 June 28, 1958.

18.   URIEL J.   Characterization of Enzymes in specific immune-precipitates.   Annals of the New York Academy of Sci. vol. 103, No. 2, May 8, 956-79, 1963.

SPECIFIC WORKING PAPER

W. Koransky

Institut für Toxikologie und Pharmakologie der Philipps-Universität, Marburg/L., Germany

Rationale for interest or concern

The data concern chlorinated cyclic hydrocarbons, viz. hexachlorocyclohexane (HCH), hexachlorobenzene (HCB), chlorophenothane (DDT), polychlorinated cyclopentadiene compounds (Aldrin) and polychlorinated biphenyls (PCBs). These organic chlorine compounds are largely resistant to the effects of oxygen, acid or heat, but less so against the effects of alkali and light. Some of them have a relatively high vapour pressure. They are all sparingly soluble in water and divide into lipoid phases of biological structures, in which their concentration continually increases under constant exposure, because redistribution occurs very slowly. Because of these properties they are built up and stored in plant and animals.

Organic chlorine compounds are eliminated by mammals partly in an unchanged state with the faeces, and partly by means of biochemical transformation processes.

The products of metabolism are excreted mainly with the urine. The following metabolic reactions produce quantitatively significant results:
- elimination of a halogen or halogenated hydrocarbon;
- introduction of hydrogen into the molecule;
- replacement of a halogen by glutathione.

The end products of the biochemical transformation processes are very often the sulphuric acid and glucuronic acid conjugates of chlorophenols and chlorophenyl mercaptan acid.

At present the question is being discussed, with regard to HCH, as to whether the insecticidal and relatively short-lived gamma isomer can be converted into the alpha and beta isomers by micro-organisms in water and soil. Both isomers, particularly the beta isomer, are chemically inert and persistent, and high levels of them are often found as environmental pollutants.

All the organic chlorine compounds mentioned above are to be found in lakes, rivers, ground and drinking water, in soil, edible plants, animal feedstuffs and food for human consumption, as well as in animal and human tissues.

These products build up through the food chain, so that when they finally reach human milk a number of substances, such as for example hexachlorocyclohexane, hexachlorobenzene, and a number of polychlorinated biphenyls are present at concentrations ten times greater than in cow's milk.

In general the organic chlorine compounds are not very toxic to mammals. In the case of insecticidal substances the main symptoms of acute poisoning, both in the mammal and in the insect, are the effects on the nervous system.

We still do not know whether these substances are chronically toxic to mammals, or what form any deleterious effects might take. There are many indications that chronic exposure is not without hazards. The absence at present of any real basis for assessment is a cogent argument in favour of taking samples from the environment now and storing them in order to determine the present position and also for research at a later date.

Some indications of possible hazards accompanying exposure to organic chlorine compounds over a number of years are provided by findings concerning the central nervous system and the liver. Practically all insecticidal organic chlorine compounds are neurotoxic. The reason for this, in terms of molecular structure, has so far not been clearly explained. Non-insecticidal HCH isomers also affect the functioning of the central nervous system under specific experimental conditions, e.g. they reduce the sensitivity of the central nervous system to spasmodic drugs.

The reason for this effect is not known. It has been proved that the presence of the HCH compounds, while they are causing these changes, is detectable in the white matter of the central nervous system (areas containing numerous nerve fibres) at high concentrations and for longer periods than in the grey matter (areas containing numerous nerve cells).

The build-up of organic chlorine compounds in this organ begins at a very early stage of its complex ontogeny. So far it has not been discovered whether this phenomenon can impair the normal development and functioning of the nervous system. One good reason for this uncertainty is that at present many of the numerous functions of the central nervous system can only be measured very imprecisely, and in some cases not at all, since neither the psychological methods nor the bio-physical or bio-chemical techniques available at present are sufficiently specific.

Important functions of the liver, unlike those of the central nervous system, can be measured with a sufficient degree of accuracy. It is known that a number of the functions of this organ are affected by organic halogen compounds. Most of the chlorinated hydrocarbons mentioned above cause an increase in the activity of microsomal oxidases, both in the liver and in a number of other organs. These enzymes play an important role in endogenous metabolism, e.g. in regulating the metabolism of steroid hormones. Induction, for instance can cause imbalances in the sexual hormones, the mineralo- and glucocorticoids which in the long term may cause permanent damage, such as fertility impairment.

There are also important indications of shifts in the triglyceride and cholesterol levels, caused by the induction effect of chlorinated hydrocarbons. These reactions could be of particular significance with regard to the formation of atheromas in human beings.

The increases caused by the chlorinated hydrocarbons in the metabolism rates of oxidizing, reducing, hydrolyzing and conjugating enzymes in the liver and other organs, accelerate the metabolism of drugs and countless other foreign substances, and can also cause shifts between toxifying and detoxifying reactions to foreign substances.

Since functional increases of varying degree are found in the different enzymes, depending on the type of inductor affecting them, this could disturb the balance between the formation of carcinogenic epoxides from cyclic hydrocarbons and the simultaneous detoxification of these oxidation products by epoxide hydratases.

A number of the organic halogen compounds mentioned above, e.g. hexachlorobenzene, at least when present in greater quantities, impair porphyrin metabolism and haem synthesis. It is conceivable, although so far this has not been investigated, that even very low concentrations of these substances, if present over a long period, may lead to porphyria or at least could be a contributory factor.

A number of the chlorinated hydrocarbons mentioned produce enlargement of the liver and possibly of a number of other organs, a condition which occurs through hyperplasia, hypertrophy and polyploidy. This process seems to be only partly reversible, but so far it has not caused any recognizable functional impairment of the organ.

Recently discussion has increased as to whether increased proliferation of cells promotes the growth of existing tumours, or more significantly whether it accelerates the development of tumorous lesions into established tumours. This question is relevant to the present situation, since hepatoma have been observed in human subjects following the use over a period of years of contraceptives which can cause increased enzyme activity and can also promote growth when administered in appropriate quantities to animals. In addition, in tests on rats and mice an increase in the occurrence of tumours, particularly of the liver, was observed following administration of DDT, HCH, PCBs, Aldrin and Dieldrin.

No precise conclusions can be drawn from the somatic changes and shifts in biochemical equilibrium so far observed, as to the effects of these processes induced by foreign substances. However, at a future date it will be possible to look for specific changes caused by these, such as a change in the rate of occurrence of tumours, endocrinological disorders, vascular changes, porphyria, etc. It is much more difficult, if at all possible at present, to establish changes in the functioning of the central nervous system. It is of prime importance that methods should be developed further before the build-up of substances observed in the central nervous system can be related to changes in its functioning. For this reason it will be particularly important to store animal and human tissue for a long period, although at the same time this makes particular demands on preservation techniques (see below).

Levels of environmental exposure, pathways for human exposure

Environmental pollution by the chlorinated hydrocarbons mentioned above has been established in many places by analysis. Data are available on water and air and also for certain basic foodstuffs, although these are by no means as complete as one could wish. However, there is a great dearth of study on the conditions governing 'carry-over' (environmental pathways). In the case of some substances, e.g. alpha- and beta- HCH and hexachlorobenzene, there is uncertainty as to the actual sources of the contamination.

In the case of a few possibly toxic effects of the substances, there is a known dose-effect relationship for laboratory animals, and these results can be extrapolated to a no-effect level. Where this was done, the threshold concentrations established were close to the concentrations observed in human subjects. At this point it becomes apparent that the contamination pathways for humans and animals must be observed further over long periods and increased efforts must be made towards the recognition of a no-effect level, so that harmful substances can, where appropriate, be eliminated from the environment at an early stage through legislation. In selecting samples particular attention should be paid to occupationally exposed persons and to considerations of sex and age and the diets of the subjects under survey. In the case of un-weaned infants a difference should be made between those fed on human milk and those fed on cow's milk.

Specimens useful and feasible for collection and analysis

The organic halogen compounds under review are distinctly lipophile substances. They therefore build up particularly in fatty tissue and organs containing a large number of lipoids, such as the central nervous system, the adrenal cortex and Harder's gland. Accumulation is also found in all cell membranes.

Whole-body autoradiography can indicate further storage. Since account must be taken of the possibility of damage to the central nervous system, and more particularly of neurological failure as well as psychical changes, it is in all probability not sufficient to keep only parts of the central nervous system for chemical investigation. It would seem to be important at least to consider the idea of preserving the whole of the human brain in such a way that it will be possible at a later date to investigate individual areas by chemical means and also to study any histological changes which may occur. In this connection neuropathologists and experts on freezing techniques should be consulted on whether conventional histological techniques or freezing techniques would be more suitable. The prime concern here is the human central nervous system, but other organs and animal tissues could also be considered. Preparatory research could include further whole-body autoradiographical examination using a small number of model substances, which might yield further criteria for selecting tissue.

It appears to me that a further interesting parameter is that of the activity of a number of enzymes, particularly those which metabolize foreign substances. Since the activity of these enzymes is closely dependent on the concentration of foreign substances and can be increased or inhibited to a large extent when these are present in great quantities, and since these enzymes also have important functions in normal metabolism, a permanent change in their basic activity can produce important functional changes in the organism in the long term. These changes cannot be established by keeping tissue samples for analysis at a later date. In this case it is necessary to use standardized techniques to measure enzyme activity both now and later, in order to be able to compare the data. The preparatory work needed to standardize methods should be done forthwith.

Over the last few years experimental cancer research has made particular efforts to identify premalignant cells in various organs, and particularly in the liver. These are cells which have already been oncogenically transformed, but have still not reached the malignant stage, although they could do so under certain conditions. It seems that it may be possible to identify these cells reliably in a few years' time using various biochemical, histological and histochemical reactions. In considering the problem of preserving tissue samples some thought should be given to this possibility of making analyses at a later date, in order to be able to correlate patterns, in the frequency of premalignant cells with contamination caused by chemical agents.

ORGANIC COMPOUNDS

F. Korte
Institut für Chemie der Technischen Universität München
8050 Freising - Weihenstephan

A specimen collection, analysis and storage program would provide for the maintenance of national collections and storage of human tissues and environmental specimens. This program would provide a centralized means for determining the current chemical composition of the various substances found in the tissues from the living environment, e.g. cadavers.

Through the sampling of tissues and the development of analytical chemical methodologies, it would be possible to identify the substances which are present in various tissues, including human, and the ascertainment over the years as to whether there is an increase or decrease in the chemical body burden.

Furthermore, when the storage of a particular chemical is found to be increasing in the various human tissues, an adequate amount of this chemical could be synthesized for studies in toxicology.   These studies will be carried out on a broad basis in order to detect any biological effect. For the evaluation of risks involved in the increasing concentration threshold-values will be established for proven harmful effects.

Safety evaluations will become necessary in early stages of the program too. Following the progress of chemical analyses it will happen that for so far unknown chemicals a hazard of high potential could be predicted from known structure activity correlations.   In these cases the program provides immediate investigations without determining any trend in the body burden for the respective chemical.

In this fashion, it would be possible to have a preventive program, to identify the source of a potentially harmful chemical and to either regulate, control, or eliminate this substance from the environment.   The program, which is two-fold, provides the possibility of going back in time for the evaluation of human tissues as well as a look into the future concerning the build-up of environmental chemicals as part of the body burden.   It is proposed that the long-term program includes animal and plant tissues to identify potential sources of human body burden, and from the ecotoxicological point of view, to help to identify endangered species in the environment.

Approaches practised so far for the detection and evaluation of environmental chemicals are non-systematic.   This is mainly due to the fact that a number of specific problems - with single chemicals - arise from random detection of their wide-spread occurrence like PCBs or HCB.   On the other hand high priority problems were arising from random finding of deleterious effects like mercury and cadmium.   Such problems had to be investigated with high priority, but following their specific aims they could not significantly contribute to the safety evaluation of total environmental chemicals. With these single chemicals investigated, however, a number of methods have been developed - both in the area of chemical analysis and structure elucidation, and in toxicology testing, which are of great use for a systematic approach.

Consequently the systematic and 'total analysis' (fingerprint) of environmental specimens for environmental chemicals should start with methods so far used with success in this field. To reach its final goal, however, all promising available methodology has to be adapted to the analysis of environmental specimens and the whole spectrum of classes of organic compounds. With special emphasis on the identification of chemicals, so far not known to occur significantly in the environment, samples have to be investigated following the scheme outlined in the program.   However, it can not be predicted which steps will provide information on the more hazardous or the higher level compounds.   With all the methodology potentially useful, and realizing the aims of the total program, it is evident that priorities based on careful judgement must be given during the progress of the investigations.

It is obvious that investigations to establish environmental safety, will first be carried out for those compounds selected from chemical investigations with already available methods.

This broad and comprehensive program needs the development of some new basic chemical and analytical methodology as well as adaptation of available methods.   Therefore, the very initial phase should cover research on the analysis of tissues by combined gas chromatography - mass spectroscopy using multichannel mass-fragmentation analysis.   The analytical approach for the whole program includes qualitative and quantitative identifications of potentially harmful chemicals with multidetection methods both according to molecular weight ranges and classes of chemicals.   Thus the methodology which will be developed will provide the means of measuring the trend of the occurrence (build-up in tissues) of single compounds and classes of compounds.   To determine the trend only for those classes of chemicals which are at a low position in the hierarchy of hazard would facilitate the long-term routine investigations.   A method for the continuous analysis of organochlorine nonpolar substances has been developed and could serve, in this program, as a model for other classes of chemicals.

The development of the analytical methodology will be stepwise, starting from the adaptation of available methods for certain chemicals, then proceeding to those classes where no methods are available to determine concentrations in the ppb range etc.   Thus it will take time to achieve the 'total analysis' of the total amount of samples.   Therefore, a long-term storage of the samples without chemical changes has to be ensured and the most practical way - storage in solvents, in oxygen-free atmosphere, deep frozen, embedded in a solid phase, or a combination of these - has to be investigated.

Furthermore, computerization of the history of the sample, its analytical data as well as methods to estimate its validity as regards representative character have to be developed.   Subcontracts with clinics, biologists, wildlife experts and food quality people will ensure the availability of the necessary numbers and sizes of samples.

Apart from the analysis which can be done with the samples on a routine basis - using the up-to-date methods - great effort will be put in development of methods to continuously improve and broaden the routine analysis.

One topic is the multielement - multimatrix analysis which provides a feasible measurement of a greater number of samples of different human tissues and of different environmental origin.   This also includes the development of the respective methods for those polar chemicals which are today excluded from analysis since no methods for extraction and clean-up are available.   The improvement of instrumental analysis, especially as regards identification of submicrogram amounts, is a predominant task for the chemists in the whole program.   In mass spectroscopy, e.g. it will be necessary to use several ion sources, like electron-impact, field desorption, chemical ionization and, where necessary, high resolution recording with computerized evaluation.   This is one condition for the identification of as many chemicals as possible.

Furthermore, nuclear magnetic resonance spectroscopy has to be adopted and used for the same purpose following the improvement of the present detection limit.   The same applies for infra-red and infra-red coupled with gas chromatography.

Samples:
To begin with, the following human and animal tissues are to be examined:

Eye

Liver

Fat

Kidney

Brain

Muscle

Samples already being stored and accessible to the program will be used together with present-day samples, provided their history is sufficiently known.

Selected plant samples (crop and wild plants) will be included.

Since the program must be valid for a wide variety of classes of organic compounds, it is impossible at this stage to suggest or select tissues to be stored.   The appropriate concept for tissue selection would be to take chemical fingerprint analyses of a variety of tissues including blood and lymphatic fluid and to decide afterwards which tissues would give representative data for most classes of environmental chemicals.

Long-term storage of samples:
Until the best and most feasible method for storing can be decided, important samples will be stored with the different methods.   If no differences between these will be found after a certain time, as regards concentration and identity of environmental chemicals, the easiest method will be used later on.

Procedure and methods to be used in the chemical investigations

Unlike inorganic analysis, identification of organic substances in biological material can not be reduced to a rigid scheme because separation of the multitude of different organic compounds by means of one standardized procedure is difficult. If one proceeds systematically, however, one should be able to perform successfully complicated organic qualitative and quantitative analyses. Inorganic components, on the other hand, can be identified according to known schemes.

Attention will be directed to obtaining identification of a maximum number of substances from the smallest possible amount of material in the course of one analytical procedure. Methods of isolation and analysis will be based on differences in molecular weight and functional groups.

PROCEDURE

The samples are homogenized under an inert gas, suspended in water and extracted with various organic solvents. The substances from the specimen are thus initially divided into:

A) Volatile components
B) Components soluble in organic solvents
C) Components soluble in aqueous medium
D) Insoluble substances

A) Volatile components are identified by means of gas chromatography in conjunction with mass spectroscopy and other methods. In this way substances or their derivatives with molecular weights up to 10,000 can be detected. A consequence is, of course, that the substances which are found by this method are those which are stable in the gas phase under the chosen conditions, e.g. temperature. Less polar compounds will be preferentially found in this group.
B) The components soluble in organic solvents are subjected to various chromatographic or distributional methods of separation. After purification, the structures are determined by means of the analytical methods to be described later. In this group one can expect to find uncharged or weakly charged compounds with molecular weights of the same order as those in Group A.
C) Water-soluble substances are to be isolated by means of ion exchange, electrophoresis, counter-current distribution, absorptive bubble separation and special chromatographic methods. In this group one expects to find those substances which are subject to hydrogen-bonding.
D) Among the insoluble substances may be found poorly soluble inorganic components or high molecular weight substances which because of extensive hydrogen bonding at neutral pH can only be solubilized with acid or base. Analysis is to be by means mentioned in C) along with derivitization.

A transformation of the substances by the tissue enzymes can generally be avoided by inactivation of the enzymes by means of heat or other methods, if one is not interested in observing such turnover. Considerable attention will be devoted to development and utilization of micromethods which enable the identification of many substances or groups particularly of foreign substances from a minimum number of samples.

STUDIES WITHIN THE FRAMEWORK OF THE SPECIMEN BANK PROGRAM
IN THE INSTITUTE OF ECOLOGICAL CHEMISTRY

A. RESULTS FROM ANALYSES OF ENVIRONMENTAL SAMPLES

Our Institute is engaged in the determination of Xenobiotica in animal and plant tissues and in soil using organochlorines as model substances. As far as studies on animal tissues are concerned, special attention is given to the different concentrations of the substances in the tissues of one organism. In this connection the following tissue types have been selected as models:

muscular meat, liver, kidney, brain and fat

Present studies are carried out on beef and pork (Table 1).

In order to detect levels and differences of chemical loads in the environment with respect to traffic and population density, plant samples from selected ecosystems were analysed. For reference purposes, two different ecosystems were chosen in the Alps far away from traffic and settlements. Two others were situated near Bavarian highways with regard to contaminanation by traffic.   The stated levels of polychlorinated biphenyls (PCBs) ranged from 0.07 to 0.17 ppm in the Alps (Fig. 2) and from 0.09 to 0.95 ppm near the highways (Fig. 3).   The mean values of the two ranges indicate a trebling by traffic.   The corresponding differences in six selected trace elements (As, Se, Sb, Hb, Sn, Br) are much less pronounced because of the very broad concentration ranges covered (Fig. 4).   These investigations yielded also some information on the choice of convenient indicator plants e.g. lichen for trace elements and tree needles for organochlorine compounds.

In another type of analysis we investigated the occurrence of special chemicals.   Fig. 5 shows results on the example of different samples analysed for hexachlorobutadiene.

Trace elements were determined in different parts of maize plants (Fig. 6) and in different cattle tissues (Fig. 8) in order to find out the best parts of a maize plant and the best target organs of cattle, respectively, for sensitive detection.   With a similar aim, eggs have been analysed e.g. for organochlorine compounds (Fig. 9).

For a rough examination of the human intake of some important trace elements with food from cereals, bread samples were analysed (Fig. 7).

Other studies should state the actual contamination of fish in Germany.   Mercury and selenium contents of German freshwater fish were compared with contents of Swedish and Japanese fish (Fig. 10).   In another investigation, methyl and total mercury in fish samples from a German river were analysed looking for a correlation with sewage influx from paper mills and communities along the river (Figs. 11 - 13).

Since solid wastes represent important sources of environmental contamination, problems related to garbage composting and solid waste deposition are under investigation.   PCB-contents in garbage, sewage sludge, and composts ranged from 0.4 to 9.7 ppm with a frequency maximum of some ppm (Fig. 14).   Soils, surface and leaching waters around solid waste deposits showed the more or less regular occurrence of a large number of organic compounds.   Ten chemicals were detected in soils (Fig. 15), eight in surface waters (Fig. 16), and about twenty in leaching waters (Fig. 17).

In addition to such routine studies by the common clean-up methods, new applications in connection with this problem will be developed, such as adsorptive bubble separation.   Known methods, too, will be adopted for these studies, e.g., counter-current distribution, chromatographic and electrochemical methods (electrophoresis).   The various methods of adsorptive bubble separation are studied with regard to their application in connection with the concentration of pesticides, enzymes and other natural constituents and foreign compounds.

Results gained so far give rise to the conclusion that selective concentration of organochlorines from animal tissues is possible.

Furthermore, palaeontologic samples are studied in connection with this problem and are compared with recent material.   The selection of suitable samples is very difficult, since only those samples can be used which are not subject to subsequent contamination, for instance by the atmosphere or ground water.   Additional difficulties exist in the preparation of petrified samples, since common methods using concentrated acids cannot be applied because of subsequent contamination.

Currently, we are trying to develop a suitable preparative method.   Samples of wood, egg shells and bones of various centuries are being examined.

B.   RESULTS OF CONTROLLED EXPERIMENTS

Residues of Environmental Chemicals in Tissues and Organs in Controlled Feeding Experiments
A series of long-term feeding experiments with laboratory animals and various ^{14}C-labeled environmental chemicals was carried out in our Institute.   Comparison of radioactive residues in tissues and organs shows, for controlled exposure, dependence of the concentration on the kind of chemical, the animal species, and the sex.

1.   **Dependence on the Kind of Chemical.**   Table 18 shows comparative data on radioactive residues in organs and tissues of rats following long-term feeding with different radiolabeled chemicals.   The daily dose was about 1 - 2 ppm in the diet, corresponding to 32 - 75 µg/animal. The application was carried out until a plateau level was reached in the body; tissue analyses were performed 1 - 3 days after the application was discontinued (Exception: the experiment with 2,4,6,2',4'-pentachlorobiphenyl, where the feeding was discontinued before a plateau level was reached).

Di-, tri- and pentachlorobiphenyl are constituents of commercial PCB-mixtures which are well-known as environmental contaminants. Chloralkylen-9 is an isopropylated 2,4'-dichlorobiphenyl and was developed as a PCB-substitute. Endrin was chosen as a representative of the cyclodiene insecticide group, and imugan as a representative of chloroaniline-derived pesticides.

The table indicates a clear analogy between chemical properties and tissue concentration or distribution. All substances applied are lipophilic and, therefore, should be accumulated preferably in the fatty tissue. However, this was observed only for the higher chlorinated biphenyls (column 1-3). These three substances show also, besides their tendency to be accumulated in abdominal and subcutaneous fat, generally a higher level in all organs than other substances, e.g. those in columns 5 and 6. Both facts are a consequence of increased chemical stability which prevents metabolism to more hydrophilic, excretable products; this results in an increased general body concentration and, above all, in high levels in the fatty tissues.

First of all, 2,4,6,2',4'-pentachlorobiphenyl which ranges between the less degradable PCBs, has the highest tissue concentrations although the experiment was discontinued before the saturation level was reached. The radioactivity in the organs was found to be only unchanged parent compound (exceptions: liver and kidneys). Furthermore, low excretion rates as well as relatively low percentages of metabolites in the excreta demonstrate that this substance is only slowly metabolized.

Endrin (column 4) is susceptible to metabolic attack by hydroxylation which results in metabolites of increased water solubility. Consequently, the highest residues are not in fat but in blood and spleen. Some tissue concentrations, however, are higher than for Chloralkylen-9.

The 2,2'-dichlorobiphenyl and imugan, also, have highest residues in blood or excretion organs (liver, kidneys), not in fat. This is in good agreement with the excretion behaviour and the high portion of metabolites in the excreted radioactivity (nearly 100%).

2.   **Dependence on the Animal Species.**   Hexachlorobenzene-^{14}C, for example, was given in a single oral dose to rats and to Rhesus monkeys (about 0.5 mg/kg body weight). Table 19 shows the tissue and organ concentrations after a 40 day excretion period.

In this experiment, the differences between tissues of rats and Rhesus monkeys are small. In some tissues, the concentrations are higher for the monkeys. This corresponds to the lower excretion rate as compared to the rat.

3.   **Sex Dependence.**   For the data listed in Tables 1 and 2, differences between male and female animals were small. However, larger differences between male and female are possible. In a long-term feeding experiment with aldrin-^{14}C, females reached the plateau level of body concentration only after 200 days (males after 53 days). This results in a much higher concentration in the abdominal fat at plateau time (females 3.5ppm, males 0.29ppm for a dosage of 0.2ppm of the diet daily).

With the set-up we use for plant metabolism studies under outdoor conditions we measure plant levels as compared to soil concentrations, e.g. with dieldrin starting 1970 with seed-treatment. In 1971, when the upper soil layer contained 0.52 ppm, we made a soil retreatment equivalent to 0.83 kg/ha. Cultivated plants have been onions 1970, cabbage turnip 1971, carrots 1972, and potatoes 1973. Four years after the first treatment, the 0 - 10 cm soil layer contained only 0.23 ppm total residues, the 10 - 20 cm soil layer 0.07 ppm, the 20 - 30 cm soil layer 0.01 ppm. Residues in potatoes were 0.009 ppm, in potato roots 1.17 ppm, in potato peels 0.05 ppm and in the leaves 0.68 ppm. Apart from the leaves where only 60% of the present radioactivity was solvent-extractable, 85-95% of the total residues could be extracted from all samples.

Looking to the residues in the 0 -10 cm soil layer, however, there is a decrease of the concentration to about one-third within one year - e.g. from 1972 to 1973 from 0.69 to 0.23 ppm. Consequently, evaporation - directly from soil or via the cultivated plants - is by far the major route of disappearance of dieldrin residues.

As regards the nature of the residues, four years after the first application, the upper soil layer contains more than 90% as dieldrin-^{14}C, about 5% as photodieldrin, and about 1% each of two unidentified compounds. Residues in peeled potatoes are also more than 90% dieldrin, about 5% photodieldrin, three and one percent respectively the two unidentified products.

TABLE 1

Rückstände chlorierter Kohlenwasserstoffe in Fleischproben

		HCB	Lindan	Heptachlor	Aldrin
Rind 1	Niere	$2{,}6 \cdot 10^{-10}$	Spur	$3{,}1 \cdot 10^{-10}$	$4{,}8 \cdot 10^{-10}$
	Hirn	$0{,}74 \cdot 10^{-10}$	n.n.	$1{,}1 \cdot 10^{-10}$	$1{,}8 \cdot 10^{-10}$
	Leber	$0{,}98 \cdot 10^{-10}$	n.n.	$0{,}73 \cdot 10^{-10}$	$1{,}8 \cdot 10^{-10}$
	Muskel	$2{,}5 \cdot 10^{-10}$	Spur	$6{,}1 \cdot 10^{-10}$	$3{,}9 \cdot 10^{-10}$
Rind 2	Niere	$3{,}8 \cdot 10^{-10}$	Spur	$9{,}5 \cdot 10^{-10}$	$7{,}8 \cdot 10^{-10}$
	Hirn	$1{,}91 \cdot 10^{-10}$	Spur	$2{,}6 \cdot 10^{-10}$	$4{,}2 \cdot 10^{-10}$
	Leber	$4{,}9 \cdot 10^{-10}$	n.n.	$13 \cdot 10^{-10}$	$64 \cdot 10^{-10}$
	Muskel	$8{,}3 \cdot 10^{-10}$	n.n.	$10{,}5 \cdot 10^{-10}$	$8{,}0 \cdot 10^{-10}$
Rind 3	Niere	$1{,}9 \cdot 10^{-10}$	Spur	$2{,}6 \cdot 10^{-10}$	$3{,}7 \cdot 10^{-10}$
	Hirn	$0{,}51 \cdot 10^{-10}$	Spur	$0{,}72 \cdot 10^{-10}$	$1{,}9 \cdot 10^{-10}$
	Leber	$1{,}2 \cdot 10^{-10}$	Spur	$3{,}9 \cdot 10^{-10}$	$2{,}7 \cdot 10^{-10}$
	Muskel	$3{,}6 \cdot 10^{-10}$	Spur	$5{,}3 \cdot 10^{-10}$	$2{,}9 \cdot 10^{-10}$
Rind 4	Niere	$3{,}3 \cdot 10^{-10}$	n.n.	$2{,}7 \cdot 10^{-10}$	$3{,}9 \cdot 10^{-10}$
	Hirn	$0{,}69 \cdot 10^{-10}$	Spur	$1{,}0 \cdot 10^{-10}$	$2{,}3 \cdot 10^{-10}$
	Leber	$2{,}8 \cdot 10^{-10}$	n.n.	$3{,}4 \cdot 10^{-10}$	$3{,}9 \cdot 10^{-10}$
	Muskel	$4{,}9 \cdot 10^{-10}$	Spur	$6{,}2 \cdot 10^{-10}$	$4{,}1 \cdot 10^{-10}$
	Fett	$4{,}6 \cdot 10^{-7}$	$0{,}2 \cdot 10^{-10}$	$0{,}27 \cdot 10^{-8}$	$0{,}12 \cdot 10^{-8}$
Rind 5	Fett	$0.3 \cdot 10^{-7}$	Spur	Spur	Spur
Rind 6	Fett	$1{,}4 \cdot 10^{-7}$	Spur	Spur	Spur
	Hirn	$0{,}9 \cdot 10^{-10}$	n.n.	n.n.	n.n.
	Muskel	$1{,}8 \cdot 10^{-10}$	n.n.	n.n.	n.n.
Schwein 1	Fett	$1{,}1 \cdot 10^{-8}$	n.n.	Spur	Spur
	Hirn	$0{,}6 \cdot 10^{-10}$	n.n.	n.n.	n.n.
	Muskel	$2{,}0 \cdot 10^{-10}$	n.n.	n.n.	n.n.
Schwein 2	Fett	$0.6 \cdot 10^{-8}$	n.n.	Spur	Spur
Schwein 3	Fett	$0.65 \cdot 10^{-8}$	Spur	Spur	Spur

Alle Angaben g Pestizide/g Gewebe

n.n. = nicht nachweisbar

Sampling near Autobahn Pfaffenhofen or Irschenberg		Sampling remote Area Alps, Tegelberg, or Hüttensee	
Plant	ppm dry weight	Plant	ppm dry weight
Moss	0.13	Moss	0.06
Heather	0.28	Heather	0.08
Raspberry leaves	0.15–0.27	Raspberry leaves	0.11
Larch leaves	0.95	Larch leaves	0.17
Rushes	0.12	Rushes	0.07
Hay	0.13	Fern	0.08–0.15
Grass	0.20–0.46	Juniper	0.07
Grass silage	0.40–0.42	Dwarf fir	0.09–0.10
Clover	0.33	Alder leaves	0.09
Mint	0.20		
Strawberry leaves	0.16–046		
Blackberry leaves	0.49		
Fir apex	0.31		
Oak foliage	0.50		
Pine leaves	0.11		
Water hemlock	0.23–0.57		

Fig. 3   Fig. 2

Figure 2

Polychlorinated Biphenyls in different plant samples from two ecosystems in the Alps.

Figure 3

Polychlorinated Biphenyls in different plant samples from two ecosystems near Bavarian highways.

Tegelberg (ppm)	As	Se	Sb	Hg	Sn	Br
Wacholdernadeln	0.02	0.0	0.03	1.9	0.04	0.56
	0.01	0.0	0.03	0.86	0.03	0.76
Himbeerblätter	0.07	0.0	0.0	0.36	0.004	58.1
Moos (Ilylocomium splendens)	0.07	0.82	0.43	0.46	12.8	
	1.29	0.44	0.28	0.0	9.1	
Fichtentriebe (diesjährig)	0.11	0.6	0.04	0.0	5.8	
Schwärzerlenblätter	0.23	0.0	0.04	0.0	0.0	12.38
	0.07	0.0	0.25	0.31	0.0	25.13
Traubenbeerblätter	0.82	0.0	0.59	0.38	0.0	25.61
	0.58	0.0	0.38	0.16	0.0	13.49

Hüttensee

	As	Se	Sb	Hg	Sn	Br
Birkenblätter	0.53	1.39	0.05	0.0	3.35	
Wacholdernadeln	0.06	0.9	0.27	0.1	14.5	
Himbeerblätter	0.07	0.4	0.09	0.0	0.0	13.0
Moos	0.06	0.04	0.92	0.0	0.02	13.3
Lärchennadeln	0.01	0.04	0.12	0.32	0.26	23.1
Heidekraut	0.16	2.67	0.10	0.0	5.57	
Brunnenkresse	0.06	0.0	0.37	2.06	0.39	116.6

Pfaffenhofen

	As	Se	Sb	Hg	Sn	Br
Haselnussblätter	0.87	0.13	0.83	0.14	0.0	71.1
	0.56	0.13	0.29	0.31	0.0	85.82
Erdbeerblätter	1.03	0.41	0.88	0.0	0.0	571.00
	0.09	0.0	0.54	0.0	0.0	298.7
Sauerkirschblätter	2.28	0.0	0.85	0.0	0.56	129.15
Binse	0.03	0.06	0.04	0.0	0.23	63.2
Wasserschierling	0.03	0.41	0.18	0.06	0.0	
Himbeerblätter	0.33	2.18	0.37	0.0	0.0	

Figure 4

Six trace elements in different plant samples from three ecosystems in the Alps

(Tegelberg and Hüttensee) and near a Bavarian Highway (Pfaffenhofen)

TABLE 5

Residues of Hexachlorobutadiene and other organohalogens
(detected with same clean-up and in same GLC run) in Food and Feed

Sample	Residue hexachloro-butadiene (ppb)	Other organohalogens
Condensed milk	4	Trichlorobenzene, pentachlorobenzene, hexachlorobenzene
Preserved milk	n.d.	n.d.
Eggs — white	n.d.	n.d.
Eggs — yolk	42	n.d.
Chicken leg	n.d.	n.d.
Turkey liver	n.d.	n.d.
Cream butter	n.d.	Dichlorobenzene, trichlorobenzene
Vegetable, margarine	33	Trichlorobenzene
Tuna	n.d.	n.d.
Oil sardines	n.d.	n.d.
Pork (abdominal muscles and fat tissue)	n.d.	Hexachlorobenzene
Minced beef	n.d.	Trichlorobutane
Ready-prepared bread-flour	n.d.	n.d.
Poultry's grain-feed	39	n.d.
Meal for laying hens	2	Tetrachloroethylene, dichlorobenzene

n.d. : none detected

Figure 6

Some trace elements in different parts of maize plants
grown near airport Munich-Riem

(ppm)	As	Se	Sb	Hg	Sn	Br
Mais-Kern 1	0.02	0.07	0.56	0.05	3.0	31.5
Mais-Blatt 1	0.23	0.8	23.2	1.00	8.3	688.0
Mais-Schutzblatt 1	0.15	0.20	0.9	0.3	43.0	194.5
Mais-Stiel 1	0.50		0.80	0.40	12.7	73.5
Mais-Blatt 2	0.4		7.1			73.0
Mais-Blatt 3	0.27		1.70		33.8	
Mais-Blatt 4	3.9		4.2	2.1	9.04	82.4
Silo-Futter	0.04	2.00	0.05	0.0	7.8	
	0.08	1.03	0.09	0.0	2.05	

Figure 7

Some trace elements in bread

(ppm)	Hg	Sb	Se	As	Br
Brot 1	0.0	0.04	0.5	0.05	8.73
Brot 2	0.05	0.0	0.0	0.0	0.25
Brot 3	0.008	0.0	0.25	0.0	2.74
Brot 4	0.0	0.004	0.03	0.01	14.07
Brot 5	0.0	0.003	0.03	0.0	17.55
Brot 6	0.0	0.0	0.0	0.0	0.34
Brot 7	0.0	0.01	0.07	0.14	1.93
Brot 8	0.0	0.007	0.13	0.05	1.65

Figure 8

Some trace elements in different cattle tissues

Rind 1	(ppm)	Hg	Se	As	Sb	Br
Fleisch		0.0	0.05	0.07	0.01	
Leber		0.0	0.12	0.04	0.01	1.02
Niere		0.0	0.49			48.92
Rind 2						
Fleisch		0.06	0.06			
Leber		1.16	0.10			13.34
Niere		3.62	0.70			
Bulle						
Leber		0.04	0.13	0.01	0.0	4.53
Niere		0.01	0.21	0.06	0.01	
Rind-Fleisch 3		0.01	0.31			
Rind-Fleisch 4		0.008	0.08			

Figure 9

Selected organochlorine compounds in eggs of birds of prey

Egg	(ppm)	PCB	DDE	HCB
1		70.6	19.0	19.0
2		286.5	116.0	17.5
3		20.3	3.3	-
4		7.0	3.5	0.2

Figure 10

Some trace elements in fish samples from Bavaria (Amper, Salzach)
compared to Japan and Sweden

Thunfisch (Japan) (ppm)	Hg	Se	As	Sb	Br
Thunfisch 1	1.08	0.14	0.02	0.02	14.73
Thunfisch 2	0.17	0.003	0.12	0.11	23.19
Thunfisch 3	0.70	0.007	0.29	0.62	0.44
Thunfisch 4	0.39	0.01	0.32	0.22	31.67
Hecht	0.55				
Hecht (Schweden) 1	0.14	0.007	0.13	0.01	4.53
Hecht (Schweden) 2	0.21	0.18	0.02	0.003	5.92
Eitel	0.17	0.19			
Amper bei Haimhausen					
Aal 1	0.06	0.17			
Leber	0.08	17.70			
Aal 2	0.04	0.24			
Leber	0.08	5.30			
Makrelenfilet	0.00	0.74	0.03	0.03	6.24
Rotauge 1	0.28	0.98			
Rotauge 2	0.26	0.26			
Rotauge 3	0.28				
Salzach **südl. Inn-Zusammenfluss**					
Forelle 1	0.08	0.24			
Forelle 2	0.07	0.39			
Nase 1	0.16	0.78			
Nase 2	0.16	0.35	0.4	0.6	Sn 4.0
(Isar) 3	0.40	2.00			

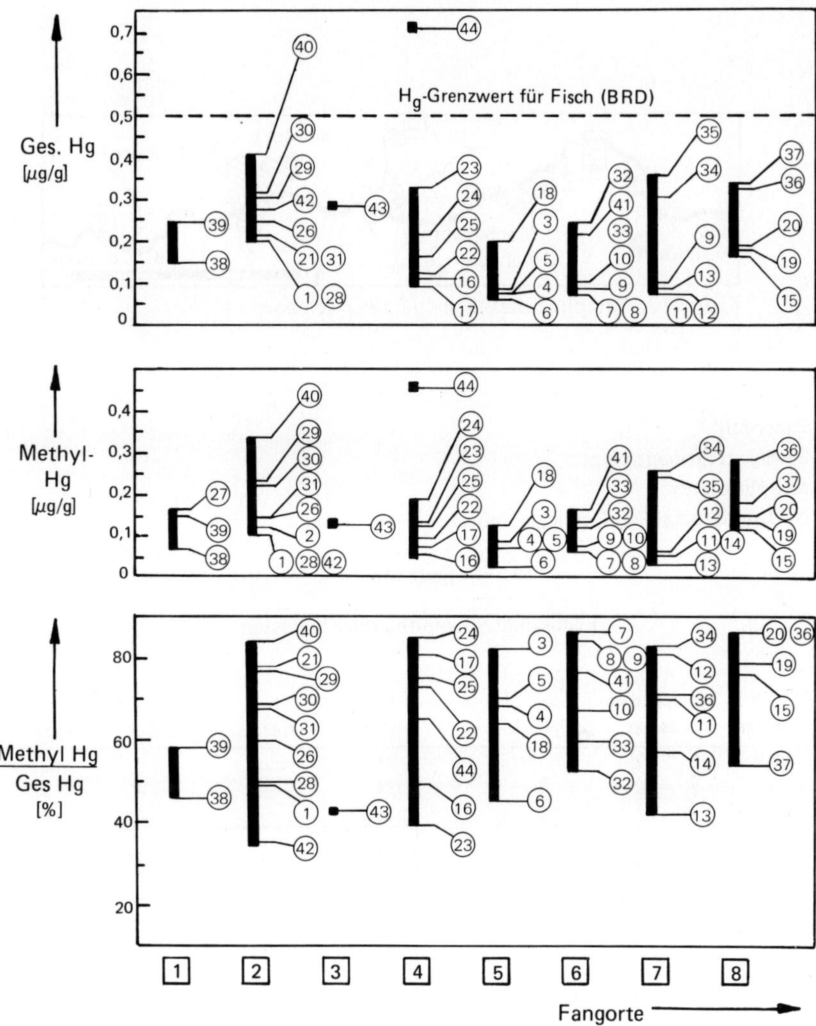

Figure 11. Total and methyl mercury contents, and methyl-to-total-mercury ratios of 44 fish samples (see Fig. 13) from 8 sampling sites along the river Schussen (see Fig. 12)

Figure 12

Sampling sites along the river Schussen

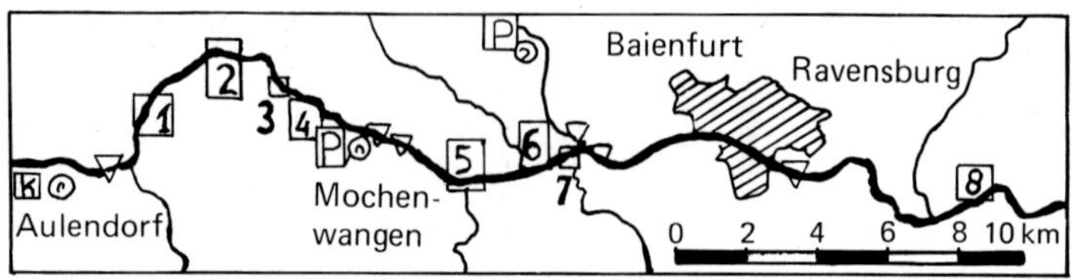

Figure 12. Sampling sites along the river Schussen

P   Paper-mill
K   Sewage treatment plant
☐   Sampling sites
△   No fish detectable (electrical fishing)

Figure 13

Fish samples from the river Schussen

Sample number	fish species	sampling site number	age (years)	sex	Sample number	fish species	sampling site number	age (years)	sex
1	trout	2	?	♀	23	tench	4	2	-
2		2	3	♀	24		4	2-3	-
3		5	1	♂	25		4	4	-
4		5	1	♂	26	roach	1	2-3	-
5		5	1	-	27	chub	1	3	-
6		5	1-2	♂	28		2	1	-
7		6	1	-	29		2	2	-
8		6	1	-	30		2	3	-
9		6	2-3	♂	31		2	4	♀
10		6	3	-	32		6	2	♂
11		7	2	-	33		6	2	♂
12		7	2	-	34		7	2	♂
13		7	2	-	35		7	4	♂
14		7	4	-	36		8	3	♂
15		8	2	-	37		8	4	♀
16	bream	4	2	-	38	barbel	1	4-5	♀
17		4	2	-	39		1	6	♀
18	eel	5	4	-	40		2	?	♂
19		8	5	-	41		6	2	♂
20		8	6	-	42	gudgeon	2	2-3	-
21	carp	2	5	♂	43	eel-pout	3	2-3	-
22		4	3	♂	44	pike	4	1-2	♂

Figure 13. Fish samples from the river Schussen

Figure 14

Polychlorinated Biphenyls (PCB) in samples of garbage and garbage compost

No	Sample	Origin	Date	pH[1]	Water[2] content %	PCB-content[3,4] (μg/g)
(1)	domestic waste	Geiselbullach	18.06.1973	6.2	47	0.5
(2)	dto.	dto.	14.06.1973	7.2	30.5	0.4
(3)	dto.	dto.	15.06.1973	7.1	31	1.0
(4)	dto.	dto.	18.06.1973	6.2	28.5	0.6
(5)	dto.	dto.	19.06.1973	7.3	24	0.7
(6)	dto.	dto.	20.06.1973	6.8	26.5	1.3
(7)	dto.	dto.	22.06.1973	7.3	28	2.2
(8)	dto.	dto.	25.06.1973	6.2	49.5	1.1
(9)	dto.	dto.	20.02.1973	5.9	43	5.9
(10)	waste	Blaubeuren	01.08.1972	-	37	9.7
(11)	waste/sewage sludge	dto.	01.08.1972	-	43.5	2.1
(12)	dto.	Schweinfurt	03.10.1972	-	45	2.5
(13)	sewage sludge	Blaubeuren	01.08.1972	-	-	2.0
(14)	dto.	Warendorf	1972	-	-	1.8
(15)	dto.	Geiselbullach	08.08.1973	7.9	-	
(16)	fresh compost	Blaubeuren	01.08.1972	-	37.5	1.9
(17)	ripe compost	Geiselbullach	20.02.1973	-	24	2.9
(18)	dto.	Blaubeuren	01.08.1972	-	31	3.8
(19)	dto.	dto.	1971	-	-	5.0
(20)	dto.	Schweinfurt	01.10.1972	-	29.5	3.7
(21)	garden soil	Blaubeuren	01.08.1972	-	26	2.5
(22)	dto.	dto.	1971	-	-	1.8
(23)	dto.	Amsterdam	01.08.1973	5.2	48	0.4

Relative standard deviation [1] 1.5 % , [2] 5 %, [3] 2.5 % , [4] related to dry weight

Figure 15

Organic contaminants in soils near solid waste deposits

in the Netherlands

SUBSTANZ	Steenwijk	Hardenberg	Heerenveen
Di-n-butylphthalat	n	n	n
Di-isooctylphthalat	n	n	n
Dichlorbiphenyl	nn	n	nn
Trichlorbiphenyl	n	n	n
Tetrachlorbiphenyl	n	n	n
Pentachlorbiphenyl	n	n	n
Hexachlorbiphenyl	n	n	nn
Hexachlorbutadien	n	n	nn
γ- Hexachlorcyclohexan	n	nn	n
Anthracen	n	nn	n

Figure 16

Organic contaminants from solid waste deposits in surface water

in the Netherlands

SUBSTANZ	Maarsden	Jutphaas
Di-n-butylphthat	12 ppm $\pm$ 5 %	5 ppm $\pm$ 5 %
Tri-n-butylphosphat	55 ppb $\pm$ 5 %	68 ppb $\pm$ 5 %
Pentachlorphenol	nn	1-2 ppb
Tetrachlorbiphenyl	nn	35 ppb $\pm$ 20 %
Pentachlorbiphenyl	nn	35 ppb $\pm$ 20 %
Hexachorbiphenyl	nn	43 ppb $\pm$ 20 %
Di-isooctylphthalat	n	n
Alkylbenzole	n	n

n : detected (ppb - range)
nn : not detectable

Figure 17

Organic contaminants from solid waste deposits in leaching water in the Netherlands

SUBSTANZ	Steenwijk II a	II b	II c	III a	III b	III c	IV a	IV b	IV c	V a	V b	V c	Hardenberg I a	I b	I c	II a	II b	II c	III a	III b	III c	IV a	IV b	IV c	Heerenveen I a	I b	I c
Di-n-butylphthalat, ppm	5	12	< 1	10	12	< 1	4	11	< 1	3			1	5	≪1	1			3	5	< 1	3	7 600b			6	
Di-isooctylphthalat	50	70	10	30	55	-	10	5	-	100			15	25	-	15			50	30	20	35	30	15		100	
Tri-n-butylphosphat	30	-	-	-	140	-	35	60	-	45			38	-	-	28			40	55	-	48	-	-		-	
Tetrachlorbiphenyl	-	-	-	-	-	-	-	35	-	-			-	-	-	-			-	-	-	-	27	-		-	
Pentachlorbiphenyl	-	-	-	-	-	-	-	-	-	48			-	-	-	-			-	-	-	-	-	-		-	
Hexachlorbiphenyl	-	-	-	-	-	-	45	-	-	53			-	-	-	-			23	-	-	45	40	-		-	
Heptachlorbiphenyl	-	-	-	-	-	-	-	-	-	-			-	-	-	-			-	-	-	-	-	-		-	
Chlorden	-	-	-	-	-	-	-	-	-	1-2			-	-	-	< 1			-	-	-	-	-	-		-	
Jonol	-	-	-	-	20	-	-	-	-	-			-	-	-	-			-	-	-	-	-	-		-	
Pentachlorphenol	-	-	-	-	-	-	-	-	< 1	-			-	-	-	< 1			-	-	-	2	1	-		-	
Tetrachloräthylen	120	-	-	60	-	-	-	-	-	-			35	-	-	-			-	-	-	-	-	-		-	
Trichloräthylen	-	-	-	-	-	-	-	-	-	-			-	-	100	-			-	-	-	-	-	-		-	
Dichlorbenzonitril	-	-	-	-	< 1	-	-	2	-	-			-	-	-	-			-	-	-	-	1	-		1	
Dimethylphenol	-	-	-	-	-	-	-	-	-	-			-	-	-	-			-	-	-	-	1-2	-		-	
Dichlornitrobenzol	-	-	-	-	< 1	-	-	5	-	-			-	-	-	-			-	3	-	-	3	-		-	
Pentachlorfluorbenzol	-	-	-	-	-	-	-	-	-	-			-	5	-	-			-	-	-	-	1			-	
Hexachlorbutadien	-	40	1	-	-	< 1	-	-	< 1	-			-	-	1-2	-			-	55	1-2	-	-	1-2		-	
n-Dodecan	35	-	-	-	-	-	-	-	-	-			-	-	-	-			-	-	-	-	-	-		-	
n-Tetradecan	30	-	-	-	-	-	-	-	-	-			-	-	-	-			-	-	-	-	-	-		-	
$C_{14}H_{25}OCl_5$-$H_{27}OCl_3$	50	-	-	-	-	-	-	-	-	-			-	-	-	-			-	-	-	-	-	-		-	
Alkylbenzole		+			+		+	+		+			+	+						+			+			+	

sampling sites : I to V

sampling dates : a : 10.12.1973   b : 01.08.1974   c : 16.12.1974

concentrations : ppb (excepted Di-n-butylphthalate ppm)

\- not detectable   +detectable (determination impossible)   relative SD 5 - 20 %

Table 18

Residues of environmental chemicals and metabolites in tissues and organs of rats
after long-term feeding (ppm, equivalent to the resp. parent compound)
Values after daily feeding (1-2 ppm in the diet) was discontinued

Organ	2,4,6,2',4'-Pentachloro-biphenyl-^{14}C	2,5,4'-Trichloro-biphenyl-^{14}C	Chloralkylen-9-^{14}C	Endrin-^{14}C	2,2'-Dichloro-biphenyl-^{14}C	Imugan-^{14}C
Liver	6.116	0.438	0.257	0.28	0.11	0.183
Lungs	11.960	0.374	0.139	0.30	0.12	0.132
Kidneys	11.883	0.692	0.451	0.29	0.23	0.053
Skin and sub-cutaneous fat	5.749	0.298	0.287	0.74	0.03	0.041
Blood	-	-	0.098	1.10	0.26	0.028
Abdominal fat	25.998	1.004	0.507	0.38	0.08	0.022
Stomach and Duodenum	-	0.443	0.104	0.67	0.13	0.019
Spleen	-	0.284	0.133	3.00	0.15	0.017
Heart	6.324	0.388	0.086	0.58	0.24	0.011
Genitals	12.692	0.389	0.261	0.97	0.07	0.008
Brain	-	0.066	-	0.25	0.03	0.004
Muscles	1.602	0.187	0.061	0.06	0.03	0.003

Table 19

Radioactive residues in tissues and organs of rats and rhesus monkeys
40 days after a single oral dose of Hexachlorobenzene-^{14}C (0.5 mg/kg body weight)
(ppm, equivalent to hexachlorobenzene)

| | Rats | | Rhesus monkeys | |
Organ	♂♂	♀♀	♂♂	♀♀
Liver	0.06	0.07	0.1	0.08
Kidneys	0.05	0.04	0.04	0.04
Heart	0.03	0.04	0.06	0.03
Gall-bladder	-	-	1.0	0.4
Bile	-	-	0.1	0.1
Spleen	0.03	0.02	0.03	0.02
Lungs	0.03	0.07	0.03	0.02
Oesophagus	-	-	0.03	0.03
Adrenal gland	0.6	0.4	0.2	0.5
Thyroid gland	0.1	0.01	0.1	0.02
Hypophysis	0.05	0.01	0.03	0.04
Thymus	0.9	1.8	1.2	1.8
Pancreas	0.04	0.08	0.04	0.05
Salivary gland	-	-	0.03	0.05
Thalamus	-	-	0.04	0.03
Hypothalamus	-	-	0.03	0.05
Lymphatic nodes	0.4	0.6	0.4	0.3
Brain	0.02	0.03	0.06	
Cerebellum	-	-	0.05	0.05
Spinal cord	0.3	1.1	0.1	0.1
Gonads	0.02	0.04	0.01	0.05
Prostata/Uterus	0.4	0.4	0.04	0.02
Urinary bladder	0.03	0.04	0.04	0.02
Stomach	0.04	0.05	0.03	0.04
Duodenum	0.1	0.1	0.08	0.04
Caecum	-	-	0.3	0.2
Colon	-	-	0.2	0.2
Small gut	0.1	0.1	0.1	0.1
Eyeball	-	-	0.04	0.06
Cornea	-	-	0.01	0.01
Lens	-	-	0.01	0.01
Optic nerve	-	-	0.1	0.1
Muscles	0.02	0.02	0.03	0.02
Tongue	-	-	0.01	0.02
Bones	0.01	0.03	0.02	0.04
Bone marrow	-	-	1.1	1.5
Skin	-	-	0.03	0.06
Abdominal fat	1.5	1.8	1.6	1.7
Subcutaneous fat	1.2	1.3	1.3	1.4
Omentum	-	-	1.7	1.5
Brown fat	-	-	1.0	1.1
Blood	0.02	0.02	0.02	0.02

SURVEY OF PESTICIDE RESIDUES AND THEIR METABOLITES IN THE GENERAL POPULATION OF THE UNITED STATES

F. Kutz and S. Strassman
Ecological Monitoring Branch, Environmental Protection Agency, Washington D.C.
and
A. Yobs
Center for Disease Control, U.S. Public Health Service, Atlanta, Georgia

Abstract

Residues of pesticides and their metabolites have been found in various tissues and body fluids of representatives of the general population of the United States, and are indicative of the environmental distribution of these chemicals. Certain organochlorine insecticides or their metabolites and polychlorobiphenyls have been detected in human adipose tissue through an annual national sampling of the general population of the United States. Results revealed that most fat samples contained measurable levels of DDT and its analogs, beta-benzene hexachloride, dieldrin, oxychlordane, heptachlor epoxide and **trans**-nonachlor. Analysis of human milk collected from selected Arkansas and Mississippi counties and of blood serum collected from other limited geographic areas also demonstrated detectable residues of these chemicals in somewhat similar patterns. Recent analytical advances permitted the analysis of urine for organophosphate insecticide metabolites, certain organochlorine pesticides, certain carbamate insecticide conjugates and selected phenoxy herbicides. Preliminary data have indicated that urine from the general population of sampled locales contained some of these chemicals.

Introduction

Residues of pesticides and their metabolites in various human tissues and body fluids have been reported by numerous investigators. These chemical residues reflect the total body burden of these pesticides and past and present exposure to them. Pesticides may gain entrance to the human body through the intestine subsequent to ingestion; through the lungs as a result of inhalation of airborne pesticide-laden dusts, vapors and aerosols; by penetration through the intact skin; and (rarely) by absorption directly into the bloodstream through broken skin.

Once within the human body, the residue is exposed to numerous metabolic pathways and other processes. In the case of certain lipophilic organochlorine pesticides, residues of the parent compound or metabolites are accumulated and stored in the lipid portion of adipose tissues. Residues of these chemicals also may be detected in the lipid portion of such fluids as milk and blood serum. Some other pesticides are rapidly metabolized in the human body to their lesser chemical components and excreted. Certain of the organophosphorous and carbamate pesticides undergo such dynamic metabolic changes. Still other chemicals are capable of passing through the human body virtually intact, and then being excreted, i.e. certain organochlorine and chlorophenoxy herbicides. There are many factors beyond the scope of this paper affecting the storage, disposition, metabolism and elimination of pesticides and associated chemicals in the human body.

From a regulatory perspective, findings of pesticide residues in humans representative of the general population provide a major element in pesticide policy decision-making. These residues are demonstrative of the extent of the environmental distribution of the particular pesticide and when coupled with laboratory animal data showing adverse biological effects, signal a potential public health hazard. In recent decisions regarding the uses of aldrin, dieldrin, heptachlor and chlordane, the Administrator of the U.S. Environmental Protection Agency cited and considered the findings of these chemicals in human tissue.

One program which examines pesticide residues and associated chemicals in human tissues and fluids is the National Human Monitoring Program for Pesticides. This program, operated by the U.S. Environmental Protection Agency, monitors on a national scale, the incidence and level of exposure to selected pesticides experienced by the general population and to identify trends in this exposure.

This paper reports findings of organochlorine insecticide residues and their metabolites in human adipose tissue collected on a national basis for fiscal years 1970 to 1974 inclusive and results from special studies performed on a more limited scope with human milk and urine. During this period of time, a fiscal year began on 1 July and extended to the end of June. For example, FY 1970 began on 1 July 1969, and ended on 30 June 1970.

MATERIALS AND METHODS

Human Adipose Tissue

Human adipose tissue was obtained through the cooperation of medical pathologists and medical examiners in geographic locations selected on the basis of an experimental survey design covering the conterminous 48 states. A proportionate, stratified-random sampling design was followed for selecting cities in which samples were collected. The population strata for the surveys conducted during fiscal years 1970, 1971 and 1972 were the four census regions as provided by the 1960 Census. For the surveys conducted during fiscal years 1973 and 1974, the population strata were the nine census divisions as defined by the 1970 Census. In each case the sampling units were cities with populations in excess of 25,000 people. The number of cities sampled in each region or division was determined based on population distribution. Cities which actually served as collecting sites were selected by randomization.

This design provided samples which would be statistically representative of the pesticide residue levels of the general population. For each collection site, an annual sample quota was established reflective of demographic distribution and allocated portionally according to the age, sex, and race distribution in the 1960 and 1970 Censuses.

Adipose tissue was collected by cooperating pathologists and medical examiners from postmortem examinations and from specimens excised surgically for therapeutic or elective reasons. Thus, tissues were received from patients having pathological conditions as well as those killed by traumatic injury. Information recorded for each tissue sample analysed included age, sex, race, and pathological diagnosis. Geographic residence was assumed to be in the general location of the hospital. Since the objective of the program was to reflect the pesticide burden in the general population, samples were not collected from patients with known or suspected pesticide poisoning, from cachectic patients, or from patients institutionalized for extended periods. Further details of the program were presented by Yobs (1971).

Adipose tissue samples were taken from unembalanced cadavers and unfixed surgical specimens. In the case of collection at postmortem, the sampling was accomplished as quickly as feasible after death, and in all instances within 24 hours. The specimens were then directly placed, without fixatives or preservatives, into clear pesticide-free glass bottles having aluminum foil-lined caps. The samples were frozen immediately and maintained in that state until analysis. After analysis, any remaining tissues were archived in frozen storage.

All chemical analyses were conducted by contract laboratories using only methodologies specified by the program. These laboratories were equipped with gas-liquid chromatographs with electron capture detectors. All laboratories were required to maintain acceptable performance levels in the interlaboratory quality assurance program, established and moderated by the EPA Environmental Toxicology Division, Research Triangle Park, N.C. This laboratory also served as technical consultants for the analytical portion of the program.

Samples were analysed for selected chlorinated hydrocarbon insecticides (Table 1), using a modified Mills-Olney-Gaither procedure. Thin layer chromatography, Coulson electrolytic conductivity detectors, microcoulometry and in some cases, combined gas chromatography-mass spectrometry were employed as confirmatory techniques. The exact analytical methods used in this program were published in manual form by Thompson (1972).

TABLE 1

List of Chemicals Detectable in Human Adipose Tissue and Milk

o,p'-DDT	Aldrin
p,p'-DDT	Dieldrin
o,p'-DDE	Heptachlor
p,p'-DDE	Heptachlor Epoxide
o,p'-DDD	Endrin
p,p'-DDD	Mirex
α-BHC	Oxychlordane
β-BHC	**trans**-Nonachlor
Lindane	Polychlorinated Biphenyls
δ-BHC	Hexachlorobenzene

The following descriptive statistics were used to characterize the data:

- Sample Size: the total number of samples analysed.
- Percent Positive: The percentage of the total number of samples which had a measurable residue of a given pesticide.
- Geometric Mean: Calculated according to the standard formula, after data had been adjusted for zero values.
- Maximum Value: The highest concentration of a given residue detected.
- Geometric Standard Deviation (-1 to +1): Equivalent areas about the geometric mean into which 68 percent of the observations fell.

In calculating these descriptive statistics, only reports of quantifiable amounts of pesticides were considered; reports of trace amounts were regarded as zero. Since these residue data tended not to be normally distributed statistically, the geometric mean was used as the most reliable measure of central tendency. All residue values were calculated on a percent lipid basis. This conversion is affected by dividing the whole tissue (wet-weight) value by the percent lipid extractable material for each specimen. This technique reduced the inherent variation in residue data attributable to differences in the lipid content of individual tissue specimens.

Human Milk

Samples of milk were collected from lactating women who resided in selected areas of Arkansas and Mississippi. Milk was manually expressed, frozen immediately after collection and held in that state until analysis. The details of this study are found in Strassman and Kutz (1976).

Human Urine

A pilot project was established during 1971 and 1972 to determine the applicability to field surveys of the general population of promising analytical procedures which measure urinary metabolites of certain organophosphate, chlorophenoxy, carbamate and organochlorine pesticides. Samples of urine were collected through the already operational procedures of the human monitoring survey utilizing the services of pathologists in hospitals or in the private practice of laboratory medicine and also from apparently normal volunteers with documented exposure to some of these pesticides. Samples from hospitals were requested from outpatients or from patients hospitalized no more than 24 hours. Samples were frozen immediately after collection in chemically clean screw-capped bottles without fixatives or preservatives and shipped packed in dry ice. Specimens were stored in a frozen state until analysis. Pesticide exposure information and clinical history were collected, if available.

Analyses for the two groups of compounds were performed on split samples in two different laboratories. The organophosphate metabolite analyses were performed according to the methods published by Shafik et al (1973a). The phenol metabolite analyses were performed according to Shafik et al (1973b). Chemicals detectable following these methods and their pesticide origin are listed in Table 2.

TABLE 2

List of Chemicals Detectable in Human Urine and their Pesticide Origin

Chemical	Pesticide Origin
Dialkyl Phosphate Method	
Dimethyl Phosphate (DMP)	
Diethyl Phosphate (DEP)	Any organophosphorous insecticide
Dimethyl Phosphothionate (DMTP)	containing these phosphates or
Diethyl Phosphothionate (DETP)	phosphothionate radicals
Dimethyl Phosphodithionate (DMDTP)	
Diethyl Phosphodithionate (DEDTP)	
Malathion	
Malathion α-monocarboxylic acid *	Malathion
Malathion dicarboxylic acid *	

TABLE 2, continued

Multi-phenol Method

Pentachlorophenol	Pentachlorophenol
Alpha-naphthol	Carbaryl
Parnitrophenol	Parathion
2,4,5-T	2,4,5-T
2,4-D*	2,4-D
Silvex*	Silvex
3,5,6-Trichloro-2-pyridonol*	Chlorpyrifos
Isopropoxyphenol*	Propoxur
Carbofuran phenol*	Carbofuran
3-Ketocarbofuran*	
2,4,5-Trichlorophenol*	2,4,5-Trichlorophenol (a disinfectant) and certain OP insecticides (a metabolite)

*   compounds not detectable during 1971-72 pilot study.

RESULTS AND DISCUSSION

Human Adipose Tissue

The results of the analysis for the organochlorine insecticide in adipose tissue are presented in Tables 3 through 8.   Although detectable in our analytical approach, residues of delta-BHC, aldrin, heptachlor and endrin were not found in general population samples.

Beta-Benzene Hexachloride (Table 3).   This residue was representative of exposure to the insecticide benzene hexachloride.   These data showed that this chemical was widely distributed at low levels in the human population during all five years.   Although there seemed to be a trend toward reduction in the quantity of residue, this was not reflected in the frequency, which remained equally high during all years.   It has been hypothesized that certain laboratory animals convert the various isomers of BHC, including lindane, to the beta configuration for storage (Kamada 1971).   If this is true in the human system, then storage of the beta isomer may be representative of exposure to all configurations of BHC.

TABLE 3

Residues of Beta-Benzene Hexachloride in Human Adipose Tissue

Survey Year	Sample Size	Percent Positive	Geometric Mean	Concentration in ppm, lipid basis Maximum Value	Geometric Standard Deviation -1	+ 1
FY 1970	1412	99.15	0.37	26.93	0.14	0.93
FY 1971	1615	99.32	0.34	9.47	0.15	0.78
FY 1972	1913	92.21	0.23	7.53	0.06	0.78
FY 1973	1095	99.18	0.26	5.76	0.10	0.61
FY 1974	898	98.55	0.21	3.05	0.08	0.55

Total DDT Equivalent (Table 4).   This conglomerate figure reflected the total burden of DDT and its analogs found in human adipose tissue.   DDT had the distinction of being stored in larger amounts than any of the other organochlorine pesticides found in adipose tissue during these five survey years.   It was detected in almost every tissue analysed.

Biochemically, DDT is dechlorinated in the human body to DDD, and then either metabolized to the water-soluble and excretable DDA, or excreted directly as DDD.   DDE storage is not appreciably derived from ingested DDT, but rather by ingestion of DDE previously formed from DDT in the environment.   Since DDE is not effectively eliminated from the body, the result is a gradual increase in the body burden of this chemical.   On the other hand, DDT would be broken down and excreted more rapidly than DDE (Morgan and Roan 1971, and Roan et al 1971).

Although the frequency of detecting these residues remained high, a trend toward the reduction in concentration was observed. This trend was apparent both in the geometric mean levels and in the area representing one geometric standard deviation. The agricultural uses of this chemical were cancelled by EPA order in late 1972. Further details of this reduction were presented by Kutz et al (1976).

TABLE 4
Residues of Total DDT Equivalent in Human Adipose Tissue

				Concentration in ppm, lipid basis			
			Average Percent			Geometric	
Survey	Sample	Percent	of Total Found	Geometric	Maximum	Standard Deviation	
Year	Size	Positive	as DDE	Mean	Value	-1	+ 1
FY 1970	1412	99.93	77.15	7.88	270.05	3.21	19.31
FY 1971	1615	99.75	79.71	7.95	207.33	3.14	20.11
FY 1972	1913	99.95	80.34	6.88	173.22	2.79	16.96
FY 1973	1095	100	81.18	5.88	329.77	2.37	14.58
FY 1974	898	99.89	83.00	4.99	89.06	1.80	13.80

Dieldrin (Table 5). Dieldrin residues were reflective of exposure to the insecticides aldrin and dieldrin. After exposure, aldrin residues are rapidly converted by the human body to dieldrin. Low levels of dieldrin residues were found in almost every tissue collected and remained appreciably unchanged during the five survey years.

TABLE 5
Residues of Dieldrin in Human Adipose Tissue

| | | | | Concentration in ppm, lipid basis | | |
| Survey | Sample | Percent | Geometric | Maximum | Geometric Standard Deviation | |
Year	Size	Positive	Mean	Value	-1	+ 1
FY 1970	1412	96.53	0.18	15.20	0.07	0.46
FY 1971	1615	99.20	0.22	2.91	0.10	0.47
FY 1972	1913	98.27	0.18	2.91	0.08	0.41
FY 1973	1094	99.00	0.18	5.64	0.08	0.38
FT 1974	898	98.89	0.15	2.21	0.06	0.32

Heptachlor Epoxide (Table 6). Residues of this chemical were representative of exposure to two pesticides, heptachlor and chlordane. This residue was also found at low levels in most of the tissues submitted to the program.

TABLE 6
Residues of Heptachlor Epoxide in Human Adipose Tissue

| | | | | Concentration in ppm, lipid basis | | |
| Survey | Sample | Percent | Geometric | Maximum | Geometric Standard Deviation | |
Year	Size	Positive	Mean	Value	- 1	+ 1
FY 1970	1412	94.76	0.09	10.62	0.03	0.25
FY 1971	1615	96.22	0.09	1.53	0.04	0.20
FY 1972	1913	90.28	0.08	1.21	0.03	0.21
FY 1973	1095	97.72	0.09	0.84	0.04	0.20
FY 1974	898	96.21	0.08	0.77	0.03	0.18

Oxychlordane (Table 7).   Oxychlordane is the mammalian metabolite of the chloro-isomers of the insecticides chlordane and heptachlor.   The capability to detect oxychlordane was introduced into our multi-residue approach during the mid-fiscal year 1971 collection year so that the FY 1972 survey was the first complete survey year for its detection.   As with its close relative heptachlor epoxide, oxychlordane residues were found with high frequencies at levels of around 0.1 ppm in adipose tissue.

Another evidence of exposure to technical chlordane and technical heptachlor has been detected within the last year.   Residues of **trans**-nonachlor have been discovered in human adipose tissue collected from the general population (Kutz et al 1976).

Residues of alpha-benzene hexachloride, lindane (gamma-benzene hexachloride) and mirex have also been detected in human adipose tissue from the general population (see Table 8).   These chemicals were found at low frequencies in most survey years.   A more detailed report on mirex has been published elsewhere (Kutz et al 1974).

TABLE 7
Residues of Oxychlordane in Human Adipose Tissue

Survey Year	Sample Size	Percent Positive	Geometric Mean	Concentration in ppm, lipid basis Maximum Value	Geometric Standard Deviation - 1	+ 1
FY 1972	1913	92.32	0.11	1.87	0.04	0.28
FY 1973	1095	98.36	0.12	1.43	0.06	0.25
FY 1974	898	98.44	0.12	1.73	0.05	0.25

TABLE 8
Organochlorine Pesticide Residues Found at Low Frequencies in Human Adipose Tissues

Chemical	Percent Positive by Survey Year FY 70	FY 71	FY 72	FY 73	FY 74
Alpha-BHC	2.05	0.12	1.99	1.64	0.45
Lindane	1.77	1.42	0.31	1.55	0.56
Mirex	(a)	(a)	0.05	0.09	0.11

(a)   Methodology to detect mirex was not introduced for a full survey year until the FY 1972 survey.

Human Milk

Residues detected in milk samples from residents of Arkansas and Mississippi are reported in Table 9.   DDT, DDE, beta-BHC, heptachlor epoxide, oxychlordane, dieldrin and **trans**-nonachlor were found.   Residues of DDT and its analogs were detected at higher concentrations than the other pesticides.   It is interesting to note that the same pesticides detected in adipose tissue in high frequencies are also found in the lipid portion of human milk.   This is not unexpected since lactation is a form of excretion.

Human Urine

Table 10 summarizes the results of the analysis of specimens from the pilot urine study. Both alkyl phosphate and phenolic derivatives were detected in some urine samples.   After entry of the biodegradable pesticide into the human body, the chemical was metabolized to its basic components.   In the case of some organophosphorous insecticides, the basic component was the dialkyl phosphate radical plus a phenolic radical, if the chemical contained a phenol structure.   In the analytical procedure, these compounds are derivatized to improve chromatographic detection.   The multi-phenol method also detected chemicals containing a chlorinated phenol structure, i.e. pentachlorophenol, 2,4,5-T, etc. Malathion detection deserves special note. Laboratory animal studies revealed that low level exposure to malathion results in the excretion of the mono- and dicarboxylic acid metabolites.   Following the analytical procedure, these two metabolites are derivatized back to the parent compound and detected as such.

TABLE 9

Organochlorine Pesticide Residues in 57 Human Whole Milk Samples
Collected from Residents of Arkansas and Mississippi

| | | Concentration in parts per million | | |
| | Percent | Arithmetic | Extreme Values | |
Pesticide	Positive	Mean	Minimum	Maximum
Total DDT equivalent*	100.0	0.34	0.02	2.76
p,p'-DDT	100.0	0.09	0.01	0.84
p,p'-DDE	100.0	0.22	0.01	1.72
β-BHC	36.8	< 0.01	trace	0.01
Dieldrin	28.1	< 0.01	trace	0.05
Heptachlor epoxide	35.1	< 0.01	trace	0.03
Oxychlordane	45.6	< 0.01	trace	0.02
trans-Nonachlor	14.1	< 0.01	trace	0.01

* Total DDT equivalent = o,p'-DDT + p,p'-DDT + 1.114 (o,p'-DDE + p,p'-DDE + o,p-DDD + p,p'-DDD)

Alkyl phosphate metabolites were found in the urine; however, only a small percentage were detected in concentrations in excess of 0.1 ppm. It should be emphasized that certain phosphates are normally present in the human body. Our current research efforts indicated that residues of DMDTP and DEDTP are less specific and that these two chemicals rapidly degrade in the human body to the other dialkyl phosphate metabolites. Residues of the other dialkyl phosphate metabolites appear to be directly attributable to pesticide exposure.

The results of the phenol method demonstrated that alpha-naphthol, a metabolite of carbaryl, paranitrophenol, a metabolite of parathion and 2,4,5-T were detected in only a few samples and usually at levels below 0.1 ppm. It is interesting to note that pentachlorophenol was found in almost all samples tested at levels below 0.1 ppm. This would indicate that most of the people sampled had some exposure to this chemical.

TABLE 10

Summary of Pesticides and their Metabolites Detected in 267 Human Urine Samples

Chemical	Percent Positive	Percent of Samples $\geq$ 0.1 ppm
Dialkyl Phosphate Method		
Dimethyl phosphate (DMP)	76.7	2.2
Diethyl phosphate (DEP)	94.0	3.4
Dimethyl phosphothionate (DETP)	70.8	7.9
Dimethyl phosphodithionate	38.2	4.5
Diethyl phosphodithionate (DEDTP)	0.4	0.4
Malathion	0.4	0
Multi-Phenol Method		
Pentachlorophenol	96.3	1.5
Alpha-naphthol	10.9	2.2
Paranitrophenol	6.7	1.9
2,4,5-T	1.5	1.5

Considerable analytical improvements have been made in the urine methods since the pilot study was completed. Based on these developments, during calendar year 1976, the National Human Monitoring Program for Pesticides embarked on a cooperative venture with the U.S. Public Health Service to estimate the exposure of the general population to other classes and types of pesticides. This survey, utilizing the Health and Nutritional Examination Survey II of the National Center for Health Statistics, entails collecting data from a scientifically selected segment of the general population. At the same time, survey personnel will collect samples of blood serum and urine from a probability sample of persons 12 to 74 years old for pesticide residue and metabolite determinations. The results of this cooperative arrangement will collect baseline data on the exposure of the general population to organophosphate, carbamate, chlorophenoxy and certain organochlorine pesticides; correlate residue and metabolite data with various medical and nutritional parameters; and collect some information on the pesticide use patterns of the general population.

LITERATURE CITED

KAMADA, T., 1971. Hygienic studies of pesticide residues. Report No. 1. Accumulation of the BHC isomers (α, β, γ and δ) in the body and the rate of urinary excretion following oral administration. Japanese Hyg. 26(4):358-364 (in Japanese).

KUTZ, F.W., A.R. YOBS, W.G. JOHNSON and G.B. WIERSMA, 1974. Mirex residues in human adipose tissue. Environmental Entomol. 3(5):882-884.

KUTZ, F.W., A.R. YOBS, S.C. STRASSMAN and J.F. VIAR Jr., 1976. Effects of reducing DDT usage on total DDT storage in humans. (manuscript in preparation).

KUTZ, F.W., G.W. SOVOCOOL, S.C. STRASSMAN and R.G. LEWIS, 1976. **Trans**-Nonachlor residues in human adipose tissue. Bull. Environ. Contamination Toxicol. 16(1):9-14.

MORGAN, D.P. and C.C. ROAN, 1971. Absorption, storage and metabolic conversion of ingested DDT and DDT metabolites in man. Arch. Environ. Health 22:301-308.

ROAN, C.C., D.P. MORGAN and E.G. PASHAL, 1971. Urinary excretion of DDA following ingestion of DDT and DDT metabolites in man. Arch. Environ. Health 22:309-315.

SHAFIK, T.M., D.E. BRADWAY, H.F. ENOS and A.R. YOBS, 1973b. Human exposure to organophosphorus pesticides. A modified procedure for the gas-liquid chromatographic analysis of alkyl phosphate metabolites in urine. Ag. Food Chem. 21:625-629.

SHAFIK, T.M., H.C. SULLIVAN and H.F. ENOS, 1973a. Multiresidue procedure for halo- and nitrophenols. Measurement of exposure to biodegradable pesticides yielding these compounds as metabolites. Ag. Food Chemistry 21:295-298.

STRASSMAN, S.C. and F.W. KUTZ, 1976. Insecticide residues in human milk from Arkansas and Mississippi. Pesticide Monitoring J. (in press).

THOMPSON, J.F. (ed), 1972. Analysis of pesticide residues in human and environmental samples. Prepared by EPA Environmental Toxicology Division, Health Effects Research Laboratory, Research Triangle Park, N.C. 27711.

YOBS, A.R., 1971. The national human monitoring program for pesticides. Pesticide Monitoring J. 5:44-46.

COLLECTION AND TRACE ELEMENT ANALYSIS OF POST-MORTEM HUMAN SAMPLES: THE WHO/IAEA RESEARCH PROGRAMME ON TRACE ELEMENTS IN CARDIOVASCULAR DISEASES

R. Masironi
World Health Organization, Geneva
and
R. M. Parr
International Atomic Energy Agency, Vienna

Summary

Heart, kidney, liver, hair, and toenails are analysed for Cd, Cr, Cu, Se and Zn. Autopsy collection is made according to a WHO protocol using a titanium knife. Tissues are immediately frozen and subsequently shipped by air to the analytical laboratory. Analysis is by neutron activation or other suitable trace analysis method according to an IAEA protocol. Pathology and analytical data are reported according to standard formats. Institutions in many countries, both developed and developing, collaborate in this programme. Statistical principles and organizational aspects, as well as cost estimates are discussed.

1. Background and Rationale

Many publications support the proposition that subjects suffering from cardiovascular diseases may have abnormal levels of several heavy metals and other trace elements in their tissues and body fluids. In an attempt to identify still unrecognized risk factors in the etiology of cardiovascular diseases, the World Health Organization and the International Atomic Energy Agency, in a joint research programme, have focussed their attention on a few trace elements which, because of their biochemical properties and as a result of the literature evidence, seem more likely to be involved in cardiocirculatory function.

Choice of Elements and of Tissues

The elements under investigation are: Cd, Cr, Cu, Se, Zn plus, as elements of secondary priority, Li, F, Si, V, Mn, Mo, Pb, Hg, I, and the major elements Ca, Mg, and Na. These elements are analysed in heart, kidneys, liver, hair and toenails. Standardized collection of autopsy specimens, as well as of clinical and pathological information on each individual donor, is done under co-ordination by WHO (see protocol in Annex 1) while trace element analyses are co-ordinated by IAEA. It was thought that decentralization and allocation of responsibilities to specialized agencies would give the best guarantee of success to the programme.

2. Collection of Tissue Specimens

The protocols adopted for use in this programme stipulate that tissues should not be collected from subjects who:
(a) are carriers of contagious diseases;
(b) are likely to have been exposed to significant amounts of heavy metals because of their occupation (e.g. metal industry, welding, mechanics, painters, etc.);
(c) have recently been treated with medicaments containing heavy metals or chelating agents (see attached list, Annex 2).

Collection from the general population is easier but is fraught with many uncertainties as to the health status of the subjects which can influence the trace element concentration in tissues. On the other hand, collection from a cohort which is well-defined in terms of age, sex and clinical history, etc., certainly gives clearer results but poses too many constraints and increases considerably the length of time needed to reach the desired number of subjects.

It is essential that the site of sampling be specified exactly. It has indeed been proved that trace element concentrations vary within adjacent areas of the same tissue (e.g. between right and left ventricle of the heart, along the hair shaft, etc., and even within a relatively homogeneous organ such as the liver). For this reason a 16mm film was produced by a WHO collaborating laboratory (The Department of Pathology, University of Geneva) to show the standard way to collect the desired tissue samples.

Ideally the subjects should all come to autopsy over a relatively short period of time (i.e. less than one year) in order to minimize the possible influence of a change in patterns of trace element pollution such as may be occurring particularly in some of the larger cities. If practical, it is recommended that they should be autopsied within six hours of death, though time after death has never, in fact, been demonstrated to have any bearing on the trace element content of tissues. Priority should be given to subjects whose residential, occupational and clinical histories can be recorded in sufficient detail. It is desirable to have equal numbers of cases of both sexes and their ages should be uniformly distributed across the life span, unless it is decided to study only one age group.

The subjects within any one group should be approximately of the same social background. If there are two or more races available for study a decision must be taken as to whether only one race should be followed up or whether the races should be studied separately.

The health status of the subjects depends on the scope of the study. In a case control study, such as the WHO/IAEA study on tissue trace element concentrations in myocardial infarction subjects as compared with healthy controls, the choice is relatively easy since myocardial infarction is usually a well-defined and easily recognisable pathological condition. The 'healthy' controls are assumed to be accident victims who were found at autopsy without this condition (and, preferably, also without other major diseases such as cancer, etc.). However, in tissue banking aimed at future determination of temporal trends in environmental pollution and in metal body burden, careful attention should be paid to the health status of subjects since many diseases have an influence on the trace element concentrations of tissues.

Selection of Tissues
In the WHO/IAEA study the samples selected for analysis include heart, liver, kidney cortex, toenails and hair. Kidney medulla was also included in the original protocols but was later deleted because the large natural variability in trace element concentrations in this tissue made the interpretation of the analytical results difficult. The organs are chosen as far as possible to exclude gross localized lesions, as well as other evident inhomogeneities and pathological portions.

Heart:
The sample is collected from the anterior wall of the left ventricle and must include essentially the greater part of the wall from outside to inside but exclude the endocardium, epicardium and any subepicardial fat. This site was chosen because the sample can thus be taken before opening the heart and thus avoids excessive contamination with blood. The interventricular septum is to be avoided because of the presence of conducting tissue.

Liver:
The sample is taken from the superior anterior surface of the right lobe after removal of the capsule and of several subjacent millimetres of tissue which contain excess fibrous material.

Kidney:
A sample of kidney cortex is taken after removal of the capsule; care must be taken to avoid the cortico-medullary junction. The sample must come from the lower pole of the left kidney. An 18 mm colour film is circulated among all WHO collaborating pathologists to show the standardized procedure to collect the above tissues.

Hair:
A lock of hair approximately the size of a matchstick is clipped from the occipital region, preferably using plastic scissors.

Toenails:
Clippings as wide as possible, and comprising at least 20 mg of material are obtained from the right and left big toes. Toenails instead of finger nails were chosen because, at least in populations normally using shoes, they are not significantly contaminated by metals and other trace elements, whereas finger nails are exposed to occupational and other kinds of everyday contamination.

Size of sample:
The size of each sample collected should be sufficient to: (a) permit analysis by less sensitive methods than neutron activation analysis and by a combination of methods if several methods are in use; (b) permit replicate analysis for quality control; (c) permit re-analysis if additional elements should later become of interest. Generally, these requirements will be satisfied if three separate one gram aliquots of the sample are collected, each being placed in a separate plastic specimen vial, or if a single 10-20 g sample is provided.

The recommended procedure:
Since the elements of interest are present in the tissues at concentrations of a few micro-

grams per gram and even much lower, great care is needed to avoid metal contamination. Handling of the samples should therefore be kept to a minimum and metal-free plastic gloves should be worn.   No chemical fixative may be used and the samples should not be pierced through with a metal instrument, nor should they be rinsed with tap water or any other medium.   The instruments used for handling the samples prior to analysis, or for cutting or breaking them into small pieces, may be a potent source of contamination unless the proper precautions are taken.   Therefore, an autopsy collection kit comprising plastic forceps, pre-cleansed plastic vials, specially prepared titanium knives, and a stone for sharpening them, are prepared at IAEA and supplied to the collaborating pathologists.   Silica or plastic knives have also been tested and found to introduce no significant contamination at least for certain elements and therefore their use is acceptable.   If it is necessary to use steel instruments these should preferably be of carbon steel rather than stainless steel.   Stainless steel instruments, for example, forceps, scalpels and scissors, could be used, but definitely not when chromium is to be analysed.   The danger of contaminating samples with chromium from stainless steel instruments and of course even more from chromium-plated instruments is well documented.   As compared with past experience with glass knives, quartz knives, or polyethylene knives such as those used in picnic sets or stiffened by cooling in liquid nitrogen, the titanium knives recently produced at IAEA are well acceptable to pathologists, have a low degree of metal contamination, can be sharpened and are easy to produce.

Although blood is not one of the tissues of primary interest in the present programme, some consideration has been given to the problems of obtaining suitably uncontaminated samples.   Blood collecting needles made from nickel or platinum on teflon mounts are commercially available and are considered to be suitable for this purpose.

An alternative procedure:

In case the collaborating pathologist is not able to follow the above procedure particularly in regard to the use of titanium knives and plastic forceps, he is recommended to remove the whole organ or a major part of it, taking care not to pierce it with any metal instrument.   It will be the responsibility of the analytical laboratory later on to remove surface contamination before selecting a part of the sample for analysis.

Storage of Specimens in the Collection Laboratory

Immediately after collection, each sample must be put in a plastic vial which is centrally supplied, closed tightly, identified and frozen at less than -15°C in a freezer where they should be kept until they can be sent to the analytical laboratory.   The samples (except hair and toenails) must arrive at the analytical laboratory in a frozen state otherwise they will be discarded. In the analytical laboratory they are stored in a frozen state while awaiting analysis.   Hair and toenails need not be frozen.   We are dealing here with short-term storage, e.g. from a few days to several months.   Longer storage periods have not been explored in the present WHO/IAEA programme.

Sample Identification

Each container is clearly marked in non-smearing ink or other suitable method with a code number followed by the letters: H (heart), L (liver), KC (kidney cortex), KM (kidney medulla), as appropriate.   Toenails and hair may be identified by TN and HR.   Attention should be paid to ensure that the label is securely fastened to the bottle and does not come off during storage and handling.   If the pathological laboratory is able to collect good, uncontaminated tissue samples, and if it also possesses good facilities for drying the samples without contamination, either under vacuum at room temperature or by freeze-drying, then an alternative procedure is to dry the samples immediately after collection, seal them in their containers, identify them with a code number and store them in a cool or refrigerated place until they can be sent for analysis.

For studies such as this involving several collecting centres, the use of a single, unambiguous, numbering system has been found to be of the greatest importance. Autopsy numbers are generally not suitable for this purpose since different centres usually have different systems and this can lead to confusion in the analytical laboratory and/or in the evaluation of the results.

Shipment of Samples

After a suitable number of samples have been collected (e.g. from at least five autopsies), they are sent to the appropriate analytical centre.   Naturally dry samples (hair and toenails) may be shipped in a simple cardboard box without any special packaging. Frozen tissue samples, however, must be shipped as follows. The containers are placed in a cardboard box or other suitable container and surrounded by at least an equal volume of dry ice. The box is then wrapped loosely with paper, packaged and despatched to the analytical laboratories without delay by air freight. More recently, temperature-controlled, insulated shipping containers have become commercially available which can be shipped back and forth for transport of frozen samples, but of course this system requires more logistics and more expense. These thermo-insulated containers permit storage of frozen material over a period of three or more days, i.e. sufficient time in which to ship samples from the pathological laboratory to the analytical laboratory.

The analytical laboratory is immediately informed in advance by cable of the flight number, airway bill number, and estimated time of arrival. The shipment must be scheduled so that the specimens do not arrive over a week-end.

Pathologist's Report

The pathologist must provide relevant information on each case autopsied by entering this information on self-copying forms which are centrally provided by the World Health Organization in triplicate sets. One copy is sent to the central co-ordinating agency for collection, i.e. WHO, the second copy is sent together with the samples to the analytical laboratory, and the third copy is retained by the pathologist for his records. A specimen autopsy information sheet is attached (Annex 3).

3. Analytical Methodology
Preparation for Analysis
Soft Tissues

The first and most important of the pre-analysis procedures is sample collection, as described above, which is usually under the responsibility of someone other than the analyst himself. Very often the person responsible for tissue collection is a busy pathologist who may not be fully aware of the hazards of metal contamination in relation to trace element analysis. However, despite the inherent dangers of this situation, there is no evidence in the current WHO/IAEA programme that it has led so far to significant errors, except possibly for blood samples particularly when they are to be analysed for chromium.

The tissue samples are kept frozen until ready for analysis, when they are allowed to thaw and are cut and handled in a glove box or laminar flow hood, using plastic forceps and titanium knives. The working surface is a clean plastic sheet or a thoroughly clean Petri dish which has been cleaned by rinsing in dilute nitric acid and demineralized water. In cases where doubts can be raised as to metal contamination at collection, the outer surfaces of the tissue specimen are removed with a plastic or a titanium knife. Of course care should be taken that the sample is not pierced with a metal tool. Samples are then freeze-dried, preferably in the irradiation container if activation analysis is used as the analytical method.

Hair

The method of choice for cleaning hair is a Soxhlet extraction of each sample with diethyl ether for two hours. This procedure removes the natural greases from the outside of the hair, but unlike other types of washing, (e.g. water, acetone, ethylalcohol or detergents) it has little effect on the major and minor elements of the hair itself.

Toenails

A washing solution comprising 90 parts of absolute ethylalcohol and 10 parts of 30 per cent H_2O_2 (in water) is used. The sample is placed in a 150 ml Ehrlenmeyer flask and washed three times with 30 ml each time of the washing solution. Each such washing step lasts two minutes with gentle shaking and is followed by decanting of the washing solution. Finally, the sample is tipped into a Hirch funnel or other suitable filtration device (e.g. a carefully cleaned plastic funnel with a ball of quartz wool pushed into the stem) and washed with 10-20 ml diethyl ether. The clippings are then removed with plastic forceps and dried in a suitably cleaned container for about 10 minutes at 60-70°C. In the case of toenails or finger nails where dirt is deeply ingrained (for instance, when collected from primitive population groups, walking barefoot), a special cleaning procedure which ensures complete cleanliness of the samples but without leaching of trace elements is carried out as follows. The samples are individually held with hard plastic forceps and are buffed using a tungsten carbide bit attached to a high speed rotary buffing tool. These samples are then individually washed for two minutes in an ultrasonic cleaner in a small test tube containing approximately 5 ml of 3 percent analytical grade hydrogen peroxide in absolute alcohol. This provides vigorous surface agitation and cleaning of the sample. The samples are then placed in polyethylene vials which had been previously cleaned by washing with dilute nitric acid and demineralized water.

Analysis

There is no single ideal method of analysis for all elements and tissues and the choice of method therefore has to be made on an element-by-element basis according to such considerations as sensitivity, matrix effects, cost, etc. In the present programme extensive use has been made of neutron activation analysis which has a number of attractive features including the fact that up to 25 or 30 elements can be analysed concurrently, some by non-destructive means which permit re-utilization of the same sample. However, other methods have also been used, particularly atomic absorption spectrophotometry, and indeed the use of several methods is to be recommended as an analytical quality control aid. The IAEA is at present engaged in a comparison of different trace analysis techniques and plans to provide some guidance on the selection of optimal methods for the assay of trace elements in biological materials. An Advisory Group meeting on this subject has recently been held in Vienna.

Quality Control

This is an essential part of the analytical procedures. The WHO/IAEA collaborating analysts follow the quality control procedures developed by a group of consultants. These involve the periodic analysis of standard reference materials and intercomparison samples of various kinds and also require that duplicate analyses be reported, if possible, from each tissue specimen together with details of all sources of analytical error known to the analyst. Further information about the methods used is available from IAEA on request.

4. Programme Design

Bio-Statistics

A most important problem is how many samples have to be collected in order to obtain a statistically significant meaningful result. According to a WHO/IAEA group of experts, in the very favourable situation where the experimental and control populations are of the same size and the standard deviation (SD) of the quantity being measured is the same in both populations, then the minimum population size needed to confirm the validity of a specified difference between the means of the two populations is as follows:

Minimum Difference to be Detected	Population Required
0.5 SD	32
0.2 SD	192
0.1 SD	768

These figures allow a 5 percent probability of the specified minimum difference occurring by chance. If the experimental and control populations are not of the same size, or are not comparable in other ways, or if the standard deviations of the two populations are not closely similar and if the two distributions or their logarithmic transforms are not normal, then the number of observations needed is larger. A difference that is not significant at the 5 percent probability level (meaning that the observed difference is likely to occur once in 20 times by chance) is, in practical terms, seldom worth using as a basis for decisions.

Data Evaluation Methods

Many trace elements are reported on the assumption that trace element concentrations in tissues conform to normal (Gaussian) distribution. This is a valid approximation for many elements particularly for some of the essential ones, but for many others the distribution is heavily skewed and therefore other more appropriate statistical methods should be applied. For instance, a logarithmic transformation is often useful and of course would lead to the determination of geometric means rather than arithmetic means. Medians rather than means can be used also. There are several methods for testing for distribution and the one commonly used in the WHO/IAEA trace element programme is the determination of the coefficient of variation (i.e. the ratio of standard variation to the mean). If this coefficient is greater than 0.12 the conventional tests based on the normal distribution are not valid. However, it is doubtful whether any but the simplest tests are relevant in the present stage of trace element studies. It must be remembered that statistics tell us about the properties of numbers — not about people, diseases or environmental problems. In view of the inevitable and often substantial errors due to sampling procedures, contamination, analytical variability, and biological variability, the mathematical models that we can make from trace element data seldom justify refined statistical analysis.

If the data are not distributed normally or lognormally (and indeed even if they are) it is advisable to use one of the distribution-free tests of significance such as Wilcoxon's sum of ranks test. It should be remembered that the widely popular student t-test and chi^2 test are valid only for normally distributed data.

Expression of Analytical Results

The concentrations of the elements should be expressed relative to both dry and wet sample weight, according to a standard format together with information on the precision of the analytical method used. A sample of data reporting format used in the WHO/IAEA programme is attached (Annex 4).

The results should be summarized in the following form:

1. Number of samples.
2. Results of tests for normal and lognormal distribution.
3. If the distribution is normal, lowest and highest values, arithmetic mean, standard deviation and median, should be given.
4. If the distribution is lognormal, lowest and highest values, geometric mean, logarithmic standard deviation, and median, should instead be given.
5. Results of tests for significance of difference between results from test and control populations.

5. **Organizational Aspects**

Existing Programme

The existing WHO/IAEA programme on Trace Elements in relation to Cardiovascular Diseases includes:

1. Central coordination of specimen collection, as well as of clinical, pathological, epidemiological data collection and evaluation of these data, including statistical and computer services, and staff, at WHO.
2. Central coordination of analytical procedures, including distribution of standard reference material, sample collection kits, titanium knives, etc.; quality control programmes, evaluation of analytical results including statistical and computer services and staff at IAEA.
3. In the case of Cd in hypertension, a well-established laboratory already active in this field (Hypertension Division, Washington University Medical School, St Louis, Missouri, USA) was designated as a WHO reference centre to: provide thermo-insulated shipping containers to all WHO collaborating pathologists in the programme; receive all tissue samples collected in various countries and shipped to the centre by air freight; check for accuracy of pathological findings and diagnoses; analyse samples for Cd.
4. A network of WHO collaborating pathologists in many countries: Hong Kong, Bulgaria, Czechoslovakia, Denmark, Greece, Israel, Singapore, Nigeria, Philippines, Sweden, Switzerland, USA, who have been collecting samples for several years in the present programme in a standardized way.
5. A network of IAEA collaborating analysts in several of the countries mentioned above, and in others as well.

Although the present WHO/IAEA programme is geared to the study of cardiovascular diseases, the services of many of the collaborating centres for sample collection and analysis could, in principle, be also used in the tissue banking exercise, if deemed necessary and if an appropriate organizational structure is set up for this purpose.

Centralized vs. decentralized approach

This depends on the scope of the programme (national or international), on the existing facilities, and on the kind of budget allocated. The present WHO/IAEA programme is decentralized, i.e. samples are collected in different countries and (except in the Cd-hypertension study) are analysed in different laboratories. There is, however, central coordination of both aspects of the programme. If the scope of the tissue banking exercise is limited to a local scale, then the central approach may be suitable, but if it is on a large international scale it might perhaps be advisable, in terms of simpler logistics, that analyses be done in the country of collection. This approach would only require a central organization to coordinate a quality control programme and a global evaluation of results. Budget, staff, laboratories and other pre-existing resources would therefore be distributed in manageable amounts between various collaborating national agencies.

In any case, besides the administrative and policy-making coordinating institution(s), it is essential that at least two technical reference centres be established, one to supervise tissue collection procedures and the other to supervise the analytical procedures. Depending on the scope of the programme, there could be national and/or international reference centres.

6.   Ethical and Legal Considerations

These are dealt with by the collaborating pathologists, who perform autopsies in accordance with the laws of the country. Problems have arisen, however, in connection with the collection of 'control' cases, which being usually cases of accidental death often are under the jurisdiction of the department of forensic medicine rather than of the pathology department. In certain countries, the pathologists collaborating with WHO in the present programme have no access to forensic cases. Under these conditions, therefore, collaboration with that particular centre had to be dropped.

Obtaining ante-mortem and post-mortem information, as well as shipment of frozen autopsy samples from one country to another using a regular airline company has never met with any problem. Nor was the WHO emblem on the containers ever needed to justify such shipments.

7.   Cost Estimates

The present WHO/IAEA programme on trace elements in cardiovascular diseases is supported only by a token amount of money that is given in the form of a technical contract to a few of the collaborating investigators, mostly to help them cover a small part of the expenses that they incur due to the additional workload caused by their collaborating in this programme. Many centres collaborate on a cost-free basis.

Of course, all collaborating investigators are senior, well-established scientists who work in laboratories where this type of research, i.e. autopsy collection and/or trace element analysis is already going on. The investigators collaborate on a scientific basis. They are an integral part of the programme, meet periodically in workshops organized by WHO and/or IAEA, and are the co-authors of WHO/IAEA reports and of other publications on this subject. Due to national and temporal monetary fluctuations a breakdown of the cost has to be worked out specifically, at the time when the tissue banking exercise is about to start, in the country or countries where the collection and analyses will be done, and depending on which elements are analysed and by which method.

Several years ago, prior to the launching of the present WHO/IAEA programme, IAEA circulated a questionnaire to a great many nuclear research centres around the world, asking which elements they could analyse and at what cost, and also whether they were interested in collaborating in this study. The report of this approach is now too old to be of use in the context of the present tissue banking plans, but it is an example of what should be done at the outset of the programme.

The present real cost of such analyses, including all direct and indirect expenses of the laboratory, is difficult to estimate. It depends, of course, on the element under consideration since some elements are easy to determine purely by instrumental means whereas others may require complicated chemical processing. In rough terms the costs probably range between U.S.\$ 5 and U.S.\$ 100 per element per sample.

WHO/IAEA code no. for this collaborating institution is: . . . .
Please write this code no. on all autopsy data sheets and on the sample containers that will be sent to you by WHO.

WHO/IAEA JOINT RESEARCH PROGRAMME ON TRACE ELEMENTS IN CARDIOVASCULAR DISEASES (AUTOPSY STUDIES)

Protocol No. 1
A study of trace elements in human tissues in relation to ischaemic heart disease
Completion time: 1 year

SUBJECTS
— Age: 45-64 years
— Sex: Male
— Cause of death: Ischaemic heart disease (ICD 1955: 420-422 or ICD 1965: 410-414)
— Controls: who died of accidental death but were otherwise free from disease.
— Number of subjects: 20 cases and 20 controls.
— DO NOT consider subjects who: — died following a contagious disease
— are known to have been significantly exposed to heavy metals because of their occupation (e.g. metal industry, welding, mechanics, painters, electro-plating etc.).
— are known to have been treated for therapeutic purposes with drugs containing heavy metals.

TISSUES (about 20 g specimens)
— Heart: sample from the **anterior wall of left ventricle** regardless of whether or not hypertrophied. In case of myocardial infarction do not collect the infarcted area but only the adjacent, non-infarcted, healthy area even if, in this case, the sample is smaller than 20 g.

— Liver: sample from **superior, anterior surface of right lobe** after removal of capsule.

— Kidney: sample from **cortex of lower pole of left kidney.** Avoid medulla and cortico-medullary junction.

— Hair (head): a lock of hair from the occipital region.
— Toenails: clippings as wide as possible from right and left large toes.
DO NOT COLLECT: kidneys or liver if they look severely diseased or damaged. Areas which contain gross localized lesions or other evident inhomogeneities. In diseased hearts it is the normal tissue area rather than the pathological area which is of interest.

Recommendations:
Avoid contamination by using plastic gloves, clean cutting instruments. Except for the cutting surfaces, do not pierce through the collected portion with a metal instrument. Do not wash the portion with water. Do not use fixatives.

Storage of specimens:
Immediately after collection each sample must be put in a plastic vial (supplied by WHO), closed tightly, identified and frozen at less than -15°C. (Hair and toenails need not be frozen). Keep frozen all the time until analysis.

Identification:
Each bottle should be identified by the autopsy number followed by the letter H (heart), L (liver), KC (kidney cortex), TN (toenails) or HR (hair) as appropriate. Non-smearing ink or a marker should be used. Make sure that the label is well glued onto the bottle, and protect it with scotch tape and an elastic band to prevent the label from becoming loose.

Shipment of Samples:
After a suitable number of samples have been collected (e.g. from at least five autopsies), they should be sent to the appropriate analytical centre. Dry samples (hair and toenails) may be shipped in a simple cardboard box without any special packaging. Frozen samples may be shipped as follows: the vials should be placed in a cardboard box or other suitable container and surrounded by at least an equal volume of dry ice. This box should then be wrapped loosely with paper and then packaged and despatched to the analytical laboratory without delay, by air freight. It is essential that the analytical laboratory be informed in advance by cable of the flight number, airway bill number and scheduled time of arrival. The specimens must arrive at the analytical centre still in a frozen state, otherwise they will be discarded.

Autopsy information:
The autopsy data sheets supplied by WHO should be completed — one copy should be sent to the analytical laboratory, one copy to Dr. R. Masironi, Cardiovascular Diseases, World Health Organization, 1211 Geneva 27, Switzerland, and one copy should be kept by the collecting pathologist for reference.

WHO/IAEA JOINT RESEARCH PROGRAMME ON TRACE ELEMENTS
IN RELATION TO CARDIOVASCULAR DISEASES

A) List of Drugs containing Cadmium, Chromium, Copper, Selenium and Zinc*

Element	Symbol	Names of drugs	Chemical formula	Names of proprietary preparations	Main uses
Cadmium	Cd	Cadmium Sulphide	CdS	Capsebon	Dermatology
Chromium	Cr	Chromium trioxide or chromic acid, or chromic anhydride	CrO_3		Dermatology
		Chromium oxide or dichromium trioxide, or chromium sesquioxide	Cr_2O_3	Chromium Sandoz	Marker for fecal output determinations in metabolic studies
		Cr-51 (as sodium chromate)			Radioisotope studies in haematology, kidney and spleen function tests
Copper	Cu	Copper sulphate or cupric sulphate	$CuSO_4 5H_2O$		Dermatology, emetic, astringent
		Cu-Zn sulphate (e.g. Dalibour cream, Sweitzer solution)			Dermatology
		Copper citrate	$C_6H_4CuO_7.2H_2O$		Dermatology
		Copper acetate	$(C_2H_3O_2)_2Cu.H_2O$		Dermatology
		Cu-64) Cu-67) As $CuCl_2$			Study of Cu metabolism and liver diseases
Selenium	Se	Selenium sulphide or disulphide	SeS_2	Lenium, Selsun, Selenol	Dermatology
		Selenium-75 (as seleno-methionine)			Radioisotope scanning tumour localization
Zinc	Zn	Zinc acetate	$(CH_3CO_2)_2Zn.2H_2O$		Emetic, eye drops
		Zinc chloride	$ZnCl_2$		Astringent, dental cement, deodorant
		Zinc sulphate	$ZnSo_4.7H_2O$	Vasozinc, zincaps, zincfrin, zincomed	Astringent, in wound healing, eye drops, mouth wash
		Zinc carbonate	$ZnCO_3$		Astringent, in dermatology
		Zinc oxide	$Zn\,O$	Calaband, Celbar, Coltapaste Eczema Cerate, Ichtopaste, Ichtaband, Noratex, Pharmakon, Quinaband, Septex cream, Tarsand, Thovaline, Uraband, Viscopaste, Zincaband	Dermatology, in creams, bandages, ointments, lotions, etc.

Element	Symbol	Names of drugs	Chemical formula	Names of proprietary preparations	Main uses
Zinc	Zn	Zinc Morrhuate Ointment (zinc oxide & cod liver oil)		Morhulin, Ung. Morrhuae Co.	Dermatology
		Zinc peroxide	ZnO_2		Disinfectant, in dermatology, wound healing
		Zinc-Bacitracin			Antibiotic
		Zinc pyrithione, Zn-pyridinethione, Zn-2-pyridinethiol-1-oxide, ZnPT, Zn bis (pyridine-2-thiol-1-oxide).	$C_{10}H_8N_2O_2S_2Zn$	Zinc Omadine Vancide ZP	As disinfectant in dermatology
		Zinc oleate	$C_{36}H_{66}O_4Zn$		Dermatology
		Zinc Stearate	$C_{36}H_{70}O_4Zn$		Dermatology
		Zinc permanganate	$Zn(MnO_4)_2.6H_2O$		Disinfectant
		Zinc propionate	$(C_3H_5O_2)_2Zn$		Antifungal in dermatology
		Zinc undecenoate or undecylenate or unde-10-enoate	$(C_{11}H_{19}O_2)_2Zn$	Mycota cream or powder, Tineafax ointment or powder.	Antifungal in dermatology

*   Taken from: Martindale — The Extra Pharmacopoeia 26th Ed. 1972.

This list does not purport to be a complete one. It is only intended as a guideline to investigators collaborating in WHO/IAEA research programme in trace elements and cardiovascular diseases.

B) List of metal-chelating agents *

Name	Formula	Synonyms	Proprietary names	Main uses in:
Acetylpenicillamine				mercury poisoning
Calcium trisodium pentetate	$C_{14}H_{18}CaN_3Na_3O_{10}$	Calcium trisodium pentahmil, Ca DTPA, calcium trisodium diethylenetriaminepentoacetic acid	Calcium Chel. 330	poisoning from lead and other heavy metals. In haemochromatosis and haemosiderosis
Desferrioxamine mesylate	$C_{25}H_{48}H_6O_8 \cdot CH_3SO_3H$	Desferrioxamine methanesulphonate; Ba-33112; DFOM mesylate; DFM mesylate; Deferoxamine mesylate; Desferrioxamine B mesylate	Desferal	iron poisoning, haemochromatosis
Dimercaprol	$C_3H_8OS_2$	Dimercap; Cimercaprolum; BAL; British Anti-Lewsite; Dimercaptopropanol	Dimercaprol (BAL)	poisoning by heavy metals having affinity for -SH groups
Diphenylthiocarbazone	$C_{13}H_{12}N_4S$	Dithizone		thallium poisoning
Disodium edetate	$C_{10}H_{14}N_2Na_2O_8 \cdot 2H_2O$	Sodium edetate Disodium dihydrogen edetate; Disodium edathamil Disodium tetracemate Tetracemindinatrium	Sequestrene NA_2 Sequestrene NA_3 Sodium Versenate Endrate Disodium	hypercalcemia, cardiac arrhythmias and peripheral vascular disorders, arteriosclerosis, diabetes, lead poisoning, ophthalmology
Edetic acid	$C_{10}H_{16}N_2O_8$	EDTA, EDTAA, Edathamil	Versene acid	same as above
Penicillamine	$C_5H_{11}NO_2S$	D-3-mercaptovaline	Cuprimine Distamine Cuprenil D-Penamine	hepatolenticular degeneration, lead poisoning, mercury poisoning, haemosiderosis, cystinuria, rheumatoid arthritis
Sodium-Calcium edetate	$C_{10}H_{12}CaN_2Na_2O_8 \cdot 2H_2O$	Natrii Calcii Edetas, Calcium disodium edathamil, Calcium disodium edetate, Calcium disodium ethylenediaminotetraacetate, Calcium EDTA	Calcium disodium versenate; Sequestrene Na_2Ca; Versene-Ca	poisoning by heavy metals, diabetes, porphyria
Sodium phytate	$C_6H_9Na_9O_{24}P_6$			hypercalcaemia, hypercalciuria
Unithiol	$C_3H_7NaO_3S_3H_2O$			poisoning by heavy metals

*   Taken from: Martindale – The Extra Pharmacopoeia 26th Ed. 1972
This list does not purport to be a complete one. It is only intended as a guideline to investigators collaborating in WHO/IAEA research programme in trace elements and cardiovascular diseases.

Project 1

Autopsy Data for WHO/IAEA Studies on Trace Elements in Heart Diseases

(describe, and tick appropriate boxes; where information is not available, write: N.A.)

Centre Code No. _______; Autopsy No. _______ and Date _______; Hours from death to autopsy_______;
Was body refrigerated? Yes ☐ No ☐; Name _____________________________; Age _______; Sex _______;
Weight (kg) _______; Height (cm) _______; Race _____________________; City of birth _____________;
Occupation _____________________; Accidental death? Yes ☐ No ☐;
If "No", was death sudden and unexpected? Yes ☐ No ☐;
Major pathol. diagnoses (underline what you consider to be immediate cause of death):

____

____

____

Myocardial infarction: acute ☐ old ☐ both ☐ none ☐; Histological observations in submitted specimens (tick first column if samples were sent to analyst; write S, M, or MK in 2nd column if vascular congestion was slight, moderate, or marked)

		Vasc. cong.	Major microscopic abnormalities, if any
Liver			
Heart			
Kidney cortex			
Kidney medulla			

Remarks on pathol. aspects (autolysis, others) _______________________________________

____

Weight of liver (g) _________; Weight of heart (g) _________; Weight of both kidneys (g) _________;
Coronary atherosclerosis (write grade of most severe lesions in each coronary according to scheme in WHO protocol):

Right _______; Left circumfl. _______; Ant. descend. _______; Post. descend. _______;
Aortic atherosclerosis: Grade _________________ (according to photographs in your possession);
Remarks on coronary and aortic atherosclerosis _______________________________________

____

Clinical findings: Diabetes?   Yes ☐   No ☐   Unknown ☐
                     Insulin required?   ☐   ☐   ☐
                     Hypertension (above 160/95)?   ☐   ☐   ☐
If female, was she on oral contraceptives?   ☐   ☐   ☐
Were drugs used which contain heavy metals? (see WHO list)   ☐   ☐   ☐
If above is "Yes", name(s) of drug(s) _______________________________________

Remarks on clinical findings ____

____

Smoking habits: unknown ☐; non-smoker ☐; more than 20 cigarettes/day ☐; 5-20/day ☐;
less the 5/day ☐; approx. No. of years smoking _______; pipe or cigars only ☐;
Were the following samples sent to analyst (tick if Yes): Hair ☐; Toenails ☐

Signature of responsible officer _______________________________________

GRADING OF AORTIC ATHEROSCLEROSIS

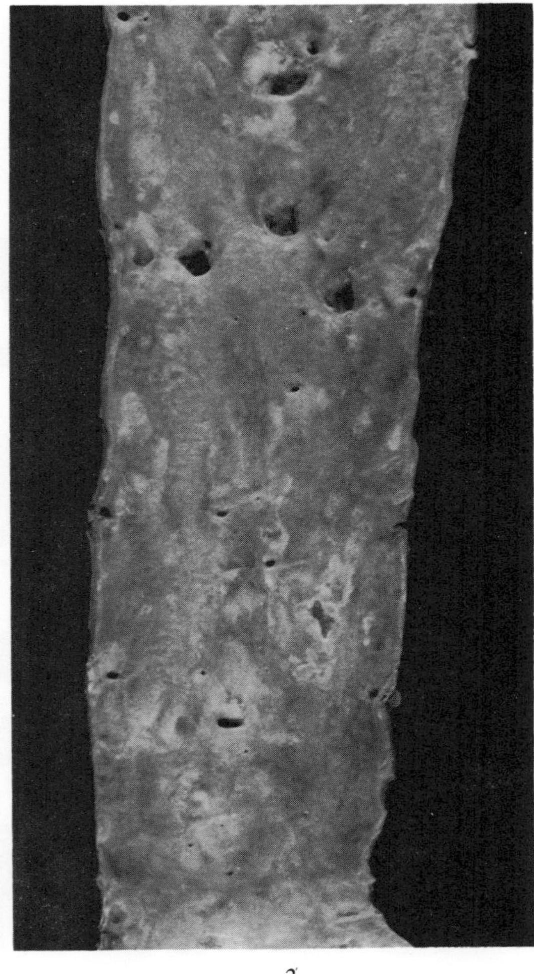

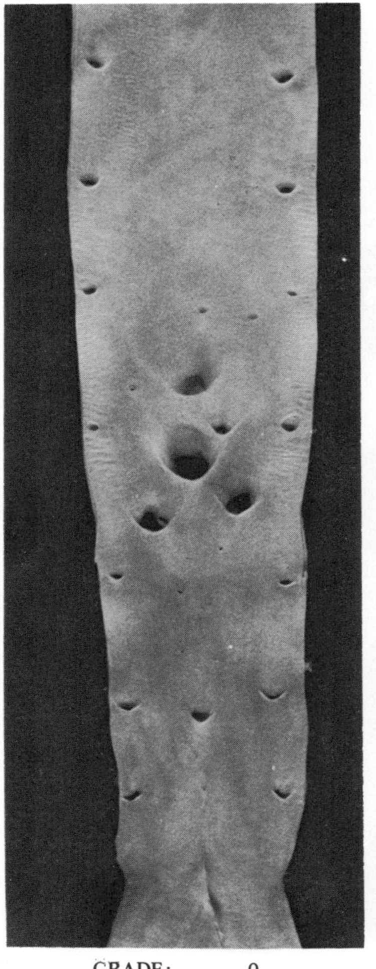

GRADE: 0   2   4

(none)   (moderate)   (severe)

GRADING OF CORONARY ARTERY STENOSIS
(based on maximum cross sectional involvement)

**GRADE N.B.: GRADES 0 AND 6 ARE AT REFERENCE POINTS
GRADES 1 TO 5 ARE BETWEEN REFERENCE POINTS**

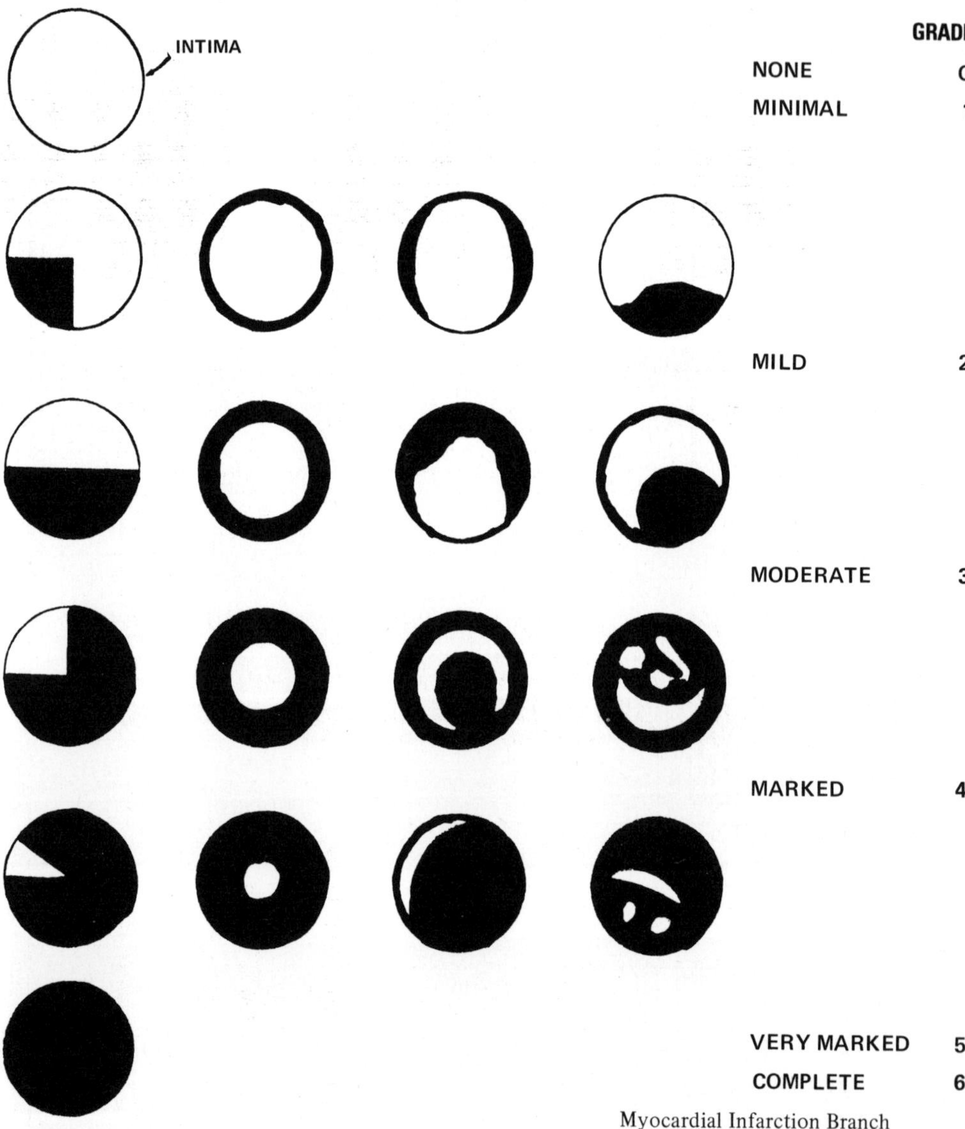

Myocardial Infarction Branch
National Heart and Lung Institute
Richard R. Liberthson, M.D.

REPORT OF ANALYSIS

WHO/IAEA JOINT RESEARCH PROGRAMME ON TRACE ELEMENTS IN CARDIOVASCULAR DISEASES

Report submitted by ___________________

Date ___________________

Analytical Lab. Code No.

Tissue				Sub-sample No.	Replicate No.	Weight of sub-sample	Wt. ratio (dry/wet)	Element	Method code	Chemical yield code No.		ERRORS		Concentration basis: 1 = wet wt; 2 = dry wt	
WHO/IAEA Code No.						1 = wet 2 = dry tissue	1 = same 2 = another 3 = total		Date of analysis	1 = measured; 2 = assumed; 3 = analysis without chemical separation				ANALYTICAL RESULTS	
of subject	Aliquot									Yield	SD	a priori	Counting statistics	Concentration	Overall SD
						(g)	(%)		Y M	(%)		SD (%)		(μg/g)	

Concentration basis columns show repeated "E" markers in the Concentration and Overall SD fields for each data row.

290

EXPLANATION OF REPORT OF ANALYSIS

Item	Example	Explanation
1	(cols 1,2) = 0 4	Analytical laboratory code no. 04
2* 2*	(cols 3,4) = 3 4 / H	Tissue: H = heart; H R = hair; K C = kidney cortex. K M = kidney medulla; L = liver; T N = toenails (see footnote)
3*	(cols 5,6,7,8,9) = 1 2 0 9 6	WHO/IAEA code No. of subject. A unique code No. for each subject studied. The first two columns (5 and 6) contain a unique specification of the project code No. (1) and of the collecting center (2). The following three columns contain the "running number" of the autopsy (see footnote).
4*	(col 10) = A	Aliquot (blank, A, B or C). (see footnote)
5	(cols 11,12) = 2	Sub-sample No. A number provided by the analyst to identify different sub-samples of the total sample for which he is reporting analytical results. Note: if part (or all) of the sample is homogenized prior to analysis all of this homogenized material is to be regarded as one sub-sample. Different aliquots of the same homogenized sub-sample are to be identified by an appropriate replicate No. (see item 6). Thus, all results for the same sub-sample should, with an ideal analytical procedure, be the same, whereas results for different sub-samples should differ to the extent that the element was inhomogeneously distributed in the sample.
6	(col 13) = 3	Replicate No. A number provided by the analyst to identify different analyses carried out on the same sub-samples (e.g. for different aliquots of homogenized material or for the same sub-sample if submitted to replicate non-destructive analysis).
7	(cols 14,15,16,17,18,19) = 0 1 2 3	Weight of the sample in grams. If the sample preparation procedure did not involve homogenization, report the actual weight of the sub-sample that was taken for analysis. Otherwise, report the total weight of material that was homogenized.
8	(col 20) = 1	A code No. to express whether the above weight (item 7) is on a wet or dry basis. (1 = wet tissue; 2 = dry tissue).
9	(cols 21,22,23,24) = 2 5 3	The ratio of dry to wet weight in percent.
10	(col 25) = 2	A code No. to express whether the above ratio (item 9) was determined by measurements on the same sub-sample, another sub-sample, or the total sample. (1 = same sub-sample, 2 = another sub-sample, 3 = total sample).
11	(cols 26,27) = Z N	Element (chemical symbol).
12	(col 28) = N	Method code. A = atomic absorption spectrophotometry; N = neutron activation analysis; F = flame photometry; E = emission spectroscopy (for other methods, leave blank but specify separately, e.g. on the back of the form).
13	(cols 29,30,31,32) = 7 4 0 1	Date of analysis (year/month).

* Items 2-4 together provide a unique specification of the sample. Normally these data (in the above example, H 2096 A) are provided by the pathologist and are written by him on the sample container. Further details can be obtained from Dr R. Parr at IAEA.

Item	Example

14

33
2

A code No. to express how the chemical yield was determined. 1 = chemical yield was measured on the same sub-sample; 2 = chemical yield was assumed from measurements on similar samples; 3 = analysis was made without chemical separation.

15

34	35	36	37	38
	8	7		6

The chemical yield expressed in percent. (If the chemical yield code No. (item 14) was 3, this field should be left blank).

16

39	40	41	42
	2		3

The standard deviation of the quantity expressed under item 15. Note: This SD normally cannot be measured directly. A reasonable estimate, based on the analyst's experience with similar samples, should therefore be quoted. (If the chemical yield code No. (Item 14) was 3, this field should be left blank).

17

43	44	45	46
	4		2

The a priori error of the analytical result expressed in terms of relative SD (o/o). For an explanation of the a priori error, see the attached Appendix.

18

47	48	49	50
	8	.	6

For activation analysis, the relative SD (o/o) arising from counting statistics. Note: for measurements near or below the limit of detection, this could have a high value. If, for this reason, there would be difficulty in reporting the value, the decimal point may be displaced or even eliminated on the report form.

e.g. write 102.6 as

1	0	3	.

or

1	0	3

19

51
1

A code No. to express whether the analytical results that follow (items 20 and 21) refer to the wet weight or the dry weight of tissue. (1 = wet weight; 2 = dry weight).

20

52	53	54	55	56	57	58
1		2	9	E	-	2

The concentration of the element in units of µg/g of wet or dry tissue (as indicated under item 19) after correction for all known systematic errors (e.g. the analytical blank). In this example the concentration is 0.0129 µg/g wet tissue. Please always quote 3 significant figures if possible. Note: for measurements at or near the limit of detection, please quote the actual value found even if this is negative. A negative number can be written as shown in the following sample:

write   - 0.0129 as

-	.	1	3	E	-	1

21

59	60	61	62	63	64	65
1		2	3	E	-	3

The overall SD of the concentration expressed in the same units as item 20. Note: items 17 and 18 added in quadrature represent the overall relative SD (o/o). It follows, therefore, that:

$$\text{item } 21 = \frac{\text{Item 20} \times \sqrt{(\text{Item 17})^2 + (\text{Item 18})^2}}{100}$$

A P P E N D I X

THE A PRIORI ERROR

A priori: based on reasoning from cause to effect; **before** analysis (as opposed to **a posteriori).**

The **a priori** error of a result is here defined as the sum in quadrature of the errors (each expressed in terms of relative SD) attributable to all sources of random variability in the measurement, except counting statistics. (The contribution of counting statistics, which is normally estimated **a posteriori**, is to be reported separately: see item 18 of the Report of Analysis).

Two features of the **a priori** error as thus defined are of note:

1. it accurately describes (after allowance for counting statistics) the degree of irreproducibility that would be found in measurements by this method of a long series of replicate samples ;

2. as a consequence of the way in which it is estimated (see below), it assists in the identification of the principal sources of the irreproducibility.

According to this definition of the **a priori** error, the investigator can never know its true value; he can only deduce and report an estimate of it. His estimate, however, serves three useful purposes, as follows:

1. It quantifies his understanding of the errors associated with his measurement in such a way that it can be tested, for example in this programme by Heydorn's quality control procedure based on the analysis of duplicate samples (see IAEA - 157, p. 186). If this estimate is found to be insufficiently accurate, he is stimulated to refine it.

2. Once the estimate is shown to be reasonably reliable, the investigator can proceed efficiently to improve the analytical technique so as to reduce the **a priori** error, if this is considered desirable (e.g. in this programme if the **a priori** error exceeds 10 o/o).

3. Provided that the estimate is shown to be reasonably reliable for a given set of measurements, the investigator is able to predict the degree of irreproducibility that would be observed in assaying another sample differing (within limits) from those he has previously analyzed (e.g. having a much lower concentration of the element in question, whereupon the variability of contamination would play a more prominent role).

The **a priori** error of each result is to be estimated by the investigator by examination in turn of each of the individual steps of the analytical procedure that yielded that result. The random variability that each of these contributes is to be evaluated, preferably on the basis of appropriate experimental measurements; these individual components of the **a priori** error (expressed in terms of relative SD) are then to be added in quadrature.

An example of this calculation, based on Table II, Report IAEA - 157, p. 182, is as follows:

	Source of error	**Component of a priori error**[1] $[\text{relative SD (o/o)}]$
A.	Elemental standard (e.g. dilution error)	0.2
B.	Sample contamination[2]	0.3
C.	Sample drying (when concentrations are expressed per unit of dry weight)	0.0 (for results on a wet weight basis)
D.	Weighing/pipetting errors	0.1
E.	Flux inhomogeneity in irradiation facility	4.2
F.	Self shielding in the standard[2]	0.0
G.	Interfering nuclear reactions[2]	0.0
H.	Chemical yield determination	1.9
I.	Impure photopeaks[2]	0.0
J.	Variations in counting geometry	0.8
K.	Instrumental errors (dead-time, etc.)	0.4
L.	γ-ray absorption in sample [2]	0.0
M.	Peak area determination	2.1
N.	Counting statistics (see IAEA-157, p. 187)	(Reported separately)

$$\text{A priori error} \quad (0.2^2 + 0.3^2 + 0.1^2 + 4.2^2 + 1.9^2 + 0.8^2 + 0.4^2 + 2.1^2)^{1/2}$$
$$5.2 \text{ o/o}$$

---

[1] The numbers quoted here are for illustrative purposes only.

[2] Normally a source of systematic error. The quantity to be listed under **a priori** error is not the systematic error itself but that random component of the systematic error that contributes to the irreproducibility of the analysis.

COMPUTER CODE FOR WHO/IAEA PROJECT No. 1 ON TRACE ELEMENTS IN CVD

Field		Columns
WHO/IAEA code		1 – 5
hours to postmortem		6 – 7
body refrigerated		8
age		9 – 10
sex		11
body wt	kg	12 – 13
height	cm	14 – 16
race		17
residence		18
occupation		19
type of death		20
cause of death		21
myocardial infarction		22
vascular congestion:		
liver		23
heart		24
KC		25
KM		26
weight of liver	gr	27 – 30
heart	gr	31 – 33
both kidneys	gr	34 – 36
grades of coronary atherosclerosis:		
right		37
left circumfl.		38
ant. desc.		39
post desc.		40
grade of aortic atherosclerosis		41
other major diseases:		
hypertension		42
cancer		43
diabetes		44
others		45
oral contraceptives		46
metal-containing drugs		47
smoker		48
years smoking		49 – 50

NB: blank = unknown

INSTRUCTIONS FOR USE OF CODE IN IAEA/WHO PROJECT No. 1

body refrigerated
1 = yes
2 = no

sex
1 = M
2 = F

race
1 = caucasoid;   2 = negroid;
3 = mongoloid;   4 = Filipino;   5 = Indian

residence
1 = native of country
2 = foreign, long-term resident
3 = foreign, recent resident

occupation
1 = significant metal exposure (industry, etc.)
2 = insignificant metal exposure (office, housewife, etc.)
3 = farmer
4 = retired
5 = unspecified "labourer" or other

type of death
1 = sudden and unexpected
2 = violent/accidental
3 = neither of these

cause of death
1 = ischaemic heart disease (410–414)
2 = other CVD
3 = non–CVD

myocardial infarction
1 = acute or recent
2 = old
3 = both
4 = none

vascular congestion
1 = S (slight);   2 = M (moderate);
3 = MK (marked)

other major diseases

hypertension	1 = yes	2 = no	
cancer	1 = yes	2 = no	
diabetes	1 = yes	2 = no	(3 = requiring insulin (4 = non requiring insulin
others	1 = yes	2 = no	

grades of coronary atherosclerosis   1 to 6

grades of aortic atherosclerosis   1 to 5

smoker
1 = non-smoking   2 = pipe/cigar only
3 = < 5 cigarettes/day
4 = 5–20/day
5 => 20/day

oral contraceptives
1 = yes   2 = no

metal-containing drugs
1 = yes   2 = no

SPECIFIC WORKING PAPER ON PESTICIDES

B. R. Ordoñez
Secretariat of Public Health and Welfare, Mexico

Summary

Pesticides, both chlorinated and phosphated organic compounds have great use in many countries. Organochlorinated pesticides are accumulated in the human body, basically in the adipose tissue, making biological monitoring programs necessary.

Many environmental contaminants surveys in blood and other tissues have been done. In the world, there are more than forty studies of pesticides in human milk already published.

Availability of human samples is not a problem in Latin America, but shipment and storage are problematic since the milk needs to be frozen. Usually there are adequate laboratory facilities for the analysis of the samples — but technical advice is needed.

The lack of representativity of the total sample collected is one of the main problems for this type of survey. The main variables are described as well as suggestions for storage of data collected from each sample donor.

The organizational aspects are discussed, in particular the problems associated with biological monitoring of pesticides in rural areas of Latin America.

Centralization of all samples for analysis, storage and data control look more practical for Latin America.

Legal regulations are, in general, less restrictive in developing countries for living human samples, but more for post-mortem specimens.

Costs for laboratory analysis are higher, compared to those of developed countries, but lower for the collection of samples. One sample collected for future reference would cost, in Mexico, U.S. $40.65 to $45.45 and $159.65 to $164.45 for Biological Monitoring including design, collection, analysis, etc.

a). Review of past and current programs

In Mexico, as in almost all the countries, especially those in Latin America, few programmes exist on biological monitoring and collection of samples for further reference, concerning pesticides.

Furthermore, it is not unusual to underestimate the studies on human tissues, giving more emphasis to the establishment of monitoring systems in the environment; systems that, on one hand, are very expensive, generally incomplete since some pollutant sources escape their surveys and, on the other hand, the collected data does not always represent what is really accumulated in the human body, because not everything found in the environment enters the human organism.

Even for a poor country, with all its limitations, a biological monitoring program is economically feasible at present as well as for the collection of future references.

Programs that could be considered of some validity, that have been effected in Latin America, concerning pesticides in human samples are those of human maternal milk done in Guatemala, a survey of approximately 40 samples, and the other in Mexico City, where a statistically valid sampling, representative of the population was taken.

b. Rationale for interest or concern

Pesticides, both chlorinated and phosphated organic compounds, as is well known, have great use in agriculture, primarily on prosperous zones or on fields of major yield. The effectiveness of pesticides in agricultural practices makes them irreplaceable.

World-wide, the greatest use of pesticides is for cotton. Particularly, of the 27,000 tons of pesticides being used annually in Mexico, 80 percent are destined for cotton crops.

Pesticides are also used on other crops such as tobacco, garden produce, rice, wheat, sorghum, sugar cane, fruits, and, to a lesser extent, on corn.

Public Health programs utilize DDT sprays in fighting malaria vectors and in smaller quantities, malathion. There is also use of pesticides in animal sanitation programs.

Relative to the tonnage used of each pesticide, the most widely used are parathion, DDT, toxophene, malathion and sevin, the former two products are imported to this country. About 20 pesticides are manufactured in Mexico; of those, DDT is exported to 14 countries, and toxophene to Central America and Colombia.

The pesticides can enter the human body through the skin, by inhalation or by absorption by the digestive tract.   Mexico, as other Latin American countries, has had accidents of acute intoxication, especially with chlorinated and phosphated organic pesticides, either because of ignorance or carelessness of those who handle them.   The damage to the nervous system by the former is the most relevant, since they do not accumulate in the tissues; on the contrary, the most important factor of the organochlorinated pesticides is their capacity to accumulate, basically in the adipose tissue.

The significance of the accumulative effects of chlorinated pesticides is still vague and under investigation.

In Latin America, the magnitude of the accumulation of chlorinated pesticides in human tissue is unknown; thus the necessity for systematic and valid studies using human samples is evident.

c. **Consideration for human sample selection, collection, containment, shipment and storage**

Studies have been made, particularly for organochlorinated pesticides in blood and human milk samples.   A review of the international scientific literature shows that more than forty studies have been done on the latter.   In Mexico, a study was conducted where six hundred milk samples of the same number of women were taken.   This represents a significant sample of the universe of the overall population in the Federal District, the country's capital.

In general, one could say that there would be little problem in obtaining any kind of human sample from the Latin American population.   The majority of the rural and urban population accept to give blood, secreta or excreta samples, if adequately sensibilized; on the other hand, it is difficult to take biopsies or post-mortem specimens.

The study of the human maternal milk is particularly effective in Latin America.   Besides the previously mentioned fact that the population would accept to donate samples, there is still a great proportion of women who still follow the practice of maternal lactation or natural baby-feeding; furthermore, the high birth rates allow for relatively large universes.

For the sample collection of the human milk, there is no need for special conditions, nor for complicated techniques, since the squeezing by the mother is the most adequate.

It is preferable to use glass flasks sufficiently big (50 ml) that these not be reused for the same study and that these be washed with special detergents, rinsed with running water and distilled water.   The glass bottles are also washed with hexane and sealed with a teflon lined cap, treated similarly as the flasks, to ensure a leakless seal and to prevent or minimize external contamination that could affect the results of the analysis.

The collected human milk samples are not treated with a chemical preservative, but are immediately stored in a portable cooler that can reach freezing temperatures, if need be, in case of delayed deliveries, or just cooled above its freezing point, if the sample will be delivered to the laboratory freezer within two hours after its collection.

The bags containing an appropriate coolant and placed inside the cooler give good results, are economical and have adequate cooling capacity when transportation distances are short and of little delays; they can even partially freeze the milk sample.   Dry ice is very useful for this purpose but it is not easy to get in Latin America, except in the bigger urban centers.

Besides the lack of dry ice, in many rural places there is no electricity, and even having it, freezers are not accessible, thus immediate transportation from the collection point to the laboratory for its storage or analysis, usually by air, is necessary.   This type of problem is very often present in rural Latin America.

To be avoided is the repeated freezing and unfreezing of the same sample, either during transportation or in the laboratory.   For this reason we prefer that once the sample is collected in a flask of suitable size, to homogenize it manually and immediately pour half of its contents into another identical flask, properly labelled.   This avoids having to unfreeze all the sample in the laboratory if two portions of the same sample are required.   For example, one portion is used for the analysis while the other remains frozen for future investigations or as a split-sample for an interlaboratory quality assurance program.

Likewise, there are areas even within urban centers where occasionally electric power system failures or black-outs occur; these can last a few hours or even days.   For this reason many laboratories have their own auxiliary power plants.   However, this desired double electric system is not always found in the Latin American laboratories, thus necessitating keeping an aliquot of the sample in another laboratory that has adequate freezers, but sufficiently separated by distance so as not to be affected by the same problem.

When a black-out happens for a short while, generally the milk sample will not unfreeze. To ensure we become aware of black-outs, especially if these occur on non-working hours or days, we decided to place in a horizontal position a milk sample that had previously been frozen in a vertical position as a control that will indicate by a change in direction of the milk's previous vertical level, to what degree the sample unfroze and the relative importance of this change in our investigation.

To store samples which will be studied in the near or long future, it is preferable in Latin America to always use freezers that operate on a double electric system; the normal and the auxiliary. Even so, it is predictable to have a decrease with time of the pesticide content in maternal milk, thus it would be desirable to find an adequate preservative.

For the present, storage of samples that will be analysed in some future date by new analytical methods — as these become available, perhaps — can best be accomplished by taking an aliquot of the sample immediately after its collection and extract the fat from the milk, the pesticides from the fat and continue with the clean-up steps of the procedure. This, along with a second aliquot of the same milk sample, can be stored in appropriate containers and conserved under subfreezing temperature for future studies.

d.   Analytical Procedures

In collecting blood or maternal milk samples, it is advantageous to take them all at the same time or within a predetermined time frame and under the same conditions or at least noting important variables if such samples are for the same study, but under different conditions. For example, we know that pesticide levels in blood change before and after childbirth and that significant changes occur in maternal milk during some lactation periods. Therefore, while the sampling programs are being designed, the population can be stratified taking into account the 'time of lactation' variable or it can be done 'a posteriori' making sure this important variable is taken into consideration. A third alternative would be to take samples only during a predetermined lactation period.

It is very important for the analysis that the samples or aliquots of these be homogeneous, since the chlorinated pesticides are found in the milk's fat. The data could be distorted if only the portion with higher fat or vice-versa is taken for the analysis.

In analysis of organochlorinated pesticide residues, gas chromatography equipped with an electron capture detector is preferred over other instruments for the determinative step. It has the following advantages over other analytical techniques: a) excellent sensitivity, detection in the picogram (10^{-12} g) is common; b) there are less interferences; c) it gives good semi-qualitative results; d) its versatility, several pesticides can be determined at the same time; e) its speed; f) its ease of handling and many others.

We believe Giuffrida's Rapid Clean-up for Chlorinated Pesticide Residue in Fats and Oils procedure, as modified by the Pesticide Center in Colorado State University, to be the better overall method taking into consideration that it has been discussed, collaborated and evaluated for many years by many investigators.

For confirmation of pesticide residues mass-spectroscopy is often preferred but this analytical tool is not recommended for Latin America because of the high cost and the difficulty in obtaining parts and services; infra-red spectroscopy is often preferred for pesticide formulations but for residue work it lacks adequate sensitivity; thin layer chromatography is the method most widely used because of its low cost, accessibility and other advantages; gas chromatography by preparing chemical derivatives of the organochlorated compounds, etc.

Standards must always be used as references to quantitate the organochlorinated compounds present in the sample. There are several types, each having its own purpose; primary standards, reference standards and technical standards.

In Mexico and generally in Latin America, reference standards are not available, therefore, they must depend on other countries as their source, such as the EPA, that can send them primary and technical standards (99.2 and 90 percent pure, respectively), whose quantitation is based on reference standards. There is a quality control in laboratories where standards are prepared, based on reference standards and, of course, there should be an internal quality control in each laboratory where the samples are analysed, with the objective that the results be valid.

Among some of the precautions not stated on the label or accompanying literature that should be taken in the preparation of standards solutions are: to weigh the standards on accurate electro-balances; prepare standard solutions whose concentrations are slightly higher than those of the working standard and check if extraneous peaks occur by GLC or if secondary spots on TLC are visible; and make sure that the declared purity on the label is applied when calculating the concentrations.

Among some of the factors to take into account in the laboratory are: a) accuracy of the analytical balances; b) purity of reactants, such as solvents, distilled water, Na_2SO_4, nitrogen, etc.; c) cleanliness of glassware and equipment; d) condition of the GC and its accessories; e) recovery data obtained by different analysts of various pesticides, etc.

e.   Program Design

The lack of representativity of the total sample collected is one of the main problems for this type of study.   Generally they are implemented without a well-designed statistically valid sampling program, at times these are too small, on occasions taken from volunteers who are more accessible or less reluctant, but in any case, a generalization can not be made with such data collected.

In Mexico City, it was possible to study a representative sample, after a geographic survey by clusters was made of the existing housing.   A census was taken on 10,000 representative families in order to know the future childbirths of the adult feminine population.   Afterwards, during a period of 6 calendar months, each home having a recent birth between the ages of 22 to 60 days, was visited and a sample of the mother's milk taken.   Not only were the socio-economic variables such as age, address, occupation, etc. of these 600 mothers documented but also from another 200 women whose homes were also visited but no sample taken either because the child died or was born dead, or a change of residence had occurred,or because bottle feeding had been preferred or because the mother did not cooperate so that afterwards we could weigh and evaluate statistically any bias of the total sample taken.

For the moment, no study has been designed for the rest of the country until we can assure ourselves adequate transportation and proper storage of the milk samples; we must also make sure that the samples are representative of the total area since in Mexico as in other Latin American countries, it is not possible to study only that segment of the population that use the hospital system for childbirth because there is a large proportion of women who do not use these services.

Invariably three items are recorded on the outside of the sample flask: case number, person's name or initials to double check, and the collection date.   These are included in the collection report as well as other important variables for each case.   The following are never omitted: address, age, socio-economic level (by means of several parameters, depending on the population being surveyed), occupation, time of residence at present address, record of previous residences, etc.   Once the pesticide levels in maternal milk are known, an analysis of possible sources of exposure is preferred by taking a subsample of those having the higher and lower levels.   In these cases an epidemiological survey is made to learn the exact use of pesticides in each home then and in the past.

Such subsequent epidemiological surveys need to be done in practically all Latin America, since contamination levels are often unknown or there is little evidence of such levels of contamination in the environment.   There are even instances, when the source of contamination is not known.

This study is difficult to realize if all the people from whom samples were taken were to be surveyed; but we think that taking a subsample — the highest and lowest levels — is feasible in Latin America and adequate to determine the origins and degrees of exposure.

Through the exchange with other foreign institutions, it is possible to standardize the information collected between the nations in question, but it would be more convenient for all concerned if an international criterion is established for such standardization.

It could be possible to store the original data collection forms but physical space frequently limits this, thus customarily, data punch cards or magnetic tapes are preferred.   In all places, more so in Latin America, it is convenient to keep the data stored by different methods in different places.   For example, originals plus cards, or cards plus magnetic tapes, or microfilms of the forms plus any of the other three procedures.   This is suggested because at times, due to various reasons, information stored in one place could be damaged or partially lost if all were kept in only one center.

The key information for the interpretation of the stored data and the criteria used should also be safely stored.

f.   Organizational Aspects

Many of the contaminants that tend to accumulate are products of new technologies and their use is wider in urban centers than in the rural environment. This is important since the realization of biological monitoring or sample collection for future reference programs in the rural environment poses a great challenge because of the difficult conditions, if not in collecting the samples, then in the transportation and storage of such.

However, the pesticide problem is important in the rural environment: therefore it is there where such programs should be implemented.   On one side, the Latin American rural population is numerically very important; on the other side, these contaminants are handled in very large quantities in this environment.   Pesticides, due to their wide use in agriculture and the fact that on occasions these are applied by aerial spraying, are probably more important as far as exposure is concerned for the rural than for the urban population.   The latter is probably less exposed to pesticides because contact is less direct and comes mainly from foods, water and household items.

In collecting the samples, it is important to use personnel of the same community that knows the local customs and knows how to sensitize the population; however, it is almost always badly qualified, thus, careful training is necessary.

The preservation of the human milk samples at the site collected presents a problem since these require to be frozen almost immediately and sent directly to another place where they can be properly stored.

With respect to samples analysis, the question of centralization versus decentralization does not arise in Latin American countries because there is almost always just one or at most two laboratories that are highly qualified to do analysis on the contaminant or group of contaminants and in particular those previously mentioned.   Regional or local laboratories are not equipped and are poorly qualified for these purposes.   They serve as concentration points for temporary storage (if necessary) and for packing and sending the samples to the central laboratory, where the analyses will be performed.   In this way, it is easier to follow one criterion, and use the same methods for the analysis of the samples.   Of course, if one or two laboratories will be responsible for the total workload, this will require an adequate and precise planning of the program, a good sampling schedule that will not overload the capacity of the laboratory and an excellent sampling design that allows to take a minimum number of samples without losing the representativity of the universe being studied.

Our experience also indicates that the processes used to concentrate the information (forms), analysis and evaluation of the results, should be done in one site so that the data can be treated uniformly.   This is done by epidemiologists and statisticians outside the laboratory, since we try for the laboratory analysis and data treatment to be done in 'double blind' form, in order to avoid personal bias.

For this reason, Mexico has established a specialized group within the Technical Council of the Subsecretariat for the Improvement of the Environment and consists of epidemiologists and statisticians, whose responsibility is to plan programs that tend to measure the effects of environmental contaminants in public health.   This group also selects surveys, plans and designs them, coordinates activities with laboratory(s) selected as the best qualified for the specific analysis, designs sampling plans and collection reports for the data to be collected, collects the samples and the data necessary, sends the samples to the laboratory, concentrates results from laboratory analyses, tabulates all analytical data according to the variables observed and prepares the final report.

The laboratory is dedicated to the reception of the samples, its preparation and analysis and prepares a report on the analytical results.   The professional personnel and qualified technicians collaborate only as consultants in the planning and in the final analysis of the results. In this manner, the limited laboratory resources available in Latin America are more efficiently used, relieving them from other planning duties, sample collection and the statistical analysis of the results that can better be performed by expert epidemiologists and statisticians.   Furthermore this guarantees the 'double blind' concept affording the study more scientific validity.

With regard to external international coordination, our experience is wide, since we have always established such with at least one other country which has greater experience on the specific biological monitoring program to be developed.   In order for the survey to be comparable we have accepted general norms: for example, keep the same variables, use the same analytical methods, use similar statistical programs to analyse data, etc.   However, there are unique aspects for each country that should be planned accordingly and these would not be the same for all. For example, the sampling of women that go to hospitals could be adequate for a developed country, but not for a developing one, since a large proportion of childbirths is done by non-institutional personnel at home. A different method is applied to design the sampling program but it must guarantee that the sample is representative.

The external coordination which we have established is basically with the United States of Amaerica (Environmental Protection Agency, Colorado States University, Public Health Services, C.D.C. of Atlanta, Georgia, etc.), but not with all of them which have implemented similar surveys. For this reason we feel it is necessary to establish at an international level, general guidelines that will enable all concerned to recognize the problem so as to find the easiest solution.

To achieve this it will be necessary to establish at that international level: a) general rules on the sampling design; b) selection of the type of human samples and contaminant(s) more adequate for the study; c) general norms for the sample collection; d) general rules and systems for the sample storage; e) appropriate analytical methodology for the laboratory; f) important variables to be observed and documented in relation to the contaminants; g) statistical treatment of the variables and results of the contaminant levels in the human samples studied; and h) criteria for storage of information.

Furthermore, as experience has shown us, it seems advisable to keep aliquots, representative of the overall samples collected, according to international standards to be established, so that these be sent to one or more reference centers at an international level, to ensure the quality of the analytical results. Independent of the above, laboratories from participating countries must be assured of having the same standards, furnished by an international laboratory or agency.

g.   Ethical and Legal Considerations

In Mexico, as in the majority of the Latin American countries, there are no laws, or these are very general, which restrict the collection of samples from living people; however, there are some legal regulations, somewhat more restrictive, for collecting post-mortem samples, but these are not always applied. In some countries, a signed authorization from a relative is required for the latter studies, but this is not the case with living human samples. Practically any study can be done with samples given voluntarily, even if no explanation is given to the individual as to the purpose or nature of the investigation.

If properly conditioned, the people easily accept to have samples drawn from them, but in most Latin American countries people are much more reluctant to give authorization for post-mortem analysis.

In Mexico, as in a good part of Latin America, each investigator applies his own discretion as to what ethical consideration he will apply in obtaining samples from living human beings, including the confidentiality of personal information and the results of the analyses. Almost always documented are the full name and address of the person from whom the sample was obtained and frequently not only are the initials written on the sample container, but also the full name, as is the sample control number, so as to verify and cross-check with the laboratory reports, the variables of each case. It is not customary to divulge specific results of any person, nor do their names appear in any publication.

It is not a common practice to pay, cash or anything, to the person from whom a sample is taken.

In Mexico, as in most countries in Latin America, no restriction exists as to transportation of human samples from one state to another; nor is there any restriction to sending quality control split-samples to reference laboratories in a foreign country, if the receiving country has no such restrictions in accepting. On the other hand, to receive samples from another country it is necessary to inform and obtain approval from the Public Health Authorities.

h.   Cost Estimates

Costs for biological monitoring programs in Latin America, compared to those from a developed country, are higher for equipment, instruments, and consumable items including reactants, than for personnel. This is generally true since the equipment has to be imported as do most of the reactants, while personnel wages, especially in regard to the less qualified, are very low. For the same reason again compared to a more developed country, sample collection could be less expensive but laboratory analysis more expensive.

Compared to all other research programs on health effects from environmental contaminants in Mexico, this project was more economical because it was planned and designed by only one group dedicated ex-professo to these duties. This was not the case with the statistical analysis of the data since this same group had to incur computer costs which are generally very high in Latin America.

Following this discussion, in the table below, is a breakdown of estimated costs per sample, based on 600 samples, for mid-1976.

ESTIMATED COSTS PER SAMPLE FOR 'BIOLOGICAL MONITORING'**
AND 'COLLECTION FOR FUTURE REFERENCE'* IN U.S. DOLLARS
FOR ORGANOCHLORINE PESTICIDES IN HUMAN MILK (BASED ON 600 SAMPLES), FOR MID-1976

Activity	Personnel	Equipment	Consumable Material	Transportation	Others	Total
1. Previous census of the working universe	$8.00	--	$0.10	$1.00	--	$9.10
2. Program design	8.00	–	0.50	–	0.50	9.00
3. Collection and Transportation	20.00	--	(a) (b) 0.70 - 1.00	(a) (b) 0.50 - 5.00	0.10	(a) (b) 21.30 - 26.10
4. Storage	(c) 1.00	$0.25 (c)	--	--	–	$1.25
(1 to 4) Subtotal*	$37.00	$0.25 (c)	(a) (b) $1.30 $1.60	(a) (b) $1.50 $6.00	$0.60	(a) (b) $40.65 $45.45
5. Laboratory Analysis	$30.00	$20.00 (d)	$35.00	–	$1.00	$86.00
6. Data Statistical Analysis	16.00	. 16.00	1.00	–	–	33.00
TOTAL (1 to 6)**	$83.00	$36.25	(a) (b) $37.30 $37.60	(a) (b) $1.50 $6.00	$1.60	(a) (b) $159.65-$164.45

*	Subtotal (1 to 4) applicable for 'Collection for future reference'.
**	Total (1 to 6) applicable for 'Biological Monitoring'.
(a)	If the study is implemented in situ by the lab.
(b)	If the study is implemented far from the lab and requires special transportation (airplane).
(c)	For a period equal to or less than 6 months.
(d)	Does not include initial investment, only the depreciation of equipment.

BIOLOGICAL SPECIMEN COLLECTION FROM HUMAN POPULATIONS FOR BIOLOGICAL MONITORING AND FUTURE REFERENCE: ORGANIC HALOGENATED COMPOUNDS

B. Paccagnella and C. Favaretti
Institute of Hygiene, University of Padova, Verona

The most relevant past and current programmes dealing with biological monitoring on human populations about organic halogenated compounds, in Italy, concern chlorinated pesticides.

An epidemiological study of long-term effects of pesticides on human health (1) was carried out on two random samples representing two rural communities: in the first one (area A) pesticides were used in larger quantities than in the second one (area B). In both these areas the consumption of organochlorine compounds was 15% of all pesticides.

First a cross-sectional study was carried out, based on gas chromatographic identification and determination of organochlorine compounds in the environment and in the fatty tissues of subjects resident in the areas.

Samples of vegetables, fruits, animal fats, hay, soil, well-water and drinking water and raw and pasteurized milk were taken and examined. Samples of surface water were drawn from the Po river and from smaller rivers and canals of the Province of Ferrara; wild birds were captured in area A.

Heptachlor epoxide, Dieldrin, TDE, DDE, o-p'-DDT, p-p'-DDT, total DDT levels were determined.

Both the populations were studied in a prospective study by clinical and biochemical tests. The clinical assessment was made at 2-year intervals after 1965.

The cross-sectional study showed that environmental pollution by organochlorine compounds was a little higher in area A than in the control area B, but this difference was not significant.

The level of storage of these compounds in fat of the people of the two areas did not differ.

The prospective study showed consistently higher morbidity in the population of area A than in the control population. Because of difficulties in correlating the storage of organochlorine pesticides in fatty and non-fatty tissues with pathology (2), some differences in morbidity may be related to the greater use of carbamates and organophosphorous compounds in area A than in area B. It is to be noted that the organization of this trial was bound to bring about behavioural changes among those involved, and in this way it has an educational value. The behavioural changes occurred mainly amoung those who handled pesticides.

As a part of the epidemiological investigation we have cited, the storage of chlorinated hydrocarbon residues in human tissues, both fatty and non-fatty, was studied in Ferrara Province (3). The samples were taken from subjects of both sexes who had had no occupational exposure to pesticides and whose age ranged from 1 to 80 years. Pesticide residues were determined by gas chromatography with electron-capture detection.

Heptachlor epoxide was present in most samples of fat and liver but in only one spleen sample, and was not detected in kidney and brain samples. HEOD was found in many samples of autopsy fat, in fewer samples of liver and biopsy fat, and in one sample each of spleen and brain.

p-p'-DDE was always present in samples of fat and liver, very often in samples of spleen, and moderately frequently in kidney and brain samples.

p-p'-TDE was found only in one sample of spleen.

o-p'-DDT was found quite often in kidney samples but seldom in the other tissues: it was never found in autopsy fat and was very seldom found in biopsy fat. p-p'-DDT was found in almost all samples of fat, in many liver and kidney samples and in a few brain and spleen samples.

DDT and its metabolites were always present at higher levels than either heptachlor epoxide or HEOD, while HCH, HHDN and heptachlor were either absent, or present in concentrations below the sensitivity of the analytical method used.

In non-fatty tissues the average levels were always less than those in fatty tissues, and liver samples and, to a lesser degree, kidney samples, showed residual concentrations higher than in other organs (spleen and brain). From comparison of the results with those from other countries it appears that higher levels of chlorinated compounds were generally present in the Ferrara population.

A lot of investigations were carried out to determine organochlorine pesticide residues in the environment. Investigations were made on vegetable foods (5, 6, 4); on animal foods (7, 8, 9); and on both vegetable and animal foods (10, 11).

Some other surveys were made on surface waters (12, 13), and on sea water (14).

The effects of radiation on the organochlorine compound residues in the foods were studied (15).

All these investigations were made without an epidemiological approach and relationship with human monitoring.

Some other studies were made on the MNFA to identify metabolic and toxicological pathways of this pesticide (16) and its residues (17).

Some investigations were carried out on PVC and particularly on problems of the pharmaceutical applications (18, 19).

Occupational involvements of lungs from PVC dust were also studied (20).

A high prevalence of bronchitis symptoms, associated or not with a spirographic deficit was found in workers occupied in the production of PVC. Smoking habits did not seem to play an important role in these results (21).

About the public health aspects, the Ministry of Health provided several regulations concerning the production, the distribution and the use of pesticides.

The use of DDT and derivatives in agriculture was restricted and that of 2,4,5-T and 2,4,5-TP is forbidden since 1970.

Special Committees were appointed to fix the residue levels of pesticides in food, following the recommendations of FAO/WHO; to provide lists of pesticides whose use needs to be regulated; to approve and register new compounds and formulae.

Furthermore, the Ministry of Health stated that all cases of acute poisoning from pesticides must be reported to the Health Authorities.

About the metabolic, toxicological aspects and pathways, some information is provided by the international literature.

Among the organochlorine pesticides, DDT was studied more than the other compounds. Its derivatives are DDD and DDE, that are accumulated, like DDT, mainly in the fatty tissues of human beings and animals. DDA is another derivative that is eliminated by stools and urine.

Aldrin becomes Dieldrin in animal liver; Heptachlor becomes heptachlor-epoxide in plants, soil and animal tissues.

DDT, Dieldrin and Endrin are accumulated with the same rhythm independently from the absorption levels; heptachlor and heptachlor-epoxide are accumulated only when the absorption levels are relatively high.

Organochlorine compounds are accumulated in non-fatty tissues, too, like liver, kidneys, muscles and so on, but in small quantities (1, 3).

Signs of activity on the enzymatic system were found in animals.

Serum Alkaline phosphate increases in rats nourished by diets with endrin (22). Serum transaminases increases in animals nourished by diets with methoxichlor (23).

Several other relationships were found between organochlorine compounds and enzymatic systems: inhibition of cholinoacetylase by DDA (24); increasing of liver sytochrone by DDT (25); inhibition of muscular LDH by o-p'-DDT, p-p'-DDD and mainly by DDT (26); reduction on utilization of vitamin A and beta-karotine by DDT (27).

Furthermore, impairments by organochlorine compounds, mainly DDT, were found in liver (28) and suprarenal bodies with change of the metabolism of steroydes (29, 30).

Reciprocal metabolic effects were found between barbiturates and organochlorine pesticides (31, 32, 33, 34, 35). Investigations on metabolic effects of organochlorine pesticides on the other toxic compounds were made: they can stimulate the production of less toxic compounds, as in the case of paraoxon (36), or that of more toxic compounds as in the case of CCl_4 (37).

Any tissue, organ, excreta or secreta could be useful and feasible for analysis and it seems rather difficult to foresee the most useful ones, mostly for future reference, because the actual and future pollutants may be stored in different parts of the body and they may damage unforeseeably different tissues, organs and apparatus (central and peripheral nervous system, cardiovascular, digestive renal apparatus, etc.); they interfere also with several metabolic patterns.

The list could start with samples of hair, kidneys, arteries, brain and nerves, placentae, blood (blood cells, serum, serum enzymatic activities), fatty tissues from cadavers (autopsy) of individuals which are dead for any cause, including early deaths from accidents.

Biopsy specimens may also be collected taking the opportunity of surgical or orthopedical operations (for instance, fatty tissues) in hospitals of different areas.

There may be differences in the concentrations of a stable compound between the tissues from a living body and a cadaver, due to dewatering process and other reasons; this must be taken into consideration.

Probably, more than one preservative method should be adopted, especially for future reference: freezing or drying, extracts homogenates, etc. even in order to stop immediately the biochemical activities. This item needs to be discussed and deeply studied.

The random pre-stratified samples of populations could be utilized only for blood, urine, hair, etc. collection; but for tissue and organ collection the only places seem to be the hospitals and the necroscopy rooms where the whole population is not statistically represented. Nevertheless, a network of 'points' carefully selected around the country or the regions in order to cover urban and rural populations of different sizes, in the northern and southern areas, in the mountains and along the coasts, on the mainland and on the islands, etc. could give reasonable and valid information taking into consideration the environmental factors, exposure estimates, etc. according to the purposes.

The existing programmes in Italy are based mainly on local and individual initiatives, but a centralized approach - all samples to selected locations for analysis, storage and data control - should be recommended and could be feasible today, particularly on a regional basis.

Of course, a conditioned international programme is also desirable, useful and feasible; the international coordination should facilitate the exchange of knowledge, the standardization of methods, the training of personnel and, finally, should improve the results.

Concerning the legal and ethical aspects, such a non-profit programme for biological monitoring could be carried out in Italy, by Universities and Public Health Institutes, without any difficulty provided the confidentiality of information is respected, and according to official agreements with the Public Health Officers, Hospitals and Anatomical Departments of the Region.

An overall estimate of costs for 'biological monitoring' and 'collection for future reference' in an Italian region - for example the Venice region - for chlorinated pesticides and for lead and mercury - could be indicated, including personnel, equipment, overheads, etc. per year, at actual rates, in Italian lire, as follows:

Design of Programme	L.	2,000,000.--
Collection and transport of samples	L.	4,000,000.--
Storage of samples	L.	3,000,000.--
Analysis of samples	L.	10,000,000.--
Data processing	L.	3,000,000.--
	L.	22,000,000.-

REFERENCES

1. PACCAGNELLA B. et al. Bull. Wld. Hlth. Org., 1971, 45, 181-99.
2. DURHAM W.F. Ann. N.Y. Acad. Sci., Vol 160, art. 1, p. 183 (1969).
3. PRATI L., R. PAVANELLO, F. GHEZZO. Bull. Wld. Hlth. Org. 1972, 46, 363-69.
4. ALESSANDRINI M.E., V. AMORMINO. Rend. Ist. Sup. San., 1954, 17, 890.

5.   ALESSANDRINI M.E., G.F. LANFORTI.   Rend. Ist. Sup. San., 1957, 20, 816.
6.   GRASSO C.   Atti Convegno Insetticidi, Firenze, 24-25 Nov. 1962.
7.   KANITZ S., G. CASTELLO.   Giorn. Ig. Med. Prev., 1966, 7, 1.
8.   BEGLIOMINI.   Arch. Vet. Ital., 1971, 22, 109-118.
9.   PESINO L.   Acta Med. Vet. 1973, 19/3-4, 253, 259.
10.   PACCAGNELLA B. et al.   Il latte, 1966, 40, 567.
11.   PACCAGNELLA B. et al.   Arch. S.Anna. 1966, 19, 357.
12.   PRATI L.   Tecnica Sanitaria, 1969, 4, 651-674.
13.   DEL VECCHIO V. et al.   N. Ann. Ig. Microb. 1970, 21, 381-451.
14.   KANITZ S.   Giornate Fitopatologiche, Cagliari, 1969.
15.   KANITZ S.   G. Ig. Med. Prev., 1971, 12, 51-59.
16.   CENCI P., G. CAVAZZINI.   Igiene Moderna, 1972, 65/3-4, 115-36.
17.   CENCI P., L. PRATI.   Atti Giornate Fitopatologiche, 1971, 27-31.
18.   SCHETTINO.   Boll. Sco. Ital. Biol. Sper., 1969, 45, 1341-4.
19.   SCHETTINO.   Boll. Soc. Ital. Biol. Sper., 1969, 45, 1337-40.
20.   SZENDE.   Med. Lav. 1970, 61, 433-6.
21.   SANNA RANDACCIO, F.   Acta Tuberc. Pneumol. Belg. 1974, 65/1, 88-92.
22.   NELSON S.C. et al.   J. Agr. Food Chem., 1956, 4, 696.
23.   TEGERIS A.S., et al.   Arch. Environm. Hlth., 1966, 13, 776.
24.   BLEIBERG M.J., et al.   Toxicol. Appl. Pharmacol., 1962, 4, 292.
25.   GREIM H., H. REMMER.   Arch. Pharmacol. Exper. Pathol., 1966, 255, 16.
26.   VELATTA V.V.   Sem. Med., 1964, 125, 2139.
27.   PHILLIPS W.E. Jr.   Canad. J. Biochem. & Physiol., 1963, 41, 1793.
28.   SCHABE U.   Arch. Exper. Pathol. Pharmakol., 1964, 249, 195.
29.   NELSON A., G. WOODWARD.   Arch. Pathol., 1949, 48, 387.
30.   BERNDT S. et al.   Arch. Pharmakol. Exper. Pathol., 1967, 256, 383.
31.   KUPFER D., L. PEETS.   Biochem. Pharmacol., 1966, 15, 573.
32.   FOUTS J.R.   Ann. N.Y. Acad. Sci. 1963, 104, 875.
33.   STRAW J.A. et al.   Proc. Soc. Exper. Pathol. Pharmakol., 1965, 118, 991.
34.   KORANSKY W. et al.   Arch. Exper. Pathol. Pharmakol., 1964, 247, 49.
35.   STREET J.C. et al.   Bull. Environ. Contam. Toxicol., 1966, 1, 6.
36.   GHAZAL A. et al.   Arch. Exper. Pathol. Pharmakol. 1964, 249, 1.
37.   MACLEAN A.E.M., E. MACLEAN.   Biochem. J., 1966, 100, 564.
38.   ANNUARIO STATISTICO ITALIANO.   1965 and 1975.
39.   AVOGARO.   Contenuto in elettroliti nel miocardio umano, nell'infarto cardiaco e nelle
miocardiosclerosi (in press).

BIOLOGICAL SPECIMEN COLLECTION FROM HUMAN POPULATIONS FOR BIOLOGICAL MONITORING AND FUTURE REFERENCE: MERCURY AND LEAD

B. Paccagnella and C. Favaretti
Institute of Hygiene, University of Padova, Verona

Among the past programmes dealing with biological monitoring on human populations, in Italy, there are lead and mercury and methyl-mercury body burdens estimated in relationship to the environmental pollution by these compounds.

1.   Mercury

A research of mercury concentration in blood and hair was carried out in a target population living on Carloforte Island (Sardinia), where fish is used in large quantities (non-occupational exposure).   High levels of mercury without symptoms and clinical impairment were found. The $84^o/o$ of total ingested mercury is absorbed as methyl-mercury.   (Paccagnella et al. 1973).

Investigations carried out in several Italian towns showed mercury levels in blood and hair much lower than in Carloforte Island.   The mercury levels in the seaside populations were higher than in other populations (Paccagnella et al 1974).

An atomic absorption spectrophotometer was used in these researches.

In the Amiata Mountain area of Tuscany a survey has examined the concentrations of mercury and selenium in the environment, in the food chain, and in human biological samples of blood, urine and hair by non-destructive neutron activation analysis. A group with occupational exposure to mercury vapour and dust, and a group of non-occupationally exposed were examined.   Results showed that the human metabolism of mercury is different from that of selenium and that selenium retention in man could be influenced by the mercury intake. (Cigna Rossi et al. 1976).   These results are not comparable with data we have cited before because of the different laboratory methods.

2.   Lead

Urinary ALA and lead values were determined in a representative sample of a population living in a rural area in Ferrara Province.   At the same time the lead concentration in the atmosphere, in a few samples of soil and water and in some food (wine, milk, vegetables) of local production was determined.   This survey gave the normal values of lead levels for rural population of northern Italy (Kumer and Luppi et al. 1974).

The pigeons were taken as an index of lead pollution in the same area and in Ferrara Centre.   Significant differences were found in erythrocytes ALA-Dehydrase activity and blood lead content among pigeons coming from these two different areas; no difference in the lead content of bones, feathers and muscles (Bucci and Cenci et al. 1974).

Erythrocyte ALA-Dehydrase activity (Secchi and Alessio 1974) and blood lead levels were determined in non-occupationally exposed, living in several Italian towns (Benvenuti and Maggio 1974).   Nevertheless, environmental pollution was not tested.

Several other studies are carried out and concern the tissues or blood and urine content of several inorganic and organic compounds in hospitalized patients, and occupational situations, but they are carried on mainly for diagnostic and treatment purposes.

In relationship to the problem of soft waters and heart disease, the electrolytes concentration in the myocardial tissue, in the infarction and in arteriosclerotic heart disease (AHD) were studied: magnesium and potassium decrease and sodium increases in the infarction; no differences in the AHD and in the normal myocardial tissue (Avogaro, in press).

No doubt on the utility of the latter studies according to the purposes they have; but they are certainly inadequate for biological monitoring, because they are unrelated to the environmental situations which must be measured to show the associations with the human indicators and they represent frequently only the sick, institutionalized, individuals.

REFERENCES

AVOGARO: Contenuto in elettroliti nel miocardio umano, nell'infarto cardiaco e nella miocardiosclerosi. (In press).

BENVENUTI and MAGGIO: I livelli di concentrazioni di piombo nel sangue dei soggetti non professionalmente esposti, abitanti in varie città italiane. Securitas, 1974, 59/7, 487-496.

BUCCI, CENCI et al: I piccioni quale test biologico di valutazione dell'inquinamento atmosferico da piombo. Ricerche a Ferrara e Ro Ferrarese. Igiene Moderna, 1974, 67/2, 129-135.

CIGNA ROSSI et al: Mercury and Selenium distribution in a defined area and in its population. Arch. Environ. Health, 1976, 31/3, 160-165.

KUMER, LUPPI et al: L'assorbimento di piombo in un campione della popolazione del Comune di Ro (Ferrara). Igiene Moderna, 1974, 67/4, 351-368.

PACCAGNELLA et al: Studio epidemiologico sul mercurio nei pesci e la salute umana in un' isola italiana del Mediterraneo. Igiene Moderna, 1973, 66, 479-503.

PACCAGNELLA and PRATI: Concentrazioni di mercurio totale nel sangue e nei capelli di persone non esposte professionalmente residenti in aree diverse dell'Italia. Igiene Moderna, 1974, 4, 369-380.

SECCHI and ALESSIO: Laboratory results of some biological measures in workers exposed to lead. Arch. Environm. Health, 1974, 29/6, 351-354.

ESTABLISHING AND OPERATING A SPECIMEN BANK
FOR ENVIRONMENTAL MONITORING

H. Rook and P. Lafleur
National Bureau of Standards, Washington D.C.   20234

Abstract

Program plans for a National Environmental Specimen Bank have been under consideration by the U.S. Environmental Protection Agency for more than five years.   The utility of such a sample storage system is clear but there are many technical aspects of long-term sample storage which have yet to be scientifically investigated.   In 1975, the National Bureau of Standards joined with the Environmental Protection Agency to study and make recommendations for acceptable methods for sampling, sample preparation and storage of various environmental matrices for both trace element and trace organic analysis.   This presentation is a summary of the current research of that cooperative program, and the program constraints imposed by scientific findings.

Introduction

For the past two years the U.S. National Bureau of Standards has been cooperating with the U.S. Environmental Protection Agency in examining sampling, storage, and analytical methods for use in archiving environmental samples for retrospective analysis.   We have been studying a number of different parameters in the sampling and sample storage areas, particularly for the determination of trace elements.   As part of this program an extensive review of presently existing sample archives in the United States was conducted in a cooperative program jointly supported by the Environmental Protection Agency, the U.S. National Science Foundation and NBS.   A survey was prepared to identify and obtain information from organizations and/or individuals that have sample archives.   Mechanics of the survey were organized and performed by the Environmental Sciences Division of the Oak Ridge National Laboratory with input from personnel of EPA, NSF and NBS.   The details of the survey may be found in reference (1).   Once the survey forms had been returned evaluation of each individual reply was performed by personnel of the NBS Analytical Chemistry Division.

The fundamental consideration of the evaluation was the suitability of the techniques used for sampling and sample handling and storage so that valid retrospective determination of the analyses of interest could be made.   The results of the evaluations indicated that although most of the collections were taken in a manner suitable for the purpose of the archivist, essentially none of these collections appear to meet the minimal conditions for valid retrospective analysis.   The results of the evaluation were reported to the Environmental Protection Agency and will be published separately by EPA.

Concomitant with the survey, a literature survey was conducted on sampling, sample handling, and storage of materials appropriate for the Bank.   This survey has been published as NBS Technical Note 929 and is available from the National Bureau of Standards (2).

The specifics of the NBS/EPA program are to study non-contaminating sampling methods, storage techniques, potential problems due to tissue variability and analytical methodology. Investigation of sampling parameters involved primarily the implements used in excising tissues (knives, forceps, etc.).   Stainless steel and various plastics are being investigated.   Storage methods being investigated include freezing at -20°C and -70°C, lyophilization and ashing techniques.   For the purposes of this study only so-called low temperature ashing (using atomic oxygen generated in an R_F field) has been used.   The results of the low temperature ashing study were reported at the International Conference on Modern Trends in Activation Analysis (3).   The effect of storage containers on various kinds of environmental samples is also being studied (4).

In discussions of archiving tissue samples for future analysis, the problem of whether to use whole tissues or a tissue homogenate has caused considerable debate.   Because of potential concentration of trace elements of interest in specific portions of highly differentiated organs, such as kidney, brain, etc., a number of investigators feel that tissue homogenates may give information that is much too general in nature.   On the other hand, in relatively non-differentiated organs, such as liver, spleen, and skeletal muscle, homogenates may be entirely satisfactory.   A study is presently under way at NBS into tissue variability problems.

The key to any monitoring program obviously is adequate analytical methodology to determine the constituent(s) of interest in samples that have been properly taken and stored. The formal portion of this program at NBS is only now beginning.

Program Design

In establishing an environmental specimen or tissue bank, a number of parameters must be considered, such as sampling and transportation problems. These include such questions as where should the samples come from geographically. For this purpose, close cooperation between the organizers of the bank and knowledgeable epidemiologists is essential to obtain the best statistical pattern. It will do little good to have several thousands of samples taken from a location only to discover that a future problem is concentrated in an area for which no archived samples are extant. While it is obviously patently impossible to sample every area in every country, it is possible to determine high risk areas. A sampling network should therefore be set up which takes into account both sample availability and potential risk.

Equally important to sampling location, is deciding what samples to take. Obviously when dealing with the effects of the environment on man, it is important that human beings be one of the species examined. In many pollutant types it will be equally important, however, to examine major food chain species, both plant and animal. The particular species may depend upon the types of analytes of interest; for example, trace elements or trace organics. However, in most cases, the sample type will be equally applicable for both types of analyte.

Of the candidate samples for inclusion in the banking system, the most important type is a soft tissue of human origin. For an environmental banking system, major organs which are used by the body to cleanse the blood stream, such as liver and kidney, are important. Also, adipose tissue is important since it concentrates many organic materials, particularly chorinated hydrocarbons. Lung tissue would be a strong candidate as an indicator of air pollution problems. Bone may be considered since it is a good concentrator for several kinds of elements, especially the heavy radionuclides. Other tissue samples might be considered depending on the specific pollutant types anticipated to be important in the future.

A second class of samples which should be considered is a single or composited food material representing a major input into the worldwide human diet. For this purpose, a food grain or composite of grains is an ideal choice. An added benefit here is that the material is readily available and relatively easy to store.

A third sample type which would indicate problems in the area of water pollution would be an accumulator of aquatic origin. Possibilities range from plankton to shark tissue. A logical choice, however, would be a shellfish bivalve, such as oysters, which passes large quantities of water through its system every day and which tends to mirror increased concentrations of many toxic pollutants.

To be complete, a sample type should be included which is a collector of atmospheric or airborne pollutant materials. A good choice here would be a lichen or moss. This material again should be readily available and readily easy to store. These four sample types are specifically discussed because of their diversity and their utility to any environmental monitoring program. One must, however, be careful with the numbers of sample types as it would be easy to swamp any banking system with too many samples.

The third important consideration, along with what samples should be taken and which ones should be taken is how the samples should be taken. It is critical to all subsequent analyses that the sample be taken in such a way that it not be contaminated. As an example, it is very easy to contaminate blood serum so grossly through normal sampling methods (such as using a stainless steel needle) that it would obviate analyses for cobalt, manganese and a number of other metals. To reduce contamination, plastic implements, such as catheters for the taking of serum and plastic or quartz knives for excising tissues should be considered for sampling. It is also very important to consider the timing of sampling. The tissues should be excised from the sample as soon as possible after death as the tissue composition may change due to 'weepage' of tissue fluids as time elapses. Considerably more study is necessary to determine the effect of this problem; it may not be too serious once these questions have been answered.

The sample container is equally important. A universal container does not appear practicable at the present time. Glass or metal containers are preferable for storage of samples to be analyzed for organic constituents, whereas plastic containers such as Teflon or high purity polyethylene are preferable for those samples to be used for trace element analyses. A potential solution may be to fast-freeze samples in the field and store them in bottles kept at dry ice or liquid nitrogen temperatures.   Contact with the container would therefore be minimal and diffusion of trace constituents from the container into the sample would be minimized.   It may be possible to store samples in a borosilicate glass, for example, for both trace elements and trace organics as long as the samples are kept frozen.   It may also be preferable to keep the samples frozen at one temperature, for example between -20° and -70°C, and prior to sub-sampling, reduce the temperature with liquid nitrogen to 77° Kelvin and then simply break off a portion of the sample for subsequent analysis.   This also takes care of any problems with the type of sampling implement used to subsample.   Obviously for differentiated organs, sampling resolution will be a problem with this technique.

Regardless of the type of storage container, a good practice would be to freeze the sample as soon as possible after it is taken, preferably at the sampling site, in dry ice or liquid nitrogen and ship it frozen to the storage destination.   At that point, the sample may be treated in a number of different ways.   It is true that freezing the sample may make histologic examination difficult and/or bacterial examination impossible, but at the present time the principal aims of the bank should be for chemical contaminants rather than biological contaminants.   Histologic examination might be done on a small portion of the tissue taken and prepared for such examination at the same time the main sample is taken.

Once the sample has been received at the banking location, it must be stored in some way such that long-term integrity is assured.   A number of possibilities present themselves.   The most obvious is freezing.   However, as is well known, freezing at the normal -20°C does result in slow sample degradation and dehydration.   Considerably more research is needed in this area but some candidate methods would be freezing at -70°C or possibly even at 77°K.   Obviously, the latter freezing requirement would be extremely expensive.   Another possibility is lyophili-zation of the samples.   The effect on trace organics obviously must be investigated, but for a number of relatively non-volatile trace organics this may be a perfectly adequate storage tech-nique.   Once the sample has been lyophilized, it may be packed in pure nitrogen or in some other inert gas, such as argon, to reduce degradation even further.   Lyophilized samples are known to be in relatively good condition as much as 20 years after the freeze-drying process.

A less desirable technique from many standpoints is that of ashing, particularly at high temperatures.   Some work has been done at NBS to evaluate the possibility of using low tem-perature ashing techniques (3).   The problem with ashing in either case is that it is only appli-cable for inorganic elements and even then at least five elements (Hg, Os, I, Br, Cl) are usually lost.   There are a number of advantages to ashing though, the most important being sample volume reduction and relatively easy storage for long periods of time.

The use of stabilizing liquids, such as formalin, gluteraldehyde or ethanol, however, is not satisfactory for a number of reasons: the possible transfer of contaminants to the sample from the container in which the sample is stored, the impurities in the fixative itself, and potential extraction of analytes of interest, particularly organics, by the liquid in which the sample is stored (5).

Trying to decide how much sample to store in the archives is a very difficult problem.   A very delicate balance must be achieved between the minimum amount of sample necessary for repetitive analyses over a long period of time to give the necessary information and the prob-lems with the volume of samples and the expense of storing such large volumes.   For this pur-pose, we must go back to the problems in deciding which samples to take and the widest spec-trum of most useful samples must be taken simply to reduce the large volume that would be required for a full-scale bank.   Obviously, one of the most important aspects of the tissue bank is the data which are available to researchers concerning those samples in the bank; where and when they were taken, the analytical results obtained at the time they were taken during a nor-mal monitoring program, and results on the samples subsequent to their placement in the bank. For this purpose, a rather elaborate data processing system would be an essential part of any such bank.

Organization and Operation

For a bank to function properly, there are a number of organizational aspects that must be considered.   One of the most important would be determining who should receive samples for analysis and distribution of the data.   Before a sample may be removed for analysis, the applicant should prove his capability for the kind of analysis that he proposes.   This capability must be demonstrated on samples which are not part of the bank (one cannot afford to allow the use of these samples for capability demonstration).   For this purpose, it would be desirable to have a number of samples for which the homogeneity has been demonstrated and a few of the major analytes of interest have been determined. For this purpose a qualified 'Board of Directors' must be selected, probably on some sort of rotating term basis, to process applications for samples, to evaluate the data, and to make sure the data are disseminated to all of the interested investigators and agencies. This information transfer could best be achieved by a regular publication from the bank containing current information of interest. Among the kinds of problems that would have to be answered are: how are samples to be submitted? Should there be a central bank that has central responsibility for the sampling and cataloging of samples, or should a number of contractor groups scattered throughout the study area take samples according to a given protocol and submit the samples to a central bank? Should there be branch banks in which samples are archived in various countries or parts of a country?

Ethical and Legal Considerations

The last difficult problem to be considered is that of ethical and legal considerations. Obviously such things as non-traceability to specific persons would be necessary. It would, however, be necessary to have associated data, such as smoking habits, age, and general state of health. It would probably be preferable to have samples as far as possible from non-diseased persons. There may also be local problems in terms of legal aspects of the transfer and storage of human tissues. Shipping plant tissues and animal tissues across international boundaries or even within a country, across state or provincial boundaries may be difficult. Such considerations will have to be taken into account prior to any serious consideration of a bank.

Costs

It is difficult to come up with a hard estimate for costs. However, an estimate has been made for a pilot program which would be done on a limited scale. This would cost approximately $700,000 per year for five years to demonstrate feasibility. For this program a limited number of samples would be taken from only one or two locations and archived. For a full program, it would probably require at least $2 million per year to operate even a modest banking problem. A more realistic estimate probably would be $5 million per year for sample archiving and data reduction.

In summary, a system for archiving samples for future analysis as part of an existing monitoring program has great potential in environmental studies. Such a banking system requires, however, careful study and meticulous operation to be credible.

REFERENCES

1. VAN HOOK, R.I. and E.E. HUBER, 'National Environmental Specimen Bank Survey' EPA Report EPA-600/1-7-006.
2. MAIENTHAL, E.J., and D.A. BECKER, 'A Survey of Current Literature on Sampling, Sample Handling, and Long Term Storage for Environmental Materials.' NBS Technical Note 929, National Bureau of Standards, Washington, D.C. 20234.
3. LUTZ, G.J. 'Volatilization Losses on Low Temperature Ashing' to be published in the Proceedings of the 5th International Conference on Modern Trends in Activation Analysis (Munich, 1976).
4. MOODY, J. and R. LINDSTROM, Selection and Cleaning of Containers for Trace Metal Analysis, to be published in Analytical Chemistry.
5. GIBBS, R.H. Jr., E. JAROSEVICH, and H.L. WINDON, Science, **184**, 475 (1974).

CONCEPTIONAL DESIGN OF AN ENVIRONMENTAL SPECIMEN BANK IN THE FEDERAL REPUBLIC OF GERMANY

F. SCHMIDT-BLEEK – P. MUHS
Federal Environmental Agency
Umweltbundesamt
Bismarckplatz 1
1000 Berlin 33

1.   PROLOGUE

"Der Deutsche Weinbau", the official publication of West Germany's wine producers recently announced a breakthrough in improved harvesting methods for grapes. A mixture of 2-chlorethylphosphoric acid and cyanamid ('VP 615') is sprayed upon the leaves just prior to harvesting time. The leaves wither away completely within a week, and consequently the grapes can be picked more efficiently. The 'cost/benefit' analysis, without social costs, shows the benefits amounting to DM 120 per hectare or roughly DM 0.01 per liter of wine; which corresponds to approximately 0.2 % reduction in retail price or alternatively 0.2 % increase in profit.

The minimum basic daily charge per person-day in German hospitals is approximately DM 120.- today.

2.   SUMMARY

This paper summarizes the major reasons for proceeding with ongoing R & D efforts and very likely adds additional projects in West Germany in order to build a foundation for allowing a governmental go/no-go decision for the permanent establishment of an Environmental Specimen Bank (ESB).

There are at least three vital services which such an ESB could render:

1.   Provide up to date information on the spread of man-made chemicals in the environment, including man;
2.   Allow extrapolations of concentration trends with respect to chemicals considered to present threats to man and his environment;
3.   'Preserve the presence' by 'fossilizing' selected environmental specimens in a repository so as to be able to analyse them for specific chemicals and histological details of urgent interest in the future originating from chemicals scavenged in past years.

Of these potential services, the third is very likely the most important since we are in no position to analyse environmental samples for all 30 000 or so man-made chemicals circulating in the environment today.

In establishing an ESB, it is to be anticipated that by far the greatest attention has to be devoted to organic pollutants and their degradation products (metabolites) rather than trace metals or their compounds. This recognition has profound ramifications upon the entire establishment and operation of an ESB.

This paper lays out the principal functional parts of an integrated ESB and indicates some areas where research is still needed. At present the assumption is made by our Agency that the exclusive collection, analysis and storage of human samples would not by itself justify the establishment of a major repository of specimens since environmental policies of the future have to take increasingly cognizance of the interdependence amongst natural systems and their continuing manipulations by man.

3.   CHEMICAL PRODUCTS AND ENVIRONMENTAL CHEMICALS

Man-made chemicals reach points of impact in two distinctly different ways : **First** they are marketed as commercial products and intentionally applied to perform pre-designed functions.   Medical specialities, detergents, pesticides, propellants, lubricants and paints may serve as examples.   Altogether, chemical industry puts in excess of 30 000 compounds on the market today, retailed in mixtures and preparations exceeding several hundreds of thousands. All over the world, more than 100 million tons of organic compounds are sold annually on the market.   In Germany more than 10 000 cleaning preparations alone are retailed today.

Figure 1 indicates the flow of chemicals through society.   The extraction of raw materials, their refinement and conversion into chemical products, the distributing and storage of the latter until they reach their destined use or consumption are all parts of a multibillion dollar   industry.   Imports add to the variety of chemical products on most domestic markets today.   It must be clearly recognized that life as we know it today could not be sustained without the designed applications of a multitude of products provided by chemical industry.

As the broad arrows pointing downward in Figure 1 indicate, each sector of the economy leaks chemicals into the environment.   And here we come to the **second** and in this case **unintentional** impacts of man-made chemicals: they enter the ecosphere as emissions and by-products from production processes and energy conversion schemes, as waste streams from all fields of consumption and in many other ways.

It is of fundamental importance to realize that while **man-made chemical products** are designed and applied to perform certain functions, these same chemicals or their decomposition products become **environmental chemicals** upon leaking into the common ecosphere, where they may attack environmental objects without purpose, in random ways, these objects having normally no means of protecting themselves against such attacks.

Figure 1 illustrates in the lower part the three main areas of effects of environmental chemicals in the ecosphere.   Air, water, and soil are still frequently perceived only as carriers of pollutants.   As Rowland's discovery of the chemical impact of fluorocarbons on ozone in 1974 has so impressively demonstrated, however, this view is no longer sufficient. — Biological objects are shown in Figure 1 to the lower left as a block separate from material assets on the lower right so as to indicate the quite different approaches in investigative research as well as in public policies for environmental protection and planning in these areas.

The distinction put forth here between chemical products and environmental chemicals will undoubtedly become of increasing importance in shaping and enforcing environmental policies in the future.   In all our efforts to develop responsible public policies we must remain aware of a simple fact which is nothing less than frightening from a normative point of view : There is no such thing as a single harmless man-made chemical from an ecological point of view and yet there will not be much, if any, future for mankind without the intentional use of chemical products.

4.   PRINCIPAL REASONS FOR THE ESTABLISHMENT OF AN ESB

At present the number and variety of environmental chemicals are such that a systematic and all-encompassing determination of their ecotoxic behaviour and discernible effects is all but impossible.   Neither is it feasible to account for their circulation (see lower part of Figure 1) and accumulation in the environment.   It seems furthermore self-evident that the same must hold for their decomposition products and metabolites.

In order to obtain more realistic information about the threats posed to man and his environment by environmental chemicals, however, it seems logical and highly desirable to consider the systematic and repetitive collection of such environmental specimens which are known to scavenge and accumulate hazardous man-made compounds from their respective environment. Examples may be sediments, oysters, plants, as well as animal and human hair, eye and umbilical cords.   Systematic and repetitive analyses over time of **comparable** samples will yield two most important types of information with respect to environmental chemicals already recognized or believed to be harmful.

1. Real-time information as to the distribution of man-made chemicals and perhaps some of their decomposition products in the environment.
2. Trends with respect to increasing threats posed by certain environmental chemicals believed to be deleterious to the environment, including man.

It seems obvious that routinely available data on water and air quality (in particular drinking water quality) can and must be correlated with the findings originating from the analysis of environmental samples such as just described.

In spite of all international efforts to investigate dose-effect relationships of various environmental chemicals it must be recognized that our sum total of knowledge in this area is still ruefully inadequate. Most health effects research got started by accidents, be these caused by DDT, Hg, Cd, Polycyclic Hydrocarbons, or CTDD. While tens of thousands of organic compounds leak into the environment, a surprisingly large part of publicly funded research is still concentrated on a few heavy metals. Today virtually no environmental law can, as it should, be based upon the quantified effects (costs) caused by the chemical and/or biological action of environmental chemicals and as a consequence no bills or laws are as yet supported by reasonable cost/benefit analyses. So far at best only a few hundred chemicals have been extensively tested for their mutagenic, carcinogenic and teratogenic effects. Standard protocols for pre-market screening of chemical products are as yet far from adequate. None of the Member States of the EEC for example has a law preventing the marketing of new chemicals with potential ecotoxic properties. The proposed directive EEC XI/ENV/236/76 will hopefully bring about some changes toward correcting this situation in the near future. Several laws in other countries, including the US Toxic Substances Control Act, signed by President Ford on 13 October 1976, should improve the control of the ubiquitous spread of harmful environmental chemicals in the long run.

Since only a fraction of the presently circulating environmental chemicals has so far been investigated with respect to their ecotoxic (and in particular chronically toxic) properties we have to expect chance discoveries of detrimental effects by environmental chemicals for many future years. And hardly one of these chemicals is now considered to be harmful or at least worthy of detailed observation.

Since 'total analyses' of environmental samples are out of the question for reasons of time and money we are coming to the **third** major function of a future ESB:
3. The long-term preservation of aliquots of such samples which were originally analysed for mapping out the present-day distribution of known harmful chemicals and interpreted to determine any trends which may exist. The possibility to analyse well preserved samples (or 'fossils' of the past) when need arises in the future for the clarification of specific problems will help greatly to develop action plans as they will then be required and also to improve public policies.

In its official Report on the Environment, dated 14 July 1976, the Government of the Federal Republic of Germany has specifically stated its intention to support the preparatory work toward establishing an environmental specimen bank.

5. **PRESENT ACTIVITIES IN THE FEDERAL REPUBLIC OF GERMANY TOWARD ESTABLISHING AN ESB**

Having recognized the potential importance of one or more ESB's, the Government of the FRG began developing plans for exploratory research late in 1974. An important impetus was provided by several ongoing R & D activities in the US which had originated in 1971 and German research proposals by F. Korte based upon these. Under the US-German environmental Agreement of 1974 detailed plans began to take shape in 1975 for a joint R & D effort. The German decision for funding 9 selected projects was reached in January 1976. The present programme covers a period of two years and calls for expenditures in excess of DM 3 million. The German research programme concentrates at present on the intake and metabolisms of selected groups of environmental chemicals recognized to be harmful (e.g., group-fingerprint analyses with multiple apparatus linkups). Up to the present time, sampling techniques, storage container examination as well as storage techniques are primarily researched at the US National Bureau of Standards in Gaithersburg (P.D. La Fleur) and co-workers under contract with the EPA (G. Goldstein).

By the end of 1976 a first comprehensive progress report on the German part of the ESB programme will be available from the Federal Environmental Agency.

The expansion of the German research efforts is currently being considered. In particular, plans call for adding detailed investigations of freeze-storing methods for selected biological samples.

The German part of the ESB programme has been designed to put the Federal Government in a position to make a no-go decision on the establishment of one or more ESB's by 1978.

The German programme is coordinated, developed, and evaluated by the Federal Environmental Agency. Funds are provided by the Federal Department for Research and Technology through an interagency agreement. Findings from a considerable number of R & D projects from the UFOPLAN (Environmental Research Plan), administered by the Federal Environmental Agency (some 500 current projects) as well as from many pertinent R & D activities sponsored by the Department of Research and Technology are also utilized to underpin the scientific and financial analysis being prepared on the ESB alternatives for the Federal Government in 1978.

6. FUNCTIONAL PARTS OF AN ESB

Figure 2 summarizes all principal aspects which must be considered while conceiving an ESB.

The major aspects are these:
6.1. Criteria for samples selection
6.2. Sampling and transportation of samples to the ESB
6.3. Sample preparation and analysis
6.4. Preparation for storage and storage techniques
6.5. Operation of an integrated ESB.

6.1. Criteria for samples selection

We should start this discussion with the recognition that one will be able to collect, analyse and store as many samples as may scientifically be desirable.

Figures 3 and 4 illustrate in a stepwise fashion the major considerations one has to weigh before making decisions as to the kinds of samples one should select for storage. From the commercial chemicals (marketing) point of view, the following sources must be considered (see Figure 1, apper part) :
6.1.1. Emissions, spills and leaks during extraction of raw materials, production processes, storage and transportation, (quantities emitted, toxicity and degradability of chemicals).
6.1.2. Quantities and types of chemical products put on the market, (compounds, mixtures and preparations, toxicity, degradability)
6.1.3. Use patterns (entry routes of chemical products into the environment, leakage probability through air and water).

There are few reliable data available at this time, satisfying the above information requirements. Implementation of the EEC directive XI/ENV/236/76 should lead to substantial progress over time at least for 6.1.2 and 6.1.3, just as the recently enacted US Toxic Substances Control Act. Attention of the reader may also be directed toward the 'OECD room document No 4' ENV/Chem, May 1976 which was submitted by the German Delegation, under the title : 'The Assessment of Environmental Chemicals'.

Figure 3 also details the principal **types** of samples, which one should consider in order to achieve a reasonably complete assessment of the distribution (and its changes) of environmental chemicals in the ecosphere (under 'Accumulation').

The procedure of selecting the most promising scavenger samples has to be guided by two more basic types of considerations :
6.1.2 the general properties of the samples (Figure 4, Sample Priorities)
6.1.3 the place of the sample in the environment relative to its proximity to man itself.

Figures 3 and 4 indicate one principal approach to narrowing down what at first is an enormous variety of different desirable samples for collection, analysis and preservation.

It may be appropriate to summarize here some specific considerations for samples.

Air and water as such are probably not worth collecting because of the volumes involved. On the other hand, it may be worth considering to collect air-filtered solids from various urban and rural areas, provided the technical concentration methods can be shown to be reproducible.

With respect to water samples the use of selected types of oysters exposed for predetermined times, both in marine and fresh waters, may be desirable. Oysters pump roughly 500 liters of water per day and are known to retain pollutants very well.

In discussing plant material, a general point of consideration should be introduced. Any establishment of an ESB is worth considering only if careful research and planning show the possibility to collect repeatedly comparable samples over a period of many years. In using biological scavenger specimens, both the type of retained pollutants and their quantities are function of the specific biological functions of the scavengers. So are the metabolic activities which will determine the remaining mixture of chemicals to be found in any specimen. Therefore the question must be answered whether or not it is mandatory to select, and breed if necessary, specific clones of plants which can be reproducibly used over a period of 20 to 30 years or more.

Animal and animal-product samples will have to be considered, some will undoubtedly be very important for the quality of the ESB (kidneys, lungs, livers, milk, milk products, honey). Barley is worldwide produced at about 170 million metric tons per year, roughly 50 % that of wheat, 3 times the amount of soybeans. Pork and beef are produced in equal amounts, about 42 million metric tons per year worldwide.

And finally we come to human samples. Figure 4 details one of the possibilities one should distinguish between human 'expendable' products such as hair, nails, placentae, umbilical cord blood, milk and other liquids on one hand and on the other hand such human tissues, the collection of which may fall under legal constraints. In the Federal Republic of Germany, written consent of the donor prior to death or by next of kin after death is sufficient to allow extraction of organs or other parts. Generally speaking, persons having died accidentally (traffic accidents) would be most desirable for collection purposes so as to obtain average healthy specimens of various ages, exposure histories and different sexes.

6.2. Sampling and samples transportation

6.2.1. The timing of sampling, the number of samples taken and the total mass needed for all foreseeable analytical purposes (including analyses after storage) have to be considered.

6.2.2. As already indicated above, the knowledge of the exposure history of the specimen is of fundamental importance, not only so as to be able to pass sound judgement on the analytical results derived from any individual sample but also because of the need to extrapolate over time by comparing the results from a number of specimens obtained and investigated over a period of time scanning 20, 30 or more years.

6.2.3. It is quite clear that very rigorous sampling protocols have to be developed and strictly adhered to. As a good number of epidemiological studies have furthermore shown, **reliable** sample collection can very likely only be achieved by trained and permanently employed personnel. This is particularly true for animal and human tissues.

We therefore foresee the use of mobile laboratories which are also equipped to do rudimentary analyses on the spot as well as sample preparation for storage and freezing.

The following experiences should be considered in connection with sample collection: all metallic cutting instruments, unless carefully prepared, leave behind the traces of heavy elements (e.g. manganese, nickel etc.). Aliquots of bulk samples have to be prepared before packaging and freezing. The fresh weight of specimens has to be carefully recorded, together with all pertinent data on age, sex, previous illnesses, social status, exposure radius, etc, of the donor.

The packaging material for transportation and for permanent storage is of particular importance. The US National Bureau of Standards has already performed a good number of studies to elucidate optimal materials. The German programme will build upon these experiences.

6.3. Sample preparation and analysis

6.3.1. Depending upon the analytical finesse required of the specimen, one can distinguish between :

a) the determination of chemical compounds in bulk samples and

b) the investigation of the histological situation of parts of specimens combined with the location of certain chemical substances.

In the first case it will probably be adequate to homogenize the sample prior to preparation for storage. Furthermore, rapid freezing techniques are most likely satisfactory. In the second case the maintenance of cell structure is of tantamount importance and experience tells that neither rapid quenching nor fast thawing of samples can generally be tolerated.

6.3.2. There is relatively little to say with respect to analytical methods and equipment. Modern techniques, adequately applied, will yield just about every sensitivity, specificity and reproducibility required. One should, however, clearly distinguish here between the routine analysis of fresh samples for the determination of the concentration of chemicals known to be harmful on one hand and on the other hand the need of such analytical procedures which will produce 'fingerprint' spectra for whole classes of compounds (which are not resolved for their individual components at the time of procurement). Such 'fingerprint' spectra should prove to be of invaluable help in evaluating time-sequence samples to observe trends of increasing (or decreasing) components with time.

6.4. Preparation for storage and storage techniques

Some of the considerations which are of importance under this heading were already discussed under 6.2.1., 6.2.3. and 6.3.1. above.

It should be stressed once more that our principal attention to environmental chemicals will have to be focused on organic compounds in the future. This will not only influence the selection of packaging materials for storage, the preparation procedures (homogenization extraction, lyophilization etc.) and analytical methodologies, this priority setting will also have a decisive influence upon the long-term storage techniques to be employed. Thus it seems inappropriate for instance to consider radiation sterilization, chemical stabilization, or high temperature ashing for most specimens to be stored. Nevertheless, all potentially applicable storage techniques will have to be explored in order to minimize storage costs for large numbers of samples over lengthy periods of time.

6.5. Operation of an integrated ESB

All things considered it must be concluded that a fully integrated operation of an ESB offers the best chance to obtain maximum services. This means that all functional parts are to be performed under full control of the installation. It is, for instance, quite impossible to have all or part of the analyses performed by outside laboratories since systematic errors tend to be laboratory specific. The reliability of an ESB operation, though, is entirely depending upon the comparability of its analytical results. In many cases the accuracy of findings will prove to be of lesser importance than the consistency of results over long periods of time.

Figure 5 illustrates the essential parts of an integrated operation as outlined above, the concept of a smallest critical mass for an ESB follows logically. According to preliminary estimates, the smallest functioning unit would require approximately :

Space: 400 m^2
Personnel: 22 (7 scientists)
Equipment: 6 million DM
operational costs/year   2.5 million DM

These figures are to be understood as highly preliminary. Such a unit could handle approximately 2000 samples per year.

7.   FURTHER POTENTIALS OF AN ESB

It may be intriguing to speculate on purposes and functions of an ESB beyond those specified above.

All highly industrialized countries, and increasingly developing nations too, have yet to come to grips with the complex problems of providing facts and figures for establishing ecological criteria as base lines for environmental impact assessments. This is as much true for human installations and activities already impacting upon the ecosphere as it is true for the pre-judgement of the future ecological consequences of plans as yet to be implemented.

We therefore contend that each country will eventually have to develop a grid-type determination and display of its 'state of the ecology' and 'permissible ecological load factors'. For these grits, a number of basic ecological data will have to be developed, and continuously updated. It is obvious that a detailed knowledge of the 'environmental chemical load factor' will be one of the most important parameters for such an information system. The uniformity and reliability of such an information network on chemical information could and may be should take its start from an ESB.

8. CONCLUSIONS

It has been shown that the establishment of one or more ESB's in the Federal Republic of Germany is seriously being considered.   R & D efforts are underway to explore the scientific feasibility, the approximate costs and other operational details so as to put the Federal Government in a position to make sound decisions within the next few years.

International cooperation in this endeavour is most desirable.   The Government of the Federal Republic of Germany is grateful for the excellent cooperation with the United States in the development of the basic knowledge necessary to implement an ESB.   The Government of the Federal Republic of Germany would welcome any additional constructive international cooperation which carries with it the prospect for helping man to enjoy life more fully on earth.

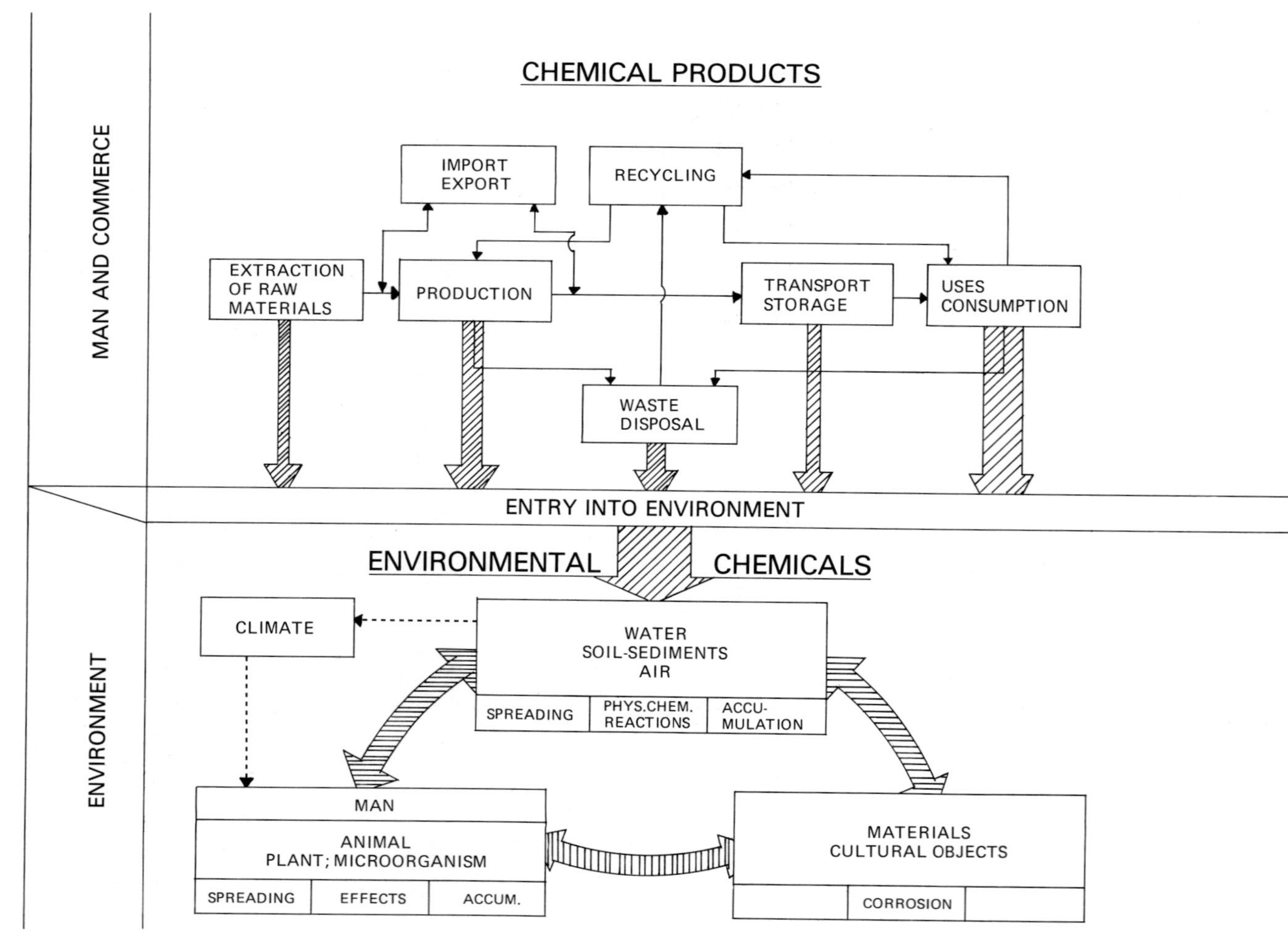

CHEMICAL PRODUCTS
MAN AND COMMERCE
IMPORT EXPORT
RECYCLING
EXTRACTION OF RAW MATERIALS
PRODUCTION
TRANSPORT STORAGE
USES CONSUMPTION
WASTE DISPOSAL
ENTRY INTO ENVIRONMENT
ENVIRONMENTAL CHEMICALS
ENVIRONMENT
CLIMATE
WATER SOIL-SEDIMENTS AIR
SPREADING
PHYS.CHEM. REACTIONS
ACCUMULATION
MAN
ANIMAL PLANT; MICROORGANISM
SPREADING
EFFECTS
ACCUM.
MATERIALS CULTURAL OBJECTS
CORROSION

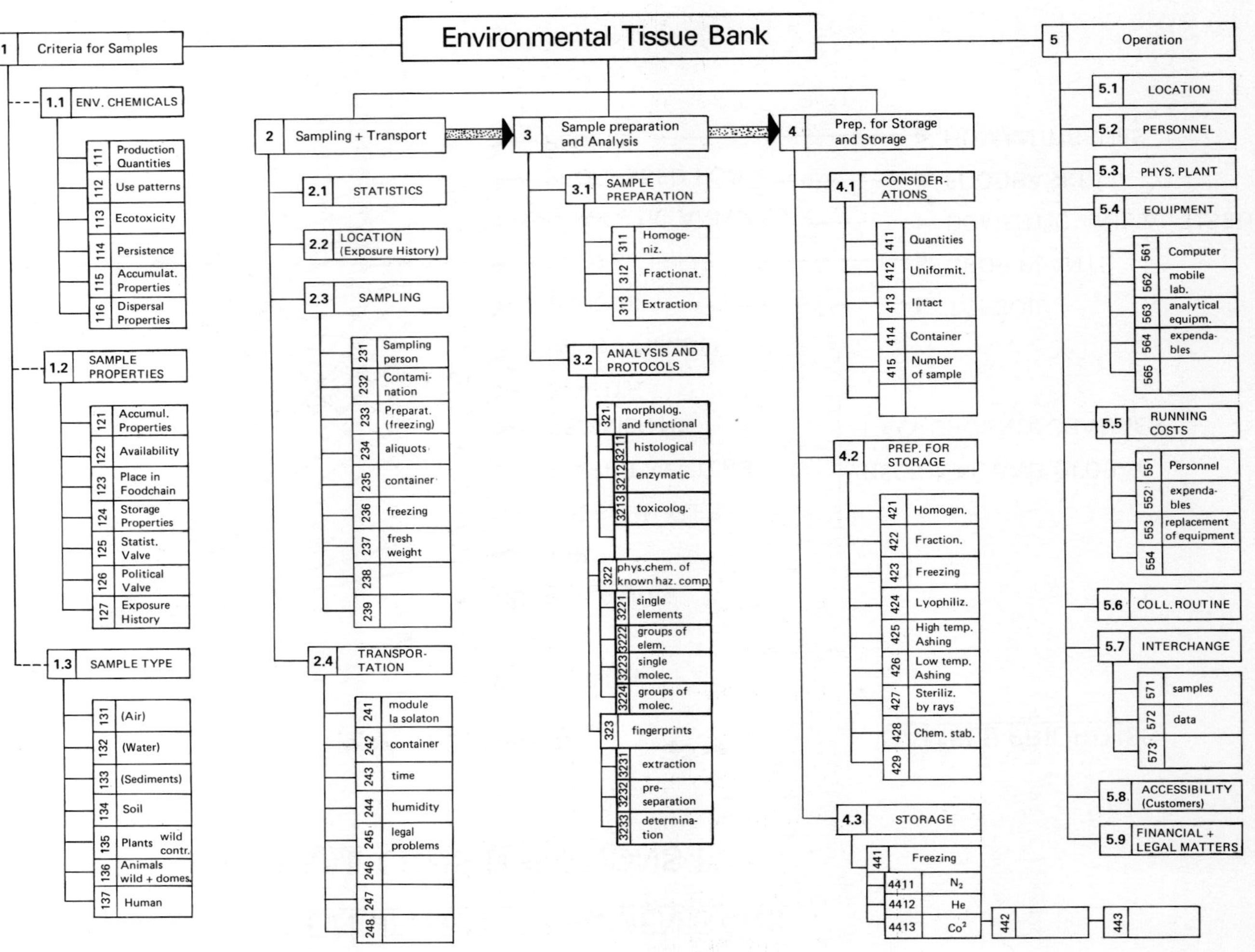

Environmental Tissue Bank

1 Criteria for Samples
1.1 ENV. CHEMICALS
111 Production Quantities
112 Use patterns
113 Ecotoxicity
114 Persistence
115 Accumulat. Properties
116 Dispersal Properties
1.2 SAMPLE PROPERTIES
121 Accumul. Properties
122 Availability
123 Place in Foodchain
124 Storage Properties
125 Statist. Valve
126 Political Valve
127 Exposure History
1.3 SAMPLE TYPE
131 (Air)
132 (Water)
133 (Sediments)
134 Soil
135 Plants wild contr.
136 Animals wild + domes.
137 Human

2 Sampling + Transport
2.1 STATISTICS
2.2 LOCATION (Exposure History)
2.3 SAMPLING
231 Sampling person
232 Contamination
233 Preparat. (freezing)
234 aliquots
235 container
236 freezing
237 fresh weight
238
239
2.4 TRANSPORTATION
241 module la solaton
242 container
243 time
244 humidity
245 legal problems
246
247
248

3 Sample preparation and Analysis
3.1 SAMPLE PREPARATION
311 Homogeniz.
312 Fractionat.
313 Extraction
3.2 ANALYSIS AND PROTOCOLS
321 morpholog. and functional
3211 histological
3212 enzymatic
3213 toxicolog.
322 phys.chem. of known haz. comp.
3221 single elements
3222 groups of elem.
3223 single molec.
3224 groups of molec.
323 fingerprints
3231 extraction
3232 pre-separation
3233 determination

4 Prep. for Storage and Storage
4.1 CONSIDERATIONS
411 Quantities
412 Uniformit.
413 Intact
414 Container
415 Number of sample
4.2 PREP. FOR STORAGE
421 Homogen.
422 Fraction.
423 Freezing
424 Lyophiliz.
425 High temp. Ashing
426 Low temp. Ashing
427 Steriliz. by rays
428 Chem. stab.
429
4.3 STORAGE
441 Freezing
4411 N2
4412 He
4413 Co2
442
443

5 Operation
5.1 LOCATION
5.2 PERSONNEL
5.3 PHYS. PLANT
5.4 EQUIPMENT
561 Computer
562 mobile lab.
563 analytical equipm.
564 expendables
565
5.5 RUNNING COSTS
551 Personnel
552 expendables
553 replacement of equipment
554
5.6 COLL. ROUTINE
5.7 INTERCHANGE
571 samples
572 data
573
5.8 ACCESSIBILITY (Customers)
5.9 FINANCIAL + LEGAL MATTERS

ENVIRONMENTAL SPECIMEN BANK

GENERAL CONSIDERATIONS I

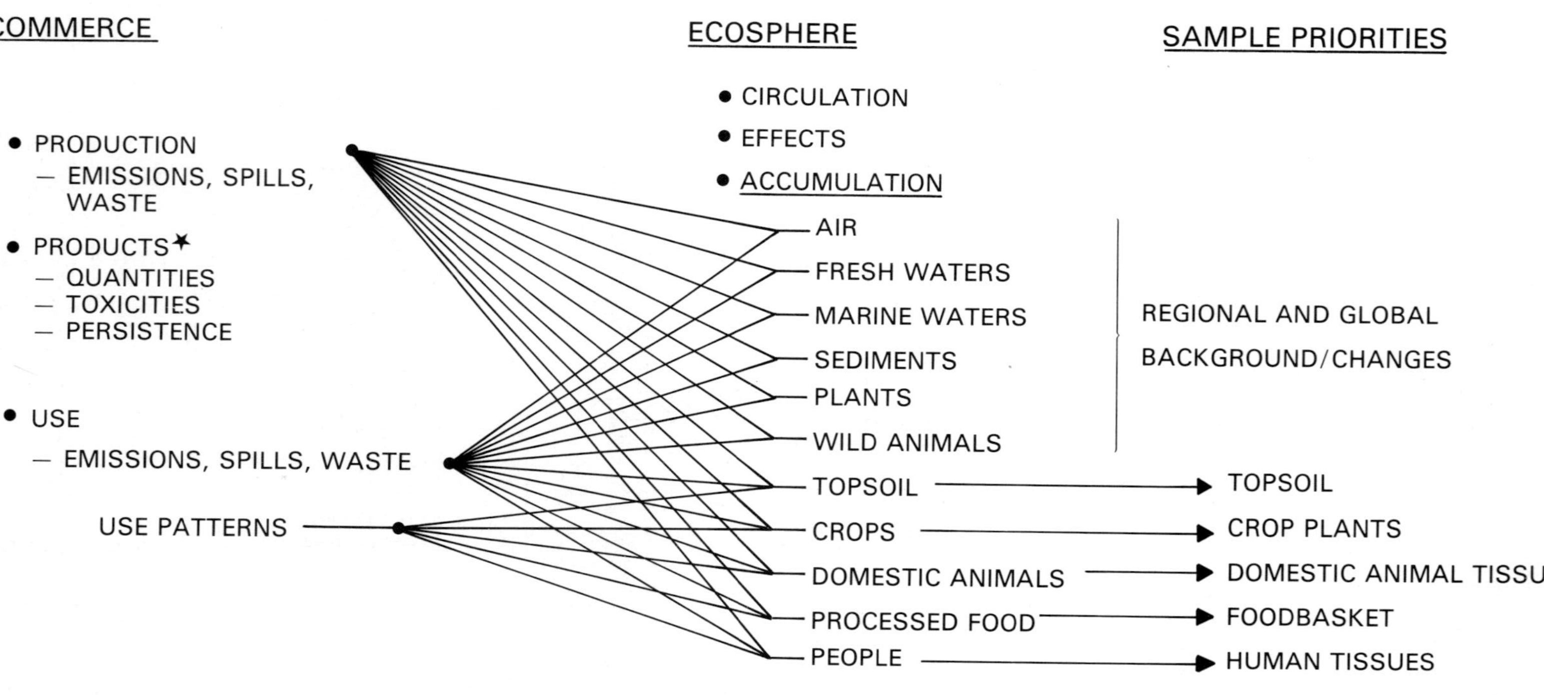

ENVIRONMENTAL SPECIMEN BANK

GENERAL CONSIDERATIONS II

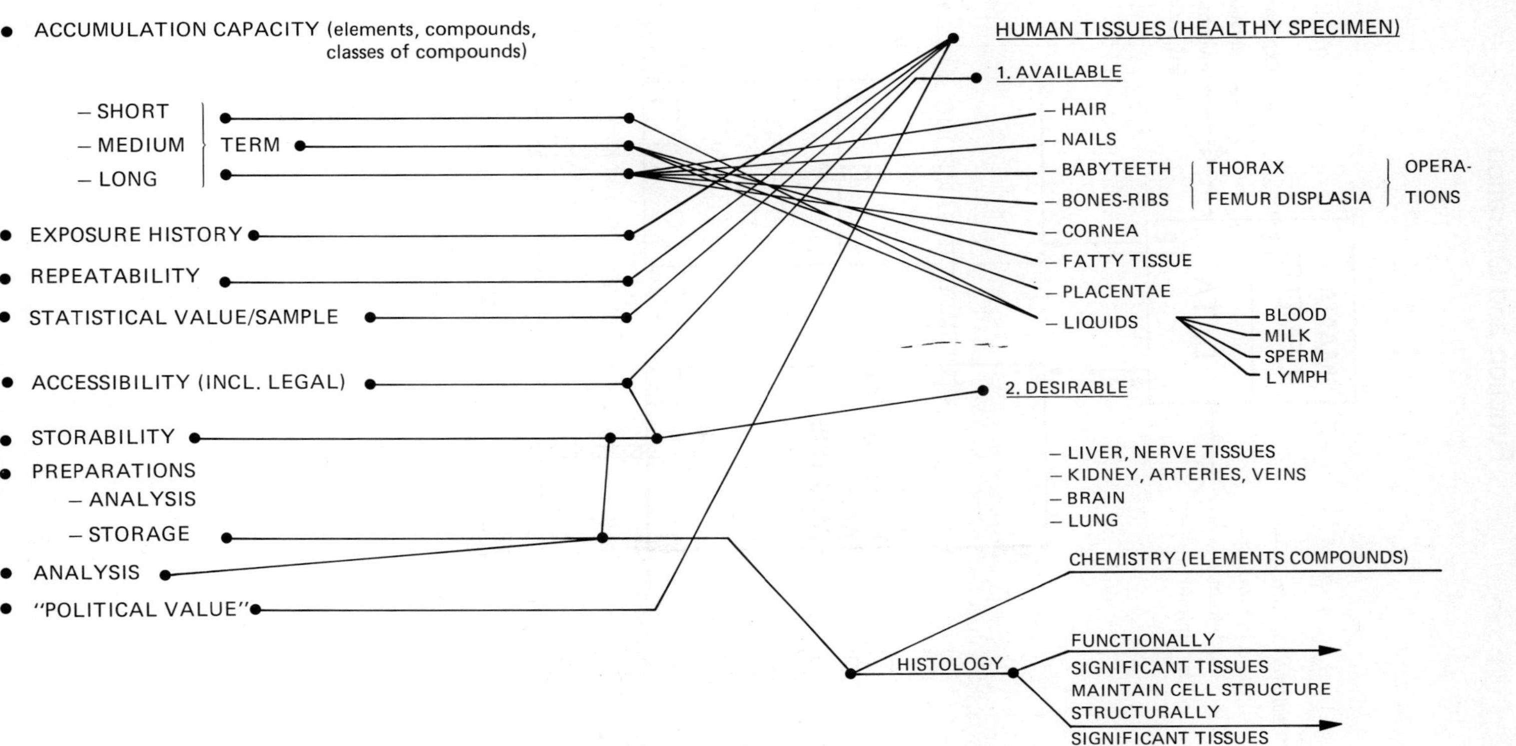

Environmental Specimen Bank
Function and Operation

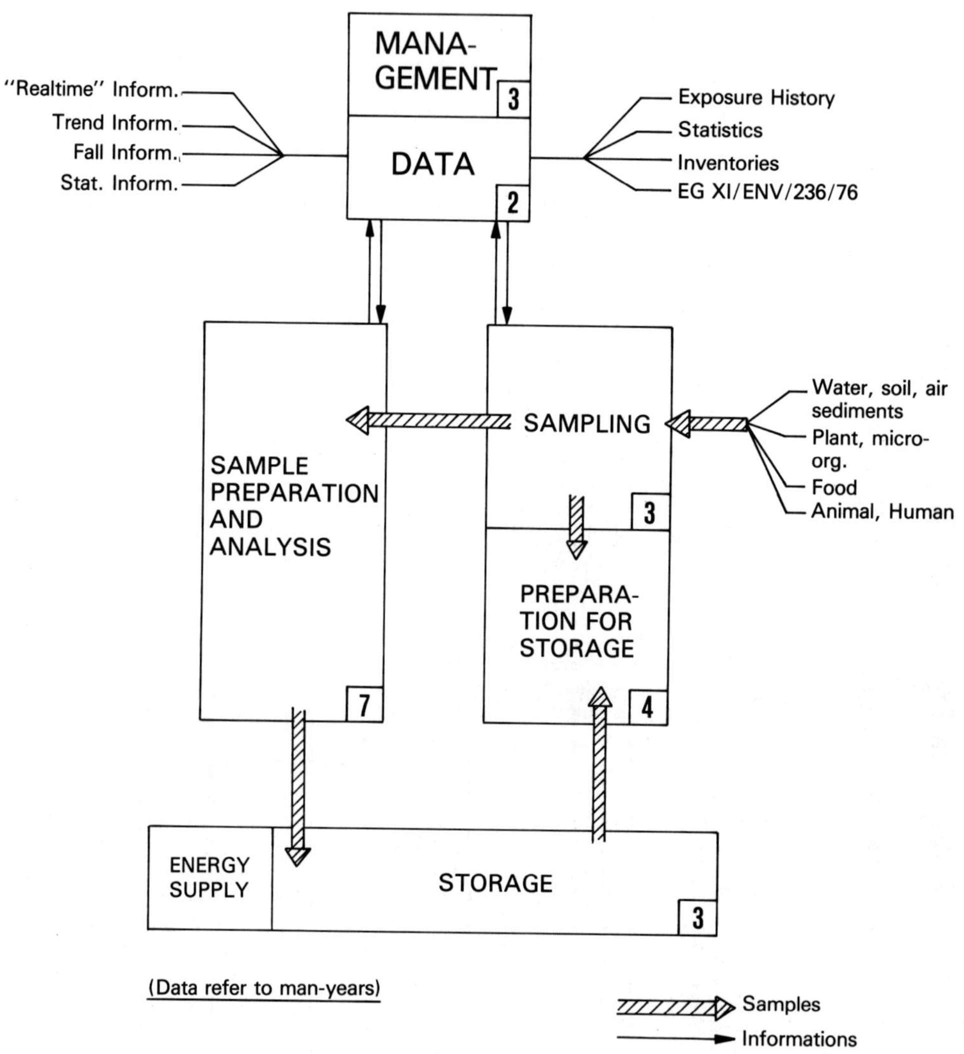

CRITICAL REVIEW OF ANALYTICAL METHODS FOR
THE DETERMINATION OF TRACE ELEMENTS IN BIOLOGICAL MATERIALS

M. Stoeppler and H. Nürnberg
Institute of Chemistry, KFA Jülich, F.R. Germany

Summary

The present situation in trace and ultratrace analysis is characterized by the frequent occurrence of severe systematic errors, as the disappointing and sometimes disastrous results of large-scale round robins have particularly demonstrated. These deficiencies in accuracy render questionable the reliability of a major amount of trace element data in various areas of environmental sciences and surveillance, including food control and occupational medicine. This general accuracy problem exists despite the fact that the tremendous advances in instrumental analysis during the last decades have made accessible, in principle, many new dimensions in trace analysis having predominant significance for environmental science and protection. The most urgent problem to be solved now is to obtain sufficiently accurate and precise data on an extended scale when the existing methods and instrumentation are utilized by the existing laboratories and their analytical staff. Certainly a necessary prerequisite is some change in the philosophy of general approach by those producing and those utilizing trace element data. The benefits without intolerable deficiencies in accuracy from highly advanced analytical instrumentation can only be gained if a comprehensive attitude on trace analytical problems is adopted, and all important working stages of a trace analytical procedure – sampling, sample storage, chemical pretreatment, instrumental measurements by the respective method, evaluation including data processing and statistics – are performed at an adequate high level of critical expertise. In this sense the principles and potentialities of the most important analytical methods for trace analysis are reviewed in a condensed manner emphasizing, based on our own long-term experiences in development and manifold applications, possible and necessary improvements in their future large-scale applications in routine environmental trace analysis.

1. Introduction

The turn of this century was characterized by a progressively intensified development of so-called instrumental analysis bringing a new dimension into analytical chemistry. Thus, trace methods became more and more accessible and indispensable for legal, medical, toxicological applications, and have gained increasing importance particularly within the last 20 years as regards environmental problems (1 - 5).

Numerous papers, dealing with recent advances, e.g. in the basic instrumental design and sensitivity and relating to new or improved multi-element methods, have appeared with nearly logarithmic growth rates up to the present day. A trend of efforts, focussed on the highest obtainable technical performance, linked with more and more improved detection limits, could be observed particularly from the middle of the forties onwards.

New methods such as neutron activation analysis and atomic absorption spectroscopy competed with basically older but recently improved approaches such as polarography, mass-, X-ray-, and emission spectroscopy, automated colorimetry and different chromatographic methods.

The instrument industry developed very sophisticated systems for the determination of trace elements and trace compounds. Thus an accelerated change from classical, e.g. manual, to instrumental methods took place. The wet, classical analysis, i.e. with gravimetric, titrimetric and colorimetric indication often based upon amplification reactions and carried out by skillful, well-trained specialized staff, in a limited number of laboratories, was replaced by methods applied in a more technical manner. At the same time equipment was introduced into numerous laboratories hitherto not experienced in trace determinations.

Though a certain amount of excellent analytical work with these methods was performed by laboratories with appropriate general analytical background, the vast increase in manufacture and sale of instruments resulted also in an immense production of mediocre data on all topics of essential and toxic elements. Unfortunately the results mentioned were often obtained by one single method which was not critically checked for systematic deviations and there was also a lack in knowledge of the possible error sources. Too many laboratories with limited experience, insufficiently trained staff, and sometimes poor additional instrumentation trusted too much upon a single advanced apparatus used in a 'black box' manner although it could be only operated successfully by analytical experts and in comparison with the results from other independent methods.

The fault of many manufacturers of analytical instruments was to ignore side problems and the urgent need for a steady and critical improvement of the knowledge on instrumental limitations. Of course, the manufacturers hoped by continuous discussion with the customers to obtain reliable suggestions on errors, creating the necessary feedback for improvements of apparatus and methods. But laboratories of the above described type — and a great percentage of customers belonged to this group — could not really contribute any valuable ideas due to their appreciable lack of experience and basic knowledge. On the other hand a number of analytical laboratories, well known for their excellent national and international standing, were frequently working away from the realistic necessities and occupied themselves by tackling particular problems connected with the further improvement of existing instrumentation, often to esoteric goals. Admittedly also methods of outstanding performance were developed and published in this context yet they could only be reproduced by the experts. Unfortunately those futuristic papers were often read by many scientists without particular experience and expertise in trace chemistry. Of course, attempts to adopt those expert approaches in their practical routine work failed frequently. Furthermore, the above mentioned kind of fundamental studies, which had doubtless the decisive merit of opening and exploring new dimensions and demonstrate the principal feasibility of new conceptions. Thus, the given values should have been considered by the customers for routine applications as guidelines only. By application to routine work they have to be carefully studied and critically adapted in all fields of research on trace elements (6, 7).

Efforts to obtain accurate data on a broad and routine scale which were started after the discovery of many contradictory results on toxic trace elements such as Pb, Cd and Hg etc. elucidated the above-discussed disastrous situation, emphasized particularly by the disappointing results of national and international round robin exercises: the experts were not very good at routine work, the routine laboratories could not reach the hitherto regarded as state of the art values of the experts. The data obtained are usually far from the expected acccuracy and precision limits (3, 7 - 18). Even at higher concentration levels unsuspected deviations are reported (19, 20).

In this review therefore the authors try to discuss the recent situation on the basis of more than 20 years experience on fundamentals of instrumental analysis and their extended applications in various fields of applied analytical and applied physical chemistry, treating in a condensed form the main potentialities and problems of modern trace analytical methods and their reliable applications.

There exist many excellent reviews on several of the before mentioned topics. The citation of only a part of them should merely be considered as an example and not as a judgement of publications not cited in the frame of this necessarily condensed contribution.

2.   Sampling and Sample Storage

The initial steps in trace and ultratrace analysis are very often responsible for erroneous results. They are the least spectacular but are the most important and most crucial stages.

Sampling has to be performed with all possible precautions with respect to contamination and also to conservation of original sample properties. All types of labware used have to be finitely low in the content of the trace elements to be analysed and clean conditions have to be established (5, 6). To obtain a reliable knowledge about contamination limits series of measurements of rinsing solutions have to be made to determine optimalized procedures for surface cleaning of sampling containers and labware and to select the material best suited to the desired purpose. From our experience (4, 6, 22 - 25, 72, 76, 77) reliable materials are quartz (suprasil^R), teflon, polyethylene, and sometimes polystyrene vessels. The storage temperature for biological samples should not exceed -50°C. For human and animal tissues, if possible taken fresh, the subsamples for later analysis should be divided at the same time and weighted and stored each in a single container. Usually one should refer to the fresh weight. If this is not possible an alternative common definition of sample weight is needed. This problem is under discussion and should be resolved as soon as possible. At present, the knowledge of storage conditions and disintegration rates of samples, particularly biological material, even at very low temperatures, has to be carefully tested to find out how long-term storage is possible and to learn about the optimal storage conditions with respect to original levels of trace elements, organometallics and organic compounds.

For various cases lyophylization followed by sterilization — as previously successfully applied to standard materials — should not be excluded for elements and some organic or organometallic compound(21). Long-term storage of aqueous solutions, e.g. potable and tap water, river and sea water, is now under study in Europe as well as in the USA. Our own research in this field has also been extensively performed during recent years on long-term reproducibility of analytical data in stored materials (4, 6, 22, 25, 26).

3. Sample Pretreatment

The preparation steps prior to analysis are manifold and numerous papers have been published and reviewed in the literature covering this item from the very important purification of re-agents (e.g. subboiling distillation of acids), to errors to be attributed to release and losses of elements from and at surfaces and to accuracy defects occurring in the various digestion and concentration (e.g. extraction) procedures (26 - 29). These procedures may introduce in the hands of inexperienced persons such a broad variety of errors that, for example, the develop-ment of a reliable digestion procedure for a respective matrix and one or more trace elements can only be performed successfully if independent methods are applied to elucidate the best conditions for minimizing all possible errors at this stage (5, 30). For standardization and rele-vant application the pretreatment procedures must be carefully checked by round robin exer-cises to obtain simple, but sufficiently accurate and precise methods to be applied in routine work (31, 32).

Furthermore, the finally chosen methods for general application must also be considered from an economical point of view.

4. Analytical Methods

We shall comment on the possibilities of the most important methods in the order from multi-via oligo- to single-element methods with respect to hitherto known applications and if neces-sary in connection with the above outlined sample pretreatment steps.

4.1 Multi-element Methods

Spark Source Mass Spectrometry is a very powerful tool for trace and ultratrace analysis with a comprehensive element coverage and a determination range down to 10^{-12} to 10^{-15} g (33, 34). Depending on the desired precision and accuracy the analysis is carried out by cor-relating the intensity of the respective element line to that of an internal matrix line or to that of the same line in a known standard or a series of standards if available.

The most accurate but time-consuming and cumbersome approach is to add known amounts of isotopes of the elements to be determined (isotope dilution).

In the last decades the method has been substantially improved by the introduction of electrical detection methods for multi- and single-element determinations (35) and computer interfacing enabling automatic evaluation of the resulting spectra and providing higher speed of analysis (36).

The method is extremely useful for fingerprint and ratio studies in the biological, environ-mental and forensic branches of science. Disadvantages are the until now relatively poor pre-cision and accuracy — with the exception of isotope dilution — the high costs for a complete system, and the dependence on reliable standards. Isotope dilution techniques could only be applied successfully if all precautions for extremely clean conditions were taken to minimize re-lease or loss of the respective elements during prior chemical preparation.

Neutron Activation with detection limits down to 10^{-14} g (or even lower in particular cases) is used for the sensitive simultaneous analysis of some 60 elements (37, 38). The prin-ciple of this method is the irradiation by a sufficiently high neutron flux of predominantly dry and undigested samples in a nuclear reactor. The resulting radioactivity of the respective radio-nuclides is then identified and quantitatively determined via the γ-spectra either directly or after chemical separation — mostly group separation — by a multichannel analyser frequently equipped now with coupled small on-line computers (39, 45).

The method is very useful for all kinds of fingerprint and ratio studies (46, 47) and offers an extraordinary approach for accurate determinations particularly in biological materials ser-ving as well to check less expensive methods as for base-line surveys.

Disadvantages are the dependence on reactor stations, the relatively high costs of irradiation facilities and γ-spectroscopic instrumentation and the problems connected with the processing of highly radioactive samples in expensive lead shielded cells. All these factors limit a broader use. Moreover, it is to be considered that this method cannot be used for the analysis of certain elements of particular biological and toxicological importance such as Pb. Also with Cd one faces difficulties. Finally the staff, applying these methods, has to be very carefully selected and trained as well from the viewpoint of radiochemical as of general ultra trace work.

Emission Spectroscopy, for decades successfully used in all research branches (48, 49), despite poor precision and accuracy, underwent recently a development which significantly enhances the signal-to-noise ratio by the introduction of plasma sources improving the detection limit drastically for about 35 elements to the 10^{-8} - 10^{-10} g range (50, 51). Due to very promising specific methods such as microwave-powered emission detectors (52), and the recently appearing computer-coupled systems it is to be expected that those methods might in the near future more and more replace at least the conventional flame atomic absorption method. At present the relatively expensive devices and not yet solved problems connected with excitation and resolving systems restrict their utilization to specialized laboratories which are able to improve commercially available instruments for trace analysis in the environmental field.

X-Ray Spectrometry, useful for single element analysis, has also significantly progressed. In the conventional wavelength - dispersive mode with the resolution of secondary emission by crystal goniometers considerable signal intensity (i.e. sensibility) is lost due to absorption. The energy-dispersive mode, however, uses a multichannel analyser for resolution and detection, thus avoiding severe losses of energy. Computerization permits in addition the simultaneous analysis of about 50 elements with detection limits down to 1 ppm or even less (49, 53, 54). Another new development is the equipment of the energy-dispersive systems with radiation sources (55), thus lowering the price for the whole unit significantly and also improving the detection limit compared with the before-mentioned versions of energy-dispersive systems.

Heavy ion-induced X-Ray Fluorescence improves the sensitivity up to about 10^{-15} g/cm^2 (56, 57) and seems to promise future applications even in ultratrace analysis.

As with other methods, X-ray fluorescence needs careful standardization and relating to conventional techniques, the application of preconcentration procedures, e.g. on ion exchanging materials such as surface accumulation. If all these factors are considered the method is, due to its good precision, very useful for fingerprints and elemental ratio studies (57). Grinding of nonhomogeneous materials may introduce contamination errors and should therefore be carefully checked.

4.2 Oligo- and Single-Element Methods

Conventional and Micro Colorimetric Methods are still in use predominantly in the ppm-range and in clinical chemistry (58). In environmental science the importance of these methods for metal constituents is decreasing, because they have no advantages compared with, for example, atomic absorption as detection approach. Only for nonmetallic compounds (e.g. iodine, nitrate, etc.) are these methods, often combined with catalytic action, still very useful.

Sometimes Gas Chromatography, for the determination of metal chelates, is successfully used (59). In environmental research this approach plays a distinct role for the determination and characterization of organomercurials after matrix-dependent clean-up procedures, particularly to distinguish between different forms of inorganic and organic mercury compounds (60, 61). The respective gas chromatographic modes seem, however, at present not to be precise enough to obtain for all matrices reliable ratios.

Polarographic and Voltammetric methods (62, 63) are of particular significance for various trace metals — Cd, Pb, Hg, Cu, Zn, As, Sb, Tl, V, etc. — and a wide variety of organic compounds of high environmental and toxicological importance. With respect to the required sensitivity advanced methods — at present mainly Pulse Polarography, in the future also very powerful 2nd order techniques (64) — are applied rather than conventional dc-polarography. While for monitoring organic traces in solutions direct measurements at various working electrodes (Hg, carbon paste) have to be made (63), the simultaneous determination of various trace metals is performed usually by different versions of Anodic Stripping voltammetry (ASV) (65, 66, 67) employing the hanging mercury drop, mercury film electrodes and the carbon paste electrode as working electrodes. The most powerful mode at present is differential pulse anodic stripping (DPASV) (22, 25, 68-77) particularly as a mercury film electrode (70-72, 76, 77).

Generally the polarographic and voltametric methods combine due to their foundation on Faraday's law — 1 mole of substance is equivalent to the enormous electrical charge of n.96500 Cb with n usually between 1 and 3 — extraordinary sensitivity with good precision and inherent accuracy. In this context it is to be emphasized also that they have the privilege to be based on a very detailed and comprehensive understanding of their physicochemical fundamentals, i.e. the kinetics and thermodynamics of electrode processes. This aspect offers for the electroanalytical expert manifold particular potentialities in trace analysis.

A further important specific property of the polarographic approach in solution trace chemistry is, however, that it is sensitive to the dissolved metal species and not only to the total elemental content. Thus, for studies on the trace metal levels (25, 67, 71, 75-77) and on their speciation (69, 73-76) in aquatic systems (inland waters, estuaries and seawater) advanced polarographic methods are frequently the definite method of choice due to the required sensitivity, the very limited amount of necessary sample pretreatment contributing significantly to established accuracy, and the specific potentialities for speciation. Employing the DPASV-mode at Hg-film electrodes detection limits of 10^{-3} µg/l, i.e. 1 ppt(!), have become accessible to routine determinations — a potentiality necessary if the normal levels of toxic trace metals dissolved in unpolluted inland waters and sea water are to be monitored with reliability (72, 76, 77).

Polarography and voltametry are also very well applicable to the determination of the elemental content of various trace metals down to the sub-ppb-range in a large variety of biological materials after prior ashing (22, 67, 68). Careful chemical pretreatment procedures eliminating contamination sources, volatization losses (e.g. by low temperature ashing (22) in oxygen plasma below 200°C) and adsorption losses (by using conditioned labware) are an indispensable prerequisite.

A general additional advantage of the polarographic approach is the relatively low price for even the most sophisticated instrumentation. The hitherto existing disadvantage in comparison to other methods of the more extended time for an analysis is now progressively disappearing with the broad introduction of automatisation and computerization into voltammetric analysis.

A further application of Mass Spectrometry as a high precision single element method down to the ng/kg-level is Isotope Dilution Mass Spectrometry with special equipment and thermal ionization techniques. This method reaches extremely accurate values and has been applied hitherto in environmental research besides the determination of isotopic composition predominantly for the analysis of lead in glacier ice, sea water, soil and tissue (6, 14, 78-80).

Disadvantages of this method are the very expensive devices, the time-consuming measurements and an extreme sensitivity to contamination. Such a method is therefore only successfully applicable if the laboratory staff is also well experienced generally in ultratrace chemistry and if other methods (e.g. flameless AAS and DPASV) are available for continuous control.

Conventional Flame and Flameless Atomic Absorption Spectroscopy (AAS) has been amply reviewed (81-83). The flameless methods requiring only milligram amounts of sample (if statistically permissible) offer extreme sensitivity down to 10^{-10} - 10^{-13} g and are applicable to the determination of about 60 elements, however, as a single element approach. Like the polarographic methods, AAS is for certain matrix types uniquely suitable for determinations of very low contents using flameless techniques with the so-called graphite tube or furnace (83) or special techniques, e.g. the cold vaporisation for Hg (24). If the samples contain large amounts of excess salts, as for instance many samples from the marine environment, prior separation of the trace metals by extraction is required to avoid interferences.

Recent developments of devices for automated sample introduction into the graphite tubes now commercially available have circumvented some former disadvantages, e.g. contamination by disposable pipette tips, improper manual dosage and a relatively low measuring capacity compared with the less sensitive but more precise flame AAS (84-87).

The first computer-controlled set-up is now under study (88).

The most obvious disadvantages of flameless AAS are spectral interferences in some critical wavelength regions and fluctuations in signal height due to hitherto not fully explained influences of the graphite composition (85, 86, 89-92). This renders it necessary to check measurements in the 10^{-9} to 10^{-12} g range for accuracy by independent methods, e.g. DPASV.

5. Final remarks

Most of the presented trace and ultratrace versions of instrumental analytical methods suffer generally from contamination or other important errors, e.g. losses due to volatisation or adsorption onto the walls of containers and vessels or onto filters. Therefore, uncritical routine procedures, if the working solutions contain the respective elements in the ng/ml to pg/ml range, may cause severe errors.

Thus, if possible, the continuous use of relevant standard materials is recommended for the reliable application of the described in principle very potent instrumental methods. If an appropriate standard is not available the running of a homogeneous sample material or a stable solution through the procedure has to be performed as often as possible to check at least random statistical fluctuations of signals and thus establish precision.

For the characterization of new or modified methods and the establishment of relative standard deviation ranges (RSD) the same sample must be run at least every day for 1-2 weeks. In this manner the long-term deviations of data become known and the resulting RSD may indicate if the method considered is precise enough for the desired purpose.

Standardization and studies on the elimination of systematic errors thus establishing accuracy must additionally be performed in routine work by the **application of at least two independent methods to the same samples or subsamples.** If this is to be carried out unbiased in the same institute its participating laboratories have to work absolutely blind (4, 93).

A last check should be made in cooperation with one or more laboratories. The performance of larger round robin exercises should be continued in the future, but as the encouraging comparisons of results from experienced and well equipped laboratories have revealed one can, only if participation is restricted to laboratories of comparable level, expect at present, with higher probability, relevant information on the achievable degree of accuracy of the respective trace analytical data. The inclusion of laboratories of significantly different levels in experience and equipment in round robins will always inherently implement the danger to miss the goal. Unfortunately a successful round robin by laboratories of high qualification will not necessarily solve the more general problem of immediately improving accuracy of the analytical output of the numerous routine laboratories trying to adopt the respective method. This fundamental problem in applied trace chemistry can be only overcome via a broad-scale rise in the level of trace analytical work due to long-term efforts in better training and education of a sufficient number of staff. Meanwhile, more laboratories with a now already sufficient standing and equipment at research centres, universities and in industry should be more encouraged by special grants and programs to direct their efforts to the numerous practical trace analytical topics which are a challenging and attractive key task to establish a relevant basis for the solution of urgent problems in environmental research and protection and in food and health control for the benefit of man.

REFERENCES

1. LAITINEN, H.A. Analyst, **99**, 1011 (1974).
2. HAMILTON, E.F. Sci. Total Environment 3, 3 (1974).
3. TOELG, G. Erzmetall, **28**, 390 (1973).
4. NUERNBERG, H.W., M. STOEPPLER, P. VALENTA. Thalassia Jugoslavica, **11**, 85 (1975).
5. HAMILTON, E.I. Sci. Total Environment 5, 1 (1976).
6. STOEPPLER, M., F. BACKHAUS, R. DAHL, M. DUMONT, H. HAGEDORN GOETZ, K. HILPERT, P. KLAHRE, H. RUETZEL, P. VALENTA, H. W. NUERNBERG. Proc. Int. Symp., Recent Advances in the Assessment of the Health Effects of Environmental Pollution, Paris, 24-28 June 1974, Commission of the European Communities, Luxembourg 1975, p.2231.
7. TOELG, G. Naturwissenschaften, **63**, 99, 1976.
8. KEPPLER, J.F., M.W. MAXFIELD, W.D. MOSS, G. TIETJEN, A.D. LINCH. Am. Ind. Hyg. Ass. Journ., 412 (1970).
9. DONOVAN, D.Th., V.M. VOUGHT, A.B. RAKOW. Arch. Environm. Health, **23**, 111 (1971).
10. HOSCHEK, R., H.J. SCHITTKE. Zbl. Arbeitsmed., 243 (1973).
11. FIORINO, J.A., R.A. MOFFITT, W.L. WOODSON, R.J. GAJON, G.E. HUSKEY, R.G. SCHOLZ. J. Ass. Offic. Anal. Chemists, **56**, 1246 (1973).

12. KJELLSTROEM, T., B. LIND, L. LINNMAN, G. NORDBERG.   Environmental Research 8, 92 (1974).
13. HEINONEN, J., O. SUSCHNY.   J. Radioanal. Chem. 20, 499 (1974).
14. Workshop participants and advisor, Meeting Report, Marine Chemistry, 2, 69 (1974).
15. BOWEN, H.J.M.   J. Radioanal. Chem. 19, 215 (1974).
16. BLACK, L.T.   J.Am.Oil Chemists Soc. 52,88 (1973).
17. LAUWERYS, R., J.P. BUCHET, H. ROELS, A. BERLIN, J. SMEETS.   Clin. Chem. 21, 551 (1975).
18. IAEA Report No. 1, Intercomparison of Trace and other Elements in Animal Muscle, H-4, June 1976.
19. KINGSFORD, M. C.D. STEVENSON, W.H.L. EDGERLEY.   New Zealand Journal of Science, 16, 895 (1973).
20. FAYE, G.H., W.S. BOWMAN, R. SUTARO.   Anal. Chim. Acta, 67, 202 (1973).
21. LAFLEUR, P.D.   J. Radioanal. Chem. 19, 227 (1974).
22. VALENTA, P., H. RUETZEL, H.W. NUERNBERG, M. STOEPPLER. Z.Anal. Chem. (in press).
23. MATTHES, W., M. STOEPPLER.   Z. Anal. Chem. 281, 141 (1976).
24. STOEPPLER, M., M. BERNHARD, F. BACKHAUS, E. SCHULTE.   Rapports et Procès-Verbaux, XXV. Congress and Plenary Assembly ICSEM, Split, October 1976.
25. VALENTA, P., L. MART, H.W. NUERNBERG, M. STOEPPLER.   Jahrbuch 'Vom Wasser', im Druck.
26. MIZUIKE, A., in Trace Analysis: Physical Methods, G.H. Morrison, ed., Interscience, New York, 1965, pp. 103-159.
27. GORSUCH, T.T.   The Destruction of Organic Matter, Pergamon, New York, 1970.
28. TOELG, G.   Talanta, 19, 1489 (1972).
29. TOELG, G.   Talanta, 21, 327 (1974).
30. ADER, D., M. STOEPPLER.   Report to IUPAC Commission on Toxicology, 1976, to be published in Clin. Chem.
31. GOJAN, R.J., J.H. GOULD, J.O. WATTS, J.A. FIORINO.   J.Assoc.Offic.Anal.Chemists 56, 876 (1973).
32. PORTER, W.K. Jr.   J. Assoc. Offic. Anal. Chemists 57, 614 (1974).
33. EVANS, C.A. Jr., G.A. MORRISON.   Appl. Spectrosc. 40, 869 (1968).
34. AHEARN, A.J., Ed.   Trace Analysis by Mass Spectrometry, Academic Press, New York, 1972.
35. BINGHAM, R.A., R.M. ELLIOTT.   Anal. Chem. 43, 43 (1971).
36. BROWN, R., P. POWERS, W.A. WOLSTENHOLME.   Anal. Chem. 43, 1076 (1971).
37. DESOETE, D., R. GIJBELS, R. HOSTE.   Neutron Activation Analysis, New York, Wiley-Interscience 1972.
38. ERDTMANN, G., H.W. NUERNBERG, in F. Korte, ed., Methodicum Chimicum, Vol. 1B, Academic Press, New York 1974, pp. 735-792.
39. SAMSAHL, K.   Sci. Total Environment, 1, 65 (1972).
40. PILLAY, K.K.S., C.C. THOMAS, Jr., C.M. HYCHE.   J. Radioanal. Chem. 20, 579 (1974).
41. ERDTMANN, G., O. ABOULWAFA.   Z. Anal. Chem. 270, 1 (1974).
42. ERDTMANN, G., O. ABOULWAFA.   Z. Anal. Chem. 272, 105 (1974).
43. DIEHL, J.F., R. SCHELENZ.   Lebensm.-Wiss. u. Technol. 8, 154 (1975).
44. STEINNES, E.   Anal. Chim. Acta, 78, 307 (1975).
45. GANDRY, A., B. MAZIERE, D. COMAR.   J. Radioanal. Chem. 29, 77 (1976).
46. FORSLEV, A.W.   J. Forensic Sciences, 11, 217 (1966).
47. ERDTMANN, G., O. ABOULWAFA, H. MERGLER, C. WEISLEDER, G. GUELDEN-BERG.   KFA-Report, Jül-Conf. 11(3), 19 (1974).
48. BEDROSIAN, A.J., R.K. SKOGERBOE, G.H. MORRISON.   Anal.Chem. 40, 854 (1968).
49. COWGILL, U.M.   Appl. Spectrosc. 27, 5 (1973).
50. MERMET, J.M., J. ROBIN.   Anal. Chim. Acta, 70, 271 (1975).
51. FASSEL, V.A., R.N. KNISELEY.   Anal. Chem., 46, 1110A (1974).
52. McCORMECK, A.J., S.S.C. TONG, W.D. COOKE.   Anal. Chem. 37, 1470 (1975).
53. RHODES, J.R., A.H. PRADZYNSKI, C.B. HUNTER, J.S. PAYNE, J.L. LINDGREN.   Environm. Sci. Technol. 6, 922 (1972).
54. LONG, R.A.   Am. Ind. Hyg. Ass. J., 33, 343 (1972).
55. WOLDSETTA, R.   X-Ray Energy Spectrometry, Burlingame, Calif. Kevex 1973.

56. JOHANSSON, T.B., R. AKSELSSON, S.A.E. JOHANSSON.   Nucl. Instrum. Methods, **84**, 141 (1970).
57. VALKOVIC, V. D. RENDIC, G.C. PHILLIPS.   Environm. Sci. Techn., **9**, 1150 (1975).
58. ROEHLE, G., G. OBERHOFFER, H. BREUER.   Dt.Ges.Klin.Chemie Mitt., 7, 32 (1976).
59. KAISER, G., E. GRALLATH, P. TSCHOEPEL, G. TOELG.   Z. Anal. Chem., **259**, 257 (1972).
60. JOHANSSON, B., R. RYHAGE, G. WESTÖÖ, Act. Chem. Scand., **24**, 6 (1970).
61. WESTÖÖ, G., Act. Chem. Scand., **21**, 1790 (1967).
62. NUERNBERG, H.W., ed.:   Electroanalytical Chemistry, J. Wiley, New York, 1974.
63. NUERNBERG, H.W., B. KASTENING, in F. Korte, ed., Methodicum Chimicum, Vol. 1A, Academic Press, New York, 1974, pp. 584-607.
64. BARKER, G.C., Proc. Anal. Div. Chem. Soc. (London) **12**, 179 (1975).
65. NEEB, R.   Inverse Polarographie und Voltammetrie, Verlag Chemie Weinheim 1969.
66. BRAININA, Kh.Z., Stripping Voltammetry in Chemical Analysis, J. Wiley, New York 1974.
67. FLORENCE, T.M.   J. Electroanal. Chem. 27. 273 (1970); **35**, 237 (1972).
68. COPELAND, T.R., H.J. CHRISTIE, R.A. OSTERYOUNG, R.K. SKOGERBOE.   Anal. Chem. **45**, 2171 (1973); **46**, 2093 (1974).
69. ERNST, R., H.A. ALLEN, K.H. MANCY, Water Research 9, 969 (1975).
70. JOENSSON, H., Z. Lebensm.-Unters. Forsch. **160**, 1 (1976).
71. NUERNBERG, H.W., Electrochim. Acta, in press.
72. VALENTA, P., L. MART, H. RUETZEL.   Electrochim. Acta, in press.
73. RASPOR, B., P. VALENTA, H.W. NUERNBERG, M. BRANICA.   Sci. Total Environment, in preparation.
74. SIPOS, L., P. VALENTA, H.W. NUERNBERG, M. BRANICA.   Marine Chemistry, in preparation.
75. NUERNBERG, H.W., P. VALENTA, in E.D. Goldberg, Ed., The Nature of Seawater, Dahlem-Konferenzen, Berlin 1975, pp. 87-136.
76. NUERNBERG, H.W., P. VALENTA, L. MART, B. RASPOR, L. SIPOS.   Z. Anal. Chem., in press.
77. NUERNBERG, H.W., L. MART, P. VALENTA, M. STOEPPLER.   Thalassia Jugoslavica, in press.
78. MUROZUMI, M., T.J. CHOW, C. PATTERSON.   Geochim. Cosmochim. Acta 33, 1247 (1969).
79. PATTERSON, C.C.   Report Concerning Public Health Hazard of Industrial Lead Pollution, 1974.
80. TERA, F., G.J. WASSERBURG.   Anal. Chem. **47**, 2214, 1974.
81. SLAVIN, W., S. SLAVIN.   Appl. Spectrosc. **23**, 421 (1969).
82. BERMAN, E.   Appl. Spectrosc. **29**, 1 (1975).
83. WELZ, B.   Atomic Absorption Spectroscopy, Verlag Chemie, Weinheim, engl. ed. 1976.
84. PICKFORD, C.J., G. ROSSI.   Analyst, **97**, 647,(1972).
85. DAHL, R., M. STOEPPLER.   Ber.d.KFA Jülich, Jül-1254, 1975.
86. STOEPPLER, M., M. KAMPEL, B. WELZ.   Z. Anal. Chem., 1976, in press.
87. STOEPPLER, M., M. KAMPEL.   Ber.d.KFA, Jülich, Nov. 1976.
88. STOEPPLER, M., D. MAECKELBURG, M. SCHULZE-FRENKING, M. KAMPEL.   Z. Anal. Chem., in preparation.
89. MAESSEN, F.J.M.J., F.D. POSMA.   Anal. Chem. **46**, 1439 (1974).
90. MASSMAN, H., S. GUEGER.   Spectrochim. Acta, 29B, 283 (1974).
91. CULVER, B.R., T. SURLES.   Anal. Chem. **47**, 920 (1973).
92. REGAN, J.G.T., J. WARREN.   Analyst, **101**, 220 (1976).
93. STOEPPLER, M., K. BRANDT, H. RUETZEL, P. VALENTA.   Sci. Total Environment, in preparation.

BIOLOGICAL MONITORING OF CHEMICAL POLLUTANTS IN THE GENERAL POPULATION IN JAPAN WITH SPECIAL REFERENCE TO CADMIUM, LEAD, AND MERCURY

K. Tsuchiya
Department of Preventive Medicine and Public Health, Keio University, Tokyo

Abstract

Biological monitoring has two purposes. First, the detection of possible effects of an environmental chemical on human health when excessive exposure to the chemical is detected at an early stage. In such a case, short-term biological monitoring is conducted in order to detect those persons whose toxic levels exceed the normal range. For this purpose, semi-quantitative determination of the chemical is adequate. The second purpose of biological monitoring is to observe changes in body burden in long-term exposure. In this case, accurate and sensitive determination of environmental chemicals in biological specimens is essential since slight decreases or increases must be detected.

For both short- and long-term biological monitoring of lead, blood is the best indicator of exposure and total body burden in living humans. Bone and aorta are pertinent post mortem specimens for long-term monitoring. Urine is the best indicator of cadmium in humans. Faeces are good for determining the level of exposure to cadmium via food. In post mortem specimens, both kidney and liver are the organs which show high accumulations of the element. Hair and blood are good indicators which reflect the exposure to or body burden of mercury. As for post mortem specimens, brain is the tissue best used for mercury monitoring. Non-human biological specimens should also be checked in both short- and long-term monitorings.

The best systematic biological monitoring is possible only by the establishment of a monitoring centre in each country. Collection and storage of specimens and data analysis and evaluation should be performed periodically by such a centre. It is recommended that such a biological monitoring centre be established associated with an already existing health organization in each country.

Introduction

Biological monitoring of chemicals such as lead, mercury, and cadmium has been conducted for many years on occupationally exposed workers in Japan. The purpose of this type of biological monitoring is to detect excessive exposure and its effects on the health of workers at an early stage. Industrial monitoring is usually performed periodically based on the laws and regulations established by the national and local governments. Regulations for the biological monitoring of pollutants in the general population have not yet been established in Japan although determinations of such pollutants as mercury, lead, and cadmium in various human specimens, including tissues and organs of autopsy cases, have been carried out in administrative investigations as well as in private research projects. However, when environmental pollution by any of these chemicals occurs or is suspected, extensive investigations of the chemical contents in various biological specimens are performed on the inhabitants involved. The following discussion is based on the considerable experience with environmental pollution which has occurred in Japan. The monitoring of industrial workers, however, is not included.

A.   Review of past and current programs

There are many studies including official administrative investigations which have been performed in Japan since environmental pollution due to mercury, lead, and cadmium has occurred in many areas in the past and present.

When methyl mercury poisoning occurred in the Minamata and Niigata areas in 1955, it was reported that hair was the best indicator of exposure with the added advantage that samples are very easy to collect. Since that time a great many studies and administrative reports have used hair from highly exposed persons as well as from those with no known high exposure for the determination of mercury content. Among the general population, it was discovered that the crews of large fishing boats (particularly those fishing tuna) and employees in restaurants specializing in the preparation of 'sushi', (a favourite in the Japanese diet, consisting of seafood and rice) and workers in fish markets showed high concentrations of mercury in hair (up to about 10 times those of the rest of the population). The monitoring of mercury in hair has been performed in polluted areas such as Minimata and Niigata. Fish is also a widely used specimen in the biological monitoring of mercury throughout Japan. Mercury contents in normal human tissues have been determined by Kitamura et al (1). However, there is no program in Japan for the storing of either hair or fish for future reference.

Biological monitoring of lead has been performed by the Tokyo metropolitan government. In 1970 and 1971, blood samples were collected from those inhabitants of Tokyo who expressed desire to be examined for possible effects of lead in the ambient air. About 3,000 subjects appeared for the examination. Since 1974, the Tokyo metropolitan government has been checking blood lead levels in school children from urban and suburban Tokyo, but these checks are arbitrary in the choice and location of subjects and small in scale. This program is still in progress.

There are approximately ten areas polluted by cadmium throughout Japan. Cadmium concentrations in urine of inhabitants from both polluted and nonpolluted areas have been determined in the past and present by the national government (2) and by numerous authors (3, 4). Cadmium concentrations in post mortem tissues and organs from coroner's autopsy cases in Tokyo have been determined by the present author (3). Two other studies similar in nature have been performed in Kobe and Kanazawa (5). Determinations of cadmium in faeces of some inhabitants from three polluted areas are now in the planning stages by the Japan Environment Agency.

A large-scale project supported by the Ministry of Health and Welfare has just been completed this year (6). The project included the determinations of chlorinated hydrocarbons such as PCB and DDT, as well as lead, cadmium, zinc, copper, mercury, chromium and other heavy metals in post mortem tissues and organs from 8 blocs throughout Japan.

The obstacles in carrying out such projects are numerous. First of all, the availability of financial sponsorship is limited. Second, a national government must have good reason for performing such determinations, and in large nationwide investigations, the coordination among the various institutes and organizations involved is often very difficult. Third, blood samples are not always easy to obtain from those persons chosen as subjects according to a study design. Fourth, when several organizations are required to cooperate in a study, analytical variations have led to difficulties in the evaluation of the results.

B.   Rationale for interest or concern and indicators of exposure or body burden

Public concern is an important factor in carrying out investigations of environmental chemicals. The inhabitants of nonpolluted areas are often not concerned with pollution by a given chemical and it sometimes becomes extremely difficult to collect samples from a control population.

Among the heavy metals, mercury, lead and cadmium are highest in priority for biological monitoring and for sample collection for future reference because of the magnitude of the use of these metals and their importance to an industrialized society.

For lead, blood is the best biological specimen for monitoring exposure in living humans, but bone or aorta are possibly the best post mortem indicators since lead in these tissues increases in an almost straight linear pattern with age. According to available data, blood lead levels in the Japanese people, particuarly children, are lower than people from the United States (7, 8).

For mercury, hair is the best indicator of exposure and accumulation of the element in the human body. Blood is also another specimen which gives a good indication of mercury exposure. However, because of its ease in collection, hair is the specimen most frequently used. Mercury levels in both the cerebrum and cerebellum correlate well with mercury levels in hair (9). For future reference, not only hair, but fish (a representative species from freshwater and from sea water) selected for age and size are also good indicator specimens since the main source of mercury intake is fish. The appropriate species would, of course, differ by country.

As for cadmium, its level in urine is the best indicator of the total body burden in living humans. However, the highest level of cadmium is always found in the renal cortex, except for those persons who suffer from renal diseases, since such persons generally show low cadmium levels in the kidney. The liver is another organ in which a great deal of cadmium accumulates. In those persons who have suffered renal changes in the past due to cadmium, the cadmium level in the liver remains high. Faeces are another good indicator of exposure to cadmium via ingestion. Rice or wheat can absorb up to 3-4 ppm cadmium when soil is highly contaminated by cadmium. These grains are good specimens which can be stored for future reference. B_2-microglobulin in urine is an indirect indicator of increased levels of cadmium exposure. However, this protein is not specific to cadmium poisoning, but increased levels are normally found among the aged. Urine may also be stored for future reference, but the storage of large volumes of urine may not be practical or economical. However, if a very sensitive RI method is used for the determination of B_2-microglobulin, only a small amount of urine is required. Also a flameless AAS method requiring only a few drops of urine has been developed for the determination of cadmium in routine analyses.

According to available data, cadmium levels in the organs and total body burden of the Japanese people in general are about three times higher than those of the Swedish people in nonpolluted areas (10).

C.   Sample collection and storage

As mentioned above in Part B, the best indicator of exposure or body burden differs by metal. However, the same biological specimen may be used for simultaneous determinations of lead, mercury, cadmium and other metals. In order to save time, space, and expense, simultaneous determination using the same sample should be considered, especially in the storage of samples for future reference. Spot sampling of both urine and faeces may include disadvantages, e.g. the spot samples may not necessarily represent the actual amount of total daily excretion of a given chemical. On the other hand, biological monitoring is performed to measure the grade of exposure or accumulation on a group basis, and this disadvantage may be made up for determining mercury concentration.

Disposable syringes for drawing blood usually contain negligible amounts of lead, mercury, or cadmium. However, special lead-free vacuum syringes are available on the market. Organ specimens preserved in formalin solution are usually not adequate for the determination of these three metals because of elution of the metals into the formalin and the possible contamination of the formalin itself from other sources before the specimens are put into it. The storage of organs in formalin is not recommended for the biological monitoring of metals even if metal-free formalin is used. To store biological specimens for short-term monitoring, the specimens should be frozen as quickly as possible after collection at temperatures below -20°C. For long-term monitoring, the specimens should be freeze dried, but the wet weight should be clearly recorded before the freeze drying procedure is carried out.

The polyethylene bottle has been widely used for the storage of biological specimens. No significant problems have been reported in its usage. Tight sealing of the bottles is, of course, necessary to prevent evaporation.

D.   Analytical procedures

According to the specific purpose of the biological monitoring, different analytical methods for a given metal can be used. For example, if the purpose of biological monitoring is to detect an excessive level of the metal, a method with low sensitivity may be used. However, if the purpose is to determine quantitative amounts in the normal range, a method with very high sensitivity and specificity and accuracy should be employed.

Since analytical procedures improve almost daily, the method, the amount of specimens required for determination, and pretreatment are and will be quite different as time progresses. Even at the present time, the pretreatment required differs according to the method used. In order to determine the contents of lead, mercury and cadmium, atomic absorption spectrometry (AAS) or flameless AAS are the best and most commonly used methods. There are several other methods suitable for the determination of lead in biological materials, e.g. anodic stripping voltametry (ASV). However, a single method should be selected for use, particularly in cases where more than one institution is involved in a common project. Even if a single method is used by several laboratories, numerous reference specimens should be kept stored so checks can be repeated by all the laboratories throughout the duration of long-term projects.

Methyl mercury in brain and hair usually makes up over 50% of the total mercury. However, according to the experience of the large-scale project of the Ministry of Health and Welfare mentioned in Part A, it seems that the determination of the total mercury is sufficient for the purpose of biological monitoring because low-level methyl mercury contents vary according to the method used. For the determination of total mercury in urine, unpretreated samples can be handled by an AAS method devised especially for the determination of total mercury which can detect levels as low as $0.2\mu g/100ml$ (11).

The sensitivity of the detection of cadmium in biological specimens by the AAS method is about 0.01 ppm. The flameless AAS method requires much smaller volumes of samples than regular AAS, but at present reports using this method are few in number. Flameless AAS for the determination of cadmium may be more frequently used in the future. Background correction is not necessary for urine, organs, and other biological specimens (except blood). The cadmium levels in blood of the general population with no known high exposure still vary greatly, most probably because of the analysis factor and because of low cadmium levels in blood which are difficult to analyse. Emission spectrography may be too costly at this time for routine biological monitoring. According to available reports, fairly good agreement of the values for urinary lead levels has been obtained among various laboratories using routine AAS after wet ashing and extraction, but sometimes there exist great discrepancies among laboratories in the results on test samples. Cadmium determinations in human organs and tissues as well as in rice and wheat have shown fairly good agreement in the results obtained from laboratories from Japan and Sweden in a cooperative study (AAS after extraction being the principal method used) (12).

E.   Program design.
1.   Living humans

Programs for biological monitoring may be quite different according to the situation, e.g. if environmental pollution is brought to the attention of the public or if it is a question of simple routine monitoring. In the case where environmental pollution is known by the public, ideally, all the inhabitants of the area should be included in the investigation. If the total population in question is too large, however, a sampling of subjects from target population should be carefully chosen according to type of pollution. Thus, in a case of lead pollution, for instance, the younger population may be more important to monitor than the older because of the higher susceptibility of the central nervous system of young children to lead. On the other hand, for cadmium, according to the experience in Japan, it is the older age groups which indicate possible renal dysfunction due to cadmium.

However, it is sometimes extremely difficult to select a target population following a program design. When a report of possible lead poisoning among the inhabitants of Tokyo appeared in the newspapers (although it was later confirmed that the report was not correct), only those people who were concerned about possible lead effects were willing to undergo a health examination. The investigators were not able to obtain samples from the inhabitants according to their study design.

Another problem in collecting blood samples is that some individuals will not participate in such a study due to fear of the hypodermic needle and some refuse on the basis that they do not wish to be 'guinea pigs'. For blood lead determinations as mentioned under Part D, there are methods such as ASV and the filter disc method using flameless AAS, but it is still difficult to obtain blood samples from children. For routine monitoring purposes, it is often difficult to obtain the cooperation of parents and children. However, in the United States thousands of children were subjects for the detection of possible lead poisoning. In these projects, ASV requiring only a few drops of blood was used. It seems that the population was very cooperative.

Concerning the information on an individual's personal history, biological specimen, and environment, age, sex, years of residence in the same location, smoking history and medical history, and in the case of lead, whether he or she has or has had pica, are important. Also in the case of lead, samples of placenta can be stored for future reference. For cadmium, the above plus cadmium concentration in rice or wheat in the area in question are important, and for mercury, mercury concentration in fish in the area plus the amount of fish consumed should be checked. It is not necessary to inquire about smoking in mercury monitoring. As mentioned above, hair samples for monitoring mercury are easy to collect, thus making it easier to follow a program design.

For continuous routine biological monitoring, it is suggested that each country establish a biological monitoring centre which selects certain areas for monitoring as necessary. The target populations should be carefully chosen following a clearly designed program and the monitoring should be performed consistently over a period of many years.

2.   Post mortem specimens

In the above-mentioned monitoring project of the Japanese Ministry of Health and Welfare, it was discovered that it is very difficult to collect post mortem specimens from younger age groups, since proportionately fewer people die young. In order to obtain the same number of specimens from all age groups, the program was designed to collect 8 specimens from each sex for each 10-year age group. In this project, Japan was divided into 8 blocs, and some blocs were unable to collect post mortem specimens from the 0–10 year-old group. In the study, specimens were taken from persons who had died of various diseases, including cancer. The report on this study includes discussion on whether these diseases affect the concentrations of heavy metals on the organs.

Ideally, post mortem specimens from coroner's autopsy cases and accidental deaths should be used to avoid possible influence of any long-term diseases on the accumulation of toxic metals, but this is often unfeasible. This is true especially in outlying regions of Japan where coroner's autopsies are often not very thorough.

F.   Organizational aspects

Since the cost of collecting and storing specimens, as well as of determining concentrations and data processing is considerable, governmental support will most probably be necessary when establishing a permanent biological monitoring centre. If biological monitoring is conducted sporadically by numerous organizations, it will not serve the purposes of long-term monitoring. In Japan, it is impossible to use information obtained from a number of different projects due to wide variations in the purposes and techniques which are particular to each program. It is important to establish a centre exclusively for the monitoring of heavy metals and other chemical substances in the environment.

It is strongly recommended that a centre for long-term biological monitoring be founded. A central organization should be formed under the auspices of an existing health institute where study design, storage of specimens for future reference, and a data bank can be accommodated. Ideally, the determinations of chemical concentrations in specimens would be carried out in a single centralized centre, but where this is impossible, they could be carried out by local health departmental or university health laboratories. However, a checking system for checking technique and analytical methods should be worked out. As mentioned previously, a 3-year biological monitoring project has just been completed in Japan. In this project, as shown below, all Japan was divided into 8 blocs. A central committee was organized to design the project and to analyse the data. In each bloc, a subcommittee, including pathologists from a university located in the bloc, officials from the local health department, and/or specialists from the Department of Public Health of the local university was formed. Determinations of environmental chemicals were performed on the local level. In the first, PCBs in human tissues (including adipose tissue of the abdomen) were determined. In the second year, DDT and BHCs, and in the third year Pb, Cd, Hg, Cu, Zn, and other trace elements were determined.

The representatives from each bloc, including technicians, were gathered together in a meeting called by the central committee prior to the start of the project. This was done in order to obtain cooperation and goodwill for the project. At this meeting the central committee determined a standardized method for the determination analyses and check samples were sent to each participating laboratory. However, upon completion of the project, it was still felt that it would have been better if all the laboratory technicians involved had undergone a special training session at a central laboratory before the start of the project. After each annual project, each bloc submitted a comprehensive written report to the central committee along with individual records and an overall analysis of the data was made by the central committee. It was sometimes difficult to evaluate the various results, it being unclear at times whether the differences were due to analytical factors or to real differences in the levels of the chemical in the samples.

Figure 1

Organization Chart for the Three-Year Project of the Ministry of Health and Welfare

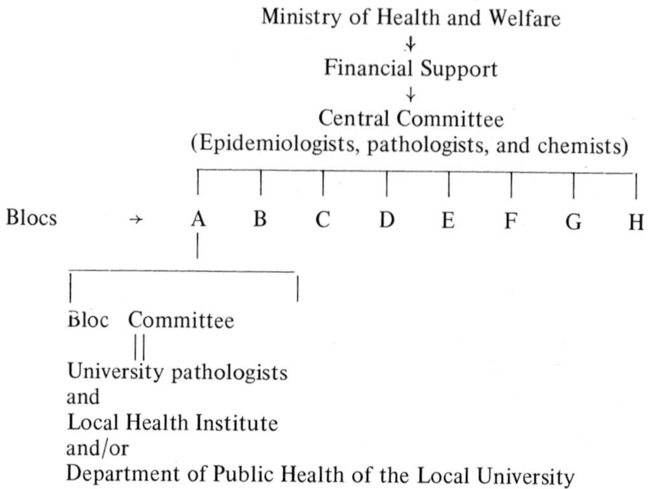

From this experience, it is clear that a centre for long-term biological monitoring should be established, and if possible have all determinations be conducted in a single laboratory affiliated with the centre. Even then, check samples should be stored over a period of years, and checks should be conducted regularly in order to insure the least amount of technical error and variation.

G. Ethical and legal considerations

In Japan, there are no laws or regulations regarding the confidentiality of information on results obtained on a group basis. (Private medical records are, of course, confidential). However, from an ethical point of view, such information should not be made public.

As already mentioned, it is sometimes difficult to obtain blood samples from living persons for various reasons. Legally it is not difficult to obtain post mortem samples, but in Japan autopsies are often not performed, especially in rural areas, for religious and other reasons. Furthermore, families of victims, e.g. Itai-Itai disease or Minamata disease victims, often refuse permission for autopsy.

There are no problems in the transportation of specimens throughout Japan and overseas. Urine, blood, and post mortem specimens have been exchanged freely with Sweden and the USA in a cooperative study.

H. Cost estimates

In Japan the cost for determining lead, mercury or cadmium is between US$10 and 20 per sample. In addition, the collection of post mortem samples costs approximately $5 per body for the extra labour on the part of autopsy assistants.

It is difficult to estimate the expense in the collection of samples for future reference. At the present time in the author's laboratory, there are 5 deep freezers containing about 3,000 specimens from about 250 cadavers. The cost for this storage is included in the routine expenses incurred by the laboratory, which are paid for by the university.

For the ideal biological monitoring centre described above, the expenses would not be so great if various governmental organizations, on both the national and local levels would contribute to the establishment and maintenance of such a centre. The centre could be organized as a division of an already existing national health institute where a staff of about 10 technicians could work and the data obtained could be analysed by an existing statistics division of the institute.   In order to obtain the necessary monies, it is important to convince the government of the necessity of this type of centre.

In the project of the Ministry of Health and Welfare, the total budget was approximately $500,000 for the 3-year period.   In the first year, 1,200 specimens from 320 cadavers were analysed for PCBs.   In the second year, about 700 specimens from 160 cadavers were analysed for DDT, BHCs and others.   In the third year, about 700 specimens were analysed for lead, mercury and cadmium, and in some specimens, other heavy metals such as copper and zinc.

Conclusion

Biological monitorings on both short· and long-term bases are very important for checking the levels of various chemical substances in the human body and for the detection of early health effects due to those chemicals.   Along with biological monitoring, environmental monitoring, including food, is essential.   Environmental monitoring is easier to carry out than biological monitoring, but for the surveillance of direct effects of environmental chemicals, the latter should not be neglected.

For short-term biological monitoring, projects organized by a private scientist or organization or by government health authorities are adequate.   However, for routine biological monitoring on a long-term basis, which is more important in terms of surveying the increase or decrease of chemical substances in humans over a period of years, a biological monitoring centre should be established in every country. Such a centre could be established as a division in an already existing government health institute and would not necessarily be inordinately costly. The citizens and government of each country must be persuaded of the importance of establishing such a centre.

REFERENCES

1.   KITAMURA, S., K. SUMINO, K. HAYADAWA and T. SHIBATA (1975).   Mercury content in 'normal' tissues.   Studies on the Health Effects of Alkylmercury in Japan.   Japan Environment Agency.
2.   HASEGAWA, Y. (1972).   Kankyo Hoken Report No. 11:13 (in Japanese).
3.   TSUCHIYA, K., Y. SEKI and M. SUGITA (1976).   Keio J. Med. 25.
4.   FRIBERG, L., M. PISCATOR, G.F. NORDBERG and T. KJELLSTROM (1974).   Cadmium in the Environment, 2nd Edition.   CRC Press, Cleveland, Ohio.
5.   SUMINO, K., K. HAYAKAWA, T. SHIBATA and S. KITAMURA (1975).   Arch.Environ. Health 30, 487.
6.   Study on the Distribution of PCB Concentrations in the Human Body.   Report of the Investigating Committee of PCB and Other Chemicals to the Japan Environment Agency (1975) (in Japanese).
7.   Airborne Lead in Perspective (1972).   Printing and Publishing Office, National Academy of Sciences, Washington, D.C.
8.   TSUCHIYA, K., T. OKUBO, M. NAGASAKI, T. MAKAJIMA, H. KAMIJO, I. MIZOGUCHI.   Biological effects of lead on school children of urban and suburban Tokyo. (To be published).
9.   TSUCHIYA, K., G. USHIYAMA, M. SUGITA and K. YASUDA (1975).   Proceedings of the 45th Annual Meeting of the Japanese Society for Hygiene, Kyoto, 2–4 April 1975 (in Japanese).
10.   TSUCHIYA, K. and S. IWAO.   Cadmium concentrations in human organs and tissues – a comparison between Japan and Sweden.   (To be published, in Japanese).
11.   HASEGAWA, N., M. NIIZEKI, R. ICHIJI and Y. SUGINO (1972).   Determination of organic and inorganic mercury by flameless AAS.   Annual Report of the Nagoya Institute of Environmental Medicine, vol. 23.
12.   Report on a 3-year cooperative research project among Japan, the United States and Sweden.   (To be published).

GENERAL ASPECTS OF BIOLOGICAL MONITORING

R.L. Zielhuis
Coronel Laboratory
University of Amsterdam

1. INTRODUCTION

This working paper discusses general aspects of Biological Monitoring (BM) in humans exposed to chemicals (and physical) factors in the ambient environment. The aspects discussed are thought to be relevant for many types of BM-programmes.

This working paper consists of a series of small working papers, each of them dealing with one aspect. The author did not try to present a review of litererature, but limited himself to points of general interest. In case examples are given, it is not meant to discuss the examples as such : they only serve to illustrate the general principles.

The paper does not discuss BM for evaluation of mutagenic or teratogenic exposures. Although this may be regarded as a very important topic, objectives, designs and methods appear to a large extent to be completely different from BM as discussed in this paper. Moreover, the author has no experience himself in this field.

2. OBJECTIVE OF BIOLOGICAL MONITORING

BM as carried out within the framework of public health has as immediate objective to provide an estimate of exposure and - indirectly - of health risk ; the ultimate objective is protection of health of population (groups).

Within the objective in general sense more specified objectives can be determined, vide Chapter 5. The actual design of each BM-programme is highly determined by the specific immediate objective.

BM in human population groups has essentially the same objective as BM in e.g. fish (Hg pollution) in plants (air pollution) : evaluation of exposure and risks.

In its original meaning the word 'monitoring' indicates a continuous or discontinuous measurement of a variable in the course of time. In actual practice BM is not always carried out periodically, if it has been proven that the exposure does not make such repeated (discontinuous) measurement necessary.   So, the question can be brought forward whether the term biological monitoring is always used in the right sense of its original meaning.

BM evaluates exposure and health risks. In practice one usually has to estimate only exposure, provided that the relation between exposure and health risk (dose-response relationship) is already fairly known (see Chapter 7).   Sometimes data on response can be added to or even take the place of data on exposure.

A BM-programme is quite different from a health screening survey : in case of health screening the objective is to detect the presence of a disease (possibly in a pre-disease phase) in individuals ; for each individual subject one has to come to a decision whether the (pre-) disease is present or not ; data on an individual subject are decisive.   In BM the distribution of data over the whole group is decisive, not the individual result as such.

3. BIOLOGICAL MONITORING (BM) VERSUS ENVIRONMENTAL MONITORING (EM)

BM indirectly estimates external environmental exposure (see Chapter 8) and health risks.   In EM one measures exposure directly, qualitatively and quantitatively (intensity, deviation).

For the following reasons BM may have to be preferred above EM:

1.   Human subjects may be exposed to one agent through contaminated air, food, water, and through tobacco smoke, cosmetics, beverages, drugs, anticaries tablets, simultaneously or subsequently, and this through various pathways (respiratory tract, gastrointestinal tract, skin), in several variations of intensity, duration and frequency.

It is extremely difficult, often even impossible to measure in a quantitatively reliable manner this total external exposure in a direct way. However, human subjects absorb and/or deposit this agent under study, and so this establishes a body burden ; the pathway and source are not relevant any longer ; the body integrates this total external exposure into one internal load (see Chapter 6). BM tries to measure or at least to estimate this internal load, qualitatively and quantitatively.

2. From the viewpoint of health protection, one is not so much interested in external exposure, but much more so in the actual internal load, as related to health risks.

3. the pharmacokinetics of a chemical agent are determined by the agent itself and by biological properties of the human organism, e.g. Pb is deposited in bone, Cd in kidney, OCI in fat, F is eliminated quickly by the kidney, asbestos remains to a large extent in the lungs. There are differences in pharmacokinetics according to age, type of respiration, inborn errors of metabolism, genetic or acquired capacity for enzyme induction, etc. BM takes into account various biological factors which determine the health risk, and so should particularly be carried out in at risk groups (Chapter 9).

4. BM allows to measure simultaneously other health parameters which are indicative for population health, e.g. Hb, cholesterol in blood.

5. BM may require much less expenditure in budget and manpower than EM in providing an adequate estimate of total exposure, particularly in case of variable simultaneous exposure through various pathways and sources, e.g. trace metals, OCI.

However, one should realize that in order to get a valid estimate of external exposure, it is not the question of either EM or BM ; both approaches may be necessary to estimate exposure and health risk (see also Chapter 7).

4. LIMITATIONS OF BIOLOGICAL MONITORING

Although BM may have great advantages over EM, one should also realize its limitations:

1. BM takes human beings as sampling units ; this may mean at least a certain inconvenience for the subjects, let alone a health risk ; it may create anxiety, emotion, etc. These aspects are discussed more fully in Chapter 14.

2. BM as routine programme can only be carried out for a limited number of environmental pollutants:
- the quantitative relationship between external exposure (to be estimated) and indices of internal exposure, and the quantitative relationship between indices of internal exposure and health risks, both on group basis, should be known beforehand (see Chapters 6 and 7).
- reliable methods to measure relevant biological parameters have to be available:
  a) presence of pollutant itself in biological specimen indicators of internal load, e.g. metals, OCI, asbestos fibres, COHb.
  b) metabolites of pollutants, e.g. TCE and TCA in case of TRI, paranitrophenol in case of some OP's, DDA and DDE in case of DDT.
  c) early and readily reversible indicators of response, e.g. ALAD in erythrocytes in case of Pb, inhibition of ChE in case of OP's.

So, if agents mainly exert a biological effect on the mucous membranes of eyes and airways, it will usually not be possible to establish biological indicators of external exposure: functional changes in lung function, subjective experience of pain in eyes or smell usually are too non-specific - in addition to being not always early and readily reversible - for the environmental pollutants under study, to provide a valid (see Chapter 11) indicator of exposure ; this applies e.g. to SO_2, H_2SO_4, NO_x, PAN, O_3, dust.

3. If external exposure is highly variable in time, and at the same time biological half life is relatively short, e.g. in case of CO, alcohol, a BM programme may fail in its objectives, unless great care is taken to guarantee a close relationship in time between the taking of samples and the expected excessive exposure.

5. CLASSIFICATION OF IMMEDIATE OBJECTIVES

1.   BM has first been developed in occupational health (OH). Also in this respect general environmental health took great advantage from previous developments in the parent discipline occupational health and hygiene.   This particularly applies for chemical and physical exposure in work - and ambient environment respectively. So, the first classification is:
1.1. BM-programme in OH-setting
1.2. BM-programme in PH-setting
In this working paper only BM-PH is discussed.

2.   One can distinguish various types of BM-programmes according to the duration of total exposure to be covered:
2.1. Agents have a short biological half life ($<$10-15 hr) or a short-term effect in biological specimens examined ; BM as indicator of recent exposure: last hours or days.
- COHb levels in non-smoking pedestrians, commuters, taxi-drivers, traffic wardens, policemen as measure of recent ambient air pollutions
- fibres in faeces of subjects with regular passing of stools, as measure of recent fibre content of food
- hydrophilic metabolites with short biological half life, e.g. DDA, can sometimes be measured instead of the more persistent pollutant itself.
2.2. Agents with a moderately long biological half life in biological specimens examined (up to 1-2 mths); BM as indicator of exposure over last months e.g.
- Pb-, Hg levels in blood
- Pb-, Hg levels in urine, possibly provocated by EDTA, BAL
2.3. Agents with a long biological half life (months) in biological specimen examined; BM as indicator of long-term - low-level exposure
- Org. chlorinated pesticides in blood, body fat
- Cd in kidney
- metals in hair
2.4. Agents with a very long biological half life or persistent effects in biological specimens examined ; BM indicates more or less total life-time exposure, e.g.
- Pb in bone, teeth
- asbestos in lungs

3.   Chemical agents reach the body through various pathways, simultaneously or subsequently, and coming from various sources.   If one knows the total exposure through other pathways (particularly if one knows this to be minimal or non-existent), then it is possible to estimate the total exposure through one pathway, with various sources contributing to it, e.g.
- metals in food and beverages when respiratory exposure is minimal, provide indicator of nutritional load
- COHb levels in non-smokers exposed to traffic exhaust, passive smoking, work in kitchen.

4.   Graded BM, in which subjects are mainly or exclusively exposed through one pathway, and mainly from one source ; one compares groups of subjects differing in exposure intensity or duration e.g.
- geographical gradient in distance from point source of specific air pollution
- gradient according to eating habits (Hg)
- gradient according to Pb-paint covered interiors of homes
- gradient according to smoking habits: Cd, COHb in blood
- gradient according to age in case of lifelong exposure ; metals in bone, asbestos fibres in lungs.

5.   Sequential BM, i.e. follow-up of the same or comparable group in the course of time, to evaluate change in total exposure, e.g.
- measuring trend in OCI concentrations in fat over subsequent years
- evaluating result of environmental protection measures (operational research), for instance the effect of reduction of local emission: metals in blood
- evaluating the effect of a new source of emission.
This type of BM may best correspond with the original meaning of the term monitoring.

This classification does not provide a set of BM-programmes, each exclusive to the other, but it indicates various immediate objectives of BM-programmes. It is necessary to state the specific objective of each programme beforehand very clearly, because it largely determines the design of the programme. The question: '**what do we want to know**' should be answered expli-
in regard to the following points:

— are we dealing with a BM-OH or BM-PH, and can present or past occupational exposure affect the data in case of BM-PH ?
— do we want to take into account long-term exposure or are we interested in recent exposure ?
— do we know the main pathway of exposure ?
— do we want to evaluate the quantitative relationship with exposure ?

The answer to these questions may determine the biological specimen to be examined, the working up of data, the choice of groups to be examined.

6.   CONCEPTS OF EXPOSURE AND DOSE

The immediate objective of BM is estimation of exposure, either external exposure or internal exposure, and so of health risks. Too often one relies merely on concentrations in inhaled air, food and on duration of exposure, and not on dose, i.e. the amount of agent taken up by the body per unit of time over a specified period of time. The same may be said for studies of elimination (exhaled air, urine). It can easily be understood that measurement of the dose of exposure is to be preferred over measurement of exposure-concentration.

The recently published book 'Effects and dose-response relationship of toxic metals', Ed. G.F. Nordberg; Elsevier Amsterdam, 1976, discusses this problem at length. In its classical sense 'dose' means amount administered to for example an experimental animal. In the context of applied toxicology dose can be defined as 'the amount or concentration of a given chemical at the site of effect'. However, measurement of this is often not possible in practice. So the dose may have to be estimated, either by EM or BM. The accuracy and precision of various estimates will depend upon the validity of sampling and analytical technology. Because the term 'dose' in BM-programmes is an estimate, it should be made as clear as possible how the dose was estimated including specific units, physical form, chemical species, time of sampling, specimen examined.

In case of BM one should have at least a limited knowledge of the pharmacokinetics of the agent under study, in order to evaluate the validity of the biological dose parameter measured in estimating (predicting) the 'amount or concentration at the effector site'. Unfortunately, this knowledge is often still very limited, so invalidating the confidence of the estimate, and sometimes even prohibiting the design of a BM-programme.

There are four concepts of exposure:

A -   **External exposure in general sense (EE)**, i.e. concentration in air, food, water, etc. and duration of exposure (T). (In case of ambient exposure skin absorption may usually be neglected). Usually it is extremely difficult to get reliable data on this total external exposure in general sense ; moreover the influence of physical activity (as distributed over the population at risk) is not taken into account ; so EM can only present a very approximative indicator of EE, and even more so of the actual dose received.

B -   **Effective external load (EL)**, i.e. the amount offered to and taken up by the body per unit of time over a period of time. In case of exposure by inhalation one has to know Ci (concentration in inhaled air), Ce (concentration in exhaled air), V (respiratory minute volume) amount of secondary ingestion, procentual absorption, in addition to duration of exposure. EL corresponds to the actual external dose, but can hardly be measured reliably in public health studies.

C -   **Internal load (IL)**, i.e. the amount present in relevant body compartments, e.g. blood, or indirectly estimated from amount (or concentration) exhaled or excreted in urine, hair, etc., in combination with duration of exposure. This amount is usually estimated from concentration in biological compartments. The total internal load is usually divided over various body compartments, particularly blood, soft tissues (organs), muscles, skin & hair, bone, fat. Depending on the agent, biological half lives in each compartment may highly differ. If the agent is deposited and consequently more or less fixed in e.g. bone (Pb), then the body burden in this compartment may be relatively large, although it hardly contributes to health risks, because it does not have an effect on bone itself.

On the other hand deposit of Cd in kidney may cause renal effects ; the same may be said for Hg or OCI in the brain. The choice of parameter (compartment) and the time relationship of sampling with exposure depend on the immediate objective of the BM programme (Chapter 5).

D - **Internal load at effector site (ILE)**, i.e. the actual 'dose' in e.g. liver, kidney, brain, that causes the relevant health effects, in combination with duration of exposure. This ED can again be estimated from the measurement of concentrations in tissues.

Biological monitoring almost never will give the most relevant parameter ILD, except maybe if the programme is based upon autopsy-studies.

The Task Group on metal accumulation (Environm. Physiol. Bioch., 1973, 3, 65-107) defined a few other concepts:

- **Critical concentration** (CC), i.e. the concentration in a cell which causes undesirable changes.

- **Critical organ concentration** (COC), i.e. the mean concentration in the organ at the time any of its cells reaches critical concentration.

In BM based upon tissue analysis organ concentrations will be measured, and compared with COC's (if known).

- **Critical organ** (COR), i.e. that particular organ which first attains its COC ; this COR is not necessarily the organ with the highest concentration.

Before designing a BM-programme one has to evaluate how the parameter measured reflects various parameters mentioned above. Often one will have to be content with approximate answers.   At least a consensus should exist about what the data gained mean in relation to exposure and to health effects (see Chapter 7).

One example of an attempt to study the relation between various indicators mentioned is given:

Hunter et al (Arch. environm. Hlth **15** (1967) 614-626, and Arch. environm. Hlth **18** (1969), 12-21) came to the following relationships for aldrin-dieldrin (HEOD):

- conc. HEOD in adipose tissue is approximately 136 (confidence limits 109-170) times the conc. in whole blood;

- dietary intake (in μg HEOD/man/day) =

$$\frac{\text{conc. in blood } (\mu g/ml)}{0.000086} \quad \text{or} \quad \frac{\text{conc. in adipose tissue } (\mu g/g)}{0.0185}$$

Dietary intake is not yet the same as EL, because procentual absorption is not taken into account ; the concentration in adipose tissue is not the same as the concentration in the effector organ (brain).   Moreover, the data are based upon long-term human volunteer study, in which exposure by inhalation or skin did not take place.

The no-effect level for HEOD conc. in blood is about 0.20μg/ml, based upon study in adult male workers ; at 0.105 μg/ml there was no sign of enzyme induction (Jager, Aldrin, dieldrin, endrin and Telodrin, Elsevier Publ. Coy, Amsterdam 1970).

7. EXPOSURE-RESPONSE RELATIONSHIPS

In toxicology one may distinguish between :

- **dose-effect relationship**, i.e. the relationship between (an estimate of) dose and the gradation of a specified parameter of effect in an individual or a population;

- **dose-response relationships**, i.e. the relationship between (an estimate of) dose and relative number (percentage, proportion) of individuals with a specified intensity (quantity) of a specified parameter (quality) of effect in a group of subjects.

Individual subjects differ in D-E-relationships both in regard to the no-effect level and slope. For a group this interindividual difference manifests itself in the D-R-relationship.

In literature both terms often are used for the same concept, which creates confusion.

As stated in Chapter 6 one should use that concept of exposure which estimates the actual dose as best as possible.   Nevertheless, one usually does not know this dose itself.   Therefore, it may be preferred to speak of **exposure-effect/response relationships** in epidemiological studies.

BM tries to estimate external exposure (EE, EL) by measuring (estimating) the internal load (IL, ILE).   A routine BM-Programme therefore has as condition that this relationship is known beforehand, or at least can be estimated beforehand.

BM has as general objective protection of health risk. This makes it necessary that in case of a routine BM-programme the exposure-response relationship also is known, or at least can be estimated beforehand.

So, before carrying out a routine BM-programme, which will serve to protect public health, it is a **prerequisite** that the following relationship is fairly well known if the BM-programme is measuring parameters of IL or ILE:

EE → (EL) → IL → (ILE) → health risks.

In some programmes one relies on measuring early subclinical indicators of response; in that case the relationship between this indicator and potential health risks should be known.

A BM-programme can also be set up with the objective to study the relationship between IL (ILE) and health risk, or between EE (EL) and IL (ILE). In that case the programme is still in a phase of research and development, and not yet in that of routine programming.

8. CLASSIFICATION OF EXTERNAL EXPOSURE

In a BM-programme members of the general population serve as sampling units; the objective is to estimate environmental exposure. In the framework of public health programmes, the possible interference with occupational exposure should be fully taken into account. However, there is no sharp distinction between occupational and "true" environmental exposure. In a recent document on "Public health risks of asbestos exposure", prepared by the author and a few other Dutch colleagues for the CEC (1976), this was demonstrated for exposure to asbestos fibres. The same applies to other environmental factors, e.g. metals, pesticides.

The following possibilities of exposure may be distinguished:

1. **Occupational exposure**
   a. **direct** occupational exposure in well-known jobs, e.g. in asbestos mines, in asbestos textile, cement and insulation board factories, and in insulation work; in case of pesticides in production and application in the field (agriculture, sanitation). It should be realized that there exists an increasing number of jobs in which exposure is not expected, and which may require an in depth history taking to be established as source of occupational exposure, e.g. in case of asbestos fibres: ironing in a laundry, stage hand; isolated jobs, carried out by one or a few individuals in a plant, whereas the main product does not or hardly contain the agent under study.
   b. **indirect** occupational exposure: the subject usually does not handle the agent himself, but works in the vicinity of such jobs, e.g. non-asbestos workers in shipbuilding; exposure to aerosols of pesticides, sprayed by (sometimes protected) workers.
   c. **natural presence of agent in the work place**: the agent is not brought there by man himself, but the work may involve exposure from natural sources, although this handling is not the objective of the job itself, e.g. agricultural workers engaged in growing tobacco on stony mountanous soil, which contains various types of asbestos.

2. **Para-occupational domestic exposure** of women married to exposed men, or of other members of the household; the agent is brought to the home environment on clothes, shoes, etc.

3. **Para-occupational exposure through leisure time activities, or second job.** There need not be a sharp distinction with circumstances in the first job. This second job may go from real wage earning jobs to hobby activities in the subjects' own home. This may also create possibilities for exposure at 2.

4. **Neighbourhood exposure**: vicinity of mines, factories, dumps, etc.. Estimation of this may be one of the objectives of a public health BM-programme.

5. **Exposure through personal habits**, e.g. use of cosmetics, beverages, use of Pb-containing hair creams, smoking. If such a habit is followed by the majority of the population as such, it may become an aspect of total environmental exposure, e.g. Pb in wine in some countries.

6.   **true environmental exposure**, through air, food, water, etc., more or less relevant for the whole group under study.

Within the population group examined, there will always be a distribution of intensities of the parameter studied.   It is necessary to evaluate carefully the various possibilities of exposure mentioned, to ensure that the data obtained are indicative for the specific external exposure situation under study.   This particularly is the case if a small number of subjects show levels highly deviating from the overall level in the group as a whole (see Chapter 9).

9.   AT RISK GROUPS

In Chapter 5 a classification of BM-programmes is given: this classification was based upon aspects of exposure (sources, duration of exposure, properties of agent).   However, the group of subjects to be studied also deserves discussion.   The choice of this group also highly determines the design of a BM-programme.

BM is one of the tools in health protection in case of environmental exposure.   So, a BM can be performed to estimate the exposure, c.q. health risks in the general population.   Several of such studies have been performed.   One recent example: in the Netherlands the RIV (Governmental Institute Public Health) measured levels of Pb, Cd, Hg, Se, As in a representative sample of military recruits: from about 1300 male subjects, about 19 years of age, blood was taken; this was examined by means of neutron activation analysis.   The sample was representative for the whole group of recruits.   One produced frequency distribution of the blood levels.   The full data have not yet been published.   The frequency distributions present a reliable indication of the internal exposure levels of male recruits in the Netherlands.   Many other examples from literature could be added.

However, it is also true that within the general population there exists a variability in exposure and in health risks; if one wants to protect health, one has to gear standards and measures to the at risk groups.

One can distinguish various possibilities for increased risk:

-- **increased exposure**, because of e.g. jobs executed in the general environment (taxi drivers, traffic police, categories 2, 3, 4, 5, of Chapter 8);
-- **differences in pharmacokinetics**, e.g. at similar exposure levels higher uptake takes place because of increased respiration, or increased absorption.   Examples: possibly increased gastro-intestinal absorption of metals in young children; increased respiration in pregnant women.   Also: decreased elimination in case of kidney disease, or increased turnover between depots and soft tissues (in case of rapidly growing children ?);
-- **differences in pharmacodynamics**: increased health effects at similar levels of estimated dose, e.g. probably increased susceptibility of haemsynthesis to lead in case of females, increased susceptibility of nervous system in embryo and infants (Hg, Pb), increased susceptibility of subjects with subclinical cardiovascular disease to CO, increased susceptibility of groups with different genetic make up (e.g. G_6 PD deficiency, sickle cell trait, thalassaemia).

An average human being does not exist, so one has to examine the extremes of the distribution curves, in respect to exposure or susceptibility, because these subgroups of the population determine the quality standards for the environment.   In each BM-programme one should carefully discuss the feasibility of the group to be examined. Too often one studies schoolchildren of 6-12 years, because they may easily be approached, whereas the real at risk group may be the toddler in case of metal exposure (increased oral exposure, different pharmacokinetics and pharmacodynamics).   In case of estimating neighbourhood exposure, adult housewives are to be preferred above adult males, because in the last case there may be intervening effects of community and occupational exposure.   One should also take into account, by means of questionnaires, data on personal habits: fish eating habits (Hg), smoking habits (Cd, Pb), use of cosmetics, alcoholics (Pb, As), contraceptive pills (Fe).

It is not possible to present general rules, because usually the local situation to be examined at the same time also determines the possibility of intervening factors, representative for the local situation.

10. PERCENTILE DISTRIBUTION

The objective of public health measures is protection of the health of those individuals and subgroups which are at risk. These groups at risk are of primary concern (Chapter 9). The data from BM-programmes should bring forward the exposure and/or health risk of these groups in particular.

The general population consists of an odd mixture of subjects with heterogeneous exposure and response (pharmacokinetics and pharmacodynamics). This particularly applies to xenobiotics, which are not essential for health, and for which the human body has no homoiostatic mechanisms to ensure a constant "milieu intérieur". It is well known that agents like non-essential metals and chlorinated pesticides are not normally (Gaussian) distributed in blood and tissue over population groups, but usually show a skewed distribution, in contrast to essential trace-elements like Co, Zn, Cu or physiologic body constituents. Moreover, in non-excessively exposed humans the levels are very low to minimal and can only increase in concentration with exposure, so there is only possibility for higher than "normal" levels. In large population groups a log-normal distribution may occur, but in subgroups of the population not even log-normality can be expected (see Chapter 13). Only in case of normal (Gaussian) or log-normal distribution, the arithmetic or geometric average together with the standard deviation define the distribution. Moreover, increasing the sample size may always yield unexpected highly deviant levels, particularly in subgroups at risk.

So, in working up the data from BM-programmes one has to examine the (log)normality of the distribution. It is fallacious to calculate arithmetic or geometric averages if (log)normality cannot be confirmed. However, in many literature reports this has not been done, with the result that it is not possible to determine the relative number (percentage) of subjects with high levels, indicating excessive exposure and/or health risk. In Chapter 7 this point has also already been emphasized: exposure-response relationships are based upon the percentage of subjects affected at different exposure levels.

Two examples from literature are given. **Gaffi** (European colloquium on problems raised by the contamination of man and his environment by persistent pesticides and organic halogenated compounds, EUR. 5196, Luxembourg 1975, page 383, Annex IV) reported on the OCI levels in body fat in various countries in the EEC; only the data on total DDT are given as an example (Table 10.1).

Table 10.1

Total DDT in body fat in ppm in the EEC

	arithmetic average	maximum	minimum
Belgium	8.18	38.00	0.30
Denmark	4.9	18.0	0.3
France	3.19	6.68	0.76
Italy	9.77	62.20	0.81
Luxembourg	9.59	27.20	1.59
The Netherlands	2.70	6.30	0.90
Un. Kingdom	2.30	9.50	0.08

It can clearly be seen that in various countries the distributions are highly skewed; it is not possible to know how many subjects actually give the sample size, so comparison between countries is even less possible. About the same arithmetic averages are given whereas at the same time the maximum levels my differ a factor 2 to 3. The Annex would have presented much more relevant information if one had calculated the percentage of subjects with e.g. >5 ppm, 10 ppm, 20 ppm, 30 ppm, or better still with the levels exceeded in 50, 10, 5 % of the population.

In his book Aldrin, dieldrin, endrin and telodrin (Elsevier 1970, page 72) **Jager** presented a review of HEOD levels in adipose tissue over the years 1961-1968; Table 10.2 gives the data for UK and USA.

This table shows that for sample sizes n > 50 the geom. averages from the UK are much less variable (0.17 - 0.23) than the arithm. averages from the USA (0.11 - 0.31). However, even if the geometric averages may yield a more valuable picture, it would have been preferred to know also the percentile distribution, e.g. percentage of subjects with > 50, 100, 150, 200 HEOD µg/g, or better still the levels exceeded in 50, 10 and 5 % of the population.

Table 10.2

HEOD levels in adipose tissue, UK and USA, in µg/g and range

	year	n	arithm. average	geom. average	range
UK	1961-62	131		0.21	0.02 - 1.20
	1963-64	66		0.21	0.02 - 1.08
	1964	100		0.23	0.02 - 1.08
	1965	101		0.23	trace- 1.80
	1966	44		0.22	0.10 - 0.73
	1966	53		0.21	-
	1965-67	248		0.17	n.d. - 1.00
	1967	18		0.27	-
	1968	29		0.10	-
USA	1961-62	28	0.15		0.02 - 0.36
	1962-63	282	0.11		n.d. - 1.00
	1964	25	0.29		0.03 - 1.15
	1964	64	0.31		0.07 - 2.82
	1965	42	0.22		n.d. - 0.70
	1965-67	146	0.22		n.d. - 0.77

These two examples could easily be multiplied with many other (in fact: most) literature data on most xenobiotics. These reports do not provide enough relevant information on the percentage of subjects at risk. The data should preferably be worked up as percentile distributions, i.e. the levels not exceeded in e.g. P_{50} (median), P_{90} and P_{95} of the population examined. Only in that case the need for concern and for action to be taken is well enough presented. Only in large sample sizes calculation of geometric averages together with standard deviation may serve as second best.

11. VALIDITY OF PARAMETERS

In BM-programmes one or a few parameters are measured to estimate external exposure and/or health risks. So, parameters examined are used as predictors, indicators of past, present or future events. The predictive validity should therefore be known (see **Zielhuis** et al, Int. Arch. Arbeitsmed. 1974, 32, 167-190).

Validity refers to the extent to which subjects in a case-control study are correctly classified as to the extent to which a situation as observed reflects the true situation. Two aspects are important:
-- sensitivity (se), i.e. the extent to which subjects who truly manifest a characteristic are so classified. A high sensitivity corresponds to a low yield of false-negatives;
-- specificity (sp), i.e. the extent to which subjects who do not manifest such a characteristic are correctly classified. A high specificity corresponds to a low yield of false-positives.

Validity can be expressed quantitatively as se + sp; maximum validity is 2.

Calculation of these indices can only be performed from individual data; usually literature reports give only grouped values, so validity cannot be evaluated.

The terms sensitivity and specificity are also applied in other concepts:
-- **analytical sensitivity**: detection level of a specific technique,
-- **analytical specificity**: absence of effects of other compounds on levels determined (high discrimination).

Improvement of detection limits and discriminative power promotes sensitivity and specificity as epidemiological concept.

Sensitivity is also used for **biological hypersusceptibility**, i.e. decreased biological threshold level; this indicates a property of exposed subjects and not of test methods.

In the paper mentioned an example is given for ALAD- and ALAU-levels as indicator of Pb > 400 ppb, based upon the result of one study (n = 135 for ALAD, n = 110 for ALAU). The validity of 50 % inhibition of ALAD for prediction of PbB > 400 ppb was 1.87 and for PpB > 700 ppb it was 1.73; for ALAU-6mg/l it was 1.35 and 1.45 respectively. This shows that ALAD is a better indicator for PbB > 400 or 700 ppb than ALAU.   Insofar as PpB may be regarded as a valid indicator for stable total external exposure over the last few months, ALAD can be used instead of PbB for indicating this external exposure in a group of subjects. In fact, this has been proposed by the EEC-Commission in its recommendation for BM in case of environmental lead exposure of the general population.

Recently **Alessio** et al (Int. Arch. Occ. Environm. Hlth, 1976, in press) have shown that FEP appears to be a valid predictor of EDTA-provocated Pb in urine, and so of metabolic available Pb; validity of FEP is higher than the validity of PbB for prediction of PbU-EDTA. So in a BM-programme FEP may be a better indicator of the internal load at the effector site than PbB.

By combining more than one biological parameter one may increase predictive validity in a BM-programme; particularly specificity will increase.

Recently **Lauwerys** et al (Int. Arch. Occ. Environm. Hlth, 1976, **36**, 275-285) suggested that on a group basis Cd in blood levels reflect total current exposure, whereas Cd in urine levels reflect body burden of Cd when exposure is low (environmental pollution) and current exposure when exposure is high (industrial pollution). This observation could have been substantiated by calculating sensitivity and specificity.

The validity of a test may be used as a criterium in selecting the most appropriate test from a set of possible tests. If the BM-programme wants to indicate most or all subjects with increased exposure or health risk, then a high sensitivity is important (low percentage of false-negatives); however this may lead to a comparatively large number of false-positives. It depends on the specific requirements of the programme, available manpower and budget and particularly on the risk one takes if the programme yields false-negatives, whether one will aim at high sensitivity or high specificity.   In health survey, particularly in screening for incipient serious diseases, sensitivity should be very high (no false-negatives), whereas a high yield of false-positives may have to be taken for granted.

In designing a BM-programme one has to observe some strict conditions:
-- One cannot determine predictive validity if the **indicator** and the **situation** to be predicted are not **exactly specified** in qualitative and possibly in quantitative terms.
-- The data should be presented as **individual data**, or at least in a percentile distribution (see Chapter 10).
-- The **methods should be exactly specified**, e.g. time of sampling in relation to exposure, method of sampling, methods of correction of rough data (in case of urine or exhaled air), accuracy and precision of analytical method.

12. BIOLOGICAL MONITORING AND STANDARD SETTING

A BM-programme results in an estimate of environmental exposure and/or health risk in the group of subjects studied, and - if this group is representative - also for the group from which the sample was drawn.   Not so much the average biological limits, but much more so the **distribution of the levels** within the sample group is of interest (see Chapter 10), not only for estimating exposure, but also for health risk, if the dose (exposure)-response relationship is adequately known. This distribution indirectly measures the **permissibility of the environment**.

Because it may be extremely difficult in case of many environmental agents to measure (or estimate) adequately the environmental exposure (see Chapter 3), the question can be raised whether health protection can be based upon the biological parameters as such, and so whether the distribution of these could also be used as a **biological quality standard** to guarantee absence of undue exposure and/or health risks for the population. In occupational health more and more biological permissible limits are being used in practice, although they have not yet achieved the status of legal standards. In public health the same development starts taking place. In 1974 **Zielhuis** (Int. Arch. Arbeitsmed. 37, 1974, 103) proposed a biological quality guide for inorganic lead, and in 1975 this proposal was to a large extent taken over by the European Economic Communities as a guide for governmental and community action. As far as known, this is the first time that a set of biological levels is going to be used as a kind of standard (still as a guide, not an official legal standard).

The author took PbB = 350 ppb as the maximum permissible limit for individuals (potentially pregnant women and infants). Because there is a large variability in internal load within population groups, one could never base a guide (standard) upon this level alone; then distributions as they actually occur in various population studies have to be taken into account. The 7-City Study from the USA (**Tepper** et al, Univ. of Cincinnati, Dept. Env. Hlth 1972) for instance showed that in groups of adult women with maximum levels of about 350 ppb at the same time 50 % had levels $\leq$ 200 ppb and 90 % $\leq$ 300 ppb; the same was seen in European population groups without undue exposure. So, it was concluded that in groups with 50 % $\leq$ 200 ppb and 90 % $\leq$ 300 ppb, levels exceeding 350 ppb are not or hardly to be expected to occur. (However, see Chapter 13).

If within a group a few individuals have a high PbB, then this is not necessarily due to general environmental exposure in the area studied, but it may be due to very local (micro-environment) excessive exposure; the presence of a few individuals with excessive PbB levels therefore cannot be accepted as indicator of a public health problem (macro-environment), although it may indicate an individual health problem. As a matter of choice, one may take the percentage of non-representative exposure to be 2 % ; this is clearly not a matter of science, but a policy decision. These 2 % should not be neglected, but approached on an individual basis. The EEC-proposal did not take over this reasoning, and required 100 % of the sample to be at or below 350 ppb. That this is an unreasonable proposal, will be discussed in Chapter 13.

So, the Biological Quality Guide for PbB-levels proposed was:
98 % $\leq$ 350 ppb; 90 % $\leq$ 300 ppb; 50 % $\leq$ 200 ppb. These percentages together could be taken as one combined guide level for estimating the permissibility of total exposure. If the distribution remains below this BQG, then the macro-environment is acceptable. If individual subjects ($\leq$ 2 %) exceed 350 ppb, then this constitutes a signal for action as to the individual micro-environment. If the group as such exceeds the BQG, then this constitutes a signal for action for the macro-environment. In **Figure 1** the proposed BQG and two hypothetical distributions A and B are given. A shows a steep incline, and particularly exceeds the BQG at high PbB levels; this indicates a **point source** within the area monitored. B shows a generally increased level of uptake throughout the **whole** area.

The proposal for a BQG for Pb is given as an example. It is easy to see that the same approach could be followed for many other environmental agents.

The **sequence of operation** for the development of a BQG is as follows:
1. Determine the relationship between the biological parameter and response (health effect).
2. Determine the acceptability of the response, and so the level of the biological parameter corresponding to the no-adverse response level.
3. Determine the distribution of biological parameters in various population groups.
4. Determine the BQG as that set of levels at which the no-adverse biological response is not exceeded.

In case the BQG proves to be exceeded, then EM has to take place:
1. Determine contributions through various routes and from various sources to the environmental load, and so to the internal load.
2. Take appropriate action as to that route and source which is mainly responsible for the uptake.

If the BQG is not exceeded, external exposure is permissible, and EM has not to be performed.

13.   SAMPLE SIZE*

In the original paper by Zielhuis (see Chapter 12) on a BQG for Pb he proposed to examine at least 50 subjects, preferably about 100.   However, this proposal on sample size was not based upon biostatistical considerations.

If one wants to examine whether the values of biological parameters in a population group do not exceed the BQG, composed of a combined set of levels for 50, 90 and 98 percent of the population, one starts to measure the biological parameter in a representative sample of the population.   The question is **how can one conclude from the values in the sample with sufficient certainty that the BQG in the population is not exceeded.**

Estimation of the percentages (with confidence intervals) of the population exceeding the BQG can be done in two ways:
-     with **parametric** methods
-     with **non-parametric** methods.

In the first case one knows or can assume a certain type of distribution for the values of the biological parameters, usually normal or log-normal; in the second case one cannot make such an assumption.   In comparison with parametric methods non-parametric methods have the disadvantages:
-     that they are less sensitive
-     that with increasing number of percentages the confidence intervals will expand. On the other hand a (log-)normal distribution is defined already with 2 parameters (mean and standard deviation).

To illustrate the problem a calculation has been made for PbB taking the BQG for Pb as proposed in Chapter 12, and using the actual data for PbB values measured in a study carried out by the Coronel Laboratory in the Netherlands in housewives, 20-45 years of age in a Dutch urban community, n = 200.   The group was divided into two samples of 50 and 150 subjects.   Actual findings in the samples are given in **Table 13.1**.

Table 13.1

Lead in blood values in housewives (in ppb),
m and s refer to log (PbB)
Number of people exceeding the BQG-levels is given

	n = 50	n = 150
range	50 - 240	40 - 240
antilog (m)	107	107
antilog (m $\pm$ s)	74 - 154	77 - 149
PbB > 200	2	5
PbB > 300	0	0
PbB > 350	0	0

In using the parametric approach we assumed for the PbB-values a log-normal distribution. We used a BQG consisting of three norms.

In using the non-parametric approach we compared a BQG of the same three norms with a BQG of one norm. We used as norms 50 % of the population < 200 ppb, 90 % of the population < 300 ppb and 98 % of the population < 350 ppb.

---

*   This chapter is based upon a contribution from H.J.A. Sallé, MSc.   ., biostatistician, Coronel Laboratory.

From our data we calculated with both methods* the 95 % upper confidence limit (P) of the percentage in the population which exceeds a certain BQG level (200, 300 and 350 ppb). The results is given in **Table 13.2.**

Table 13.2

Upper confidence limits (P) of the percentage of the population
which exceeds a certain BQG level
Comparison of the parametric and the non-parametric method
Those percentages which do not fulfil the BQG are given in brackets

BQG percentage	level (ppb)	percentage allowed to exceed the level	parametric BQG with 3 norms		non-parametric BQG with 3 norms		BQG with 1 norm	
			n = 50	n = 150	n = 50	n = 150	n = 50	n = 150
50 %	$\leq$ 200	50 %	12.6 %	6.4 %	14.7 %	8.1 %	12.1 %	6.9 %
90 %	$\leq$ 300	10 %	2.1 %	0.5 %	7.9 %	2.7 %	5.9 %	2 %
98 %	$\leq$ 350	2 %	0.9 %	0.1 %	(7.9) %	(2.7) %	(5.9) %	2 %

This table shows that in using the non-parametric method, we are not 95 % confident to state that the BQG of three norms is fulfilled even if we use a sample size n = 150, because for PbB = 350 ppb P = 2.7 %, which is larger than 2 %. In using the parametric method one is at least 95 % confident that the BQG is fulfilled even if we use the sample size n = 50, because all confidence limits derived are lower than the percentages allowed for the population (e.g. 0.9 % < 2 %, 2.1 % < 10 %, 12.6 % < 50 %). However if one should have found higher PbB values in the actual study an increased sample size would have been necessary to enable a judgement.

Another way of presenting the non-parametric method is given in **table 13.3.** Here we calculated the maximum number of people with PbB above the BQG in the sample such that we can state with 95 % confidence that the population fulfils the BQG.

---

* For the parametric method we used the approximation:

$$T_{1-P/100} = \left(\frac{\log (\text{BQG-level}) - m}{s} - \frac{t\,0.975}{\sqrt{n}} \right) \sqrt{\frac{x^2\,0.025}{n-1}}$$

where: m and s are mean and standard deviation of log PbB in a sample with size n;
t 0.975: 0.975 fractile of the Student-distribution with (n−1) df
$x^2$0.025 : 0.025 fractile of the x^2-distribution with (n−1)df; P is the calculated percentage.
For the non-parametric method P is the upper confidence limit in binomial sampling with α = 0.05 and α = 0.05/3.

Table 13.3

Maximum number of people with PbB-BQG in a sample (size n)
such that it can be stated with 95 % confidence that the population fulfils the BQG.

In parenthesis the number of people which may be expected in the sample with PbB
above the BQG level if the population just fulfils the BQG.

	percentage of the population not allowed to exceed the BQG-level	n = 50	n = 150
BQG with	50 %	18 (25)	64 (75)
	90 %	1 (5)	8 (15)
one norm	98 %	- (1)	0 (3)
BQG with	50 %	17 (25)	61 (75)
	90 %	0 (5)	7 (15)
three norms	98 %	- (1)	- (3)

This table just as table 13.2 shows that we cannot state (with a confidence > 95 %) that in the population a BQG of three norms is fulfilled, even with a sample size n = 150. Also the table reveals the more strict requirements for the sample in regard to the population. If n = 150 then one should have no subject (and not 3) exceeding 350 ppb, to be confident that PbB = 350 ppb (one level only) is not exceeded in the population by more than 2 %; in a sample n = 50, only one subject is allowed to exceed PbB = 350 ppb (one level only) and not 5 subjects as one could surmise from 10 % of 50. The discrepancy between the number allowed in the sample and the number to be expected if the population just fulfils the BQG increases strongly with the higher percentages (from 50 to 98 %), whereas with increasing sample size the discrepancy decreases.

Comparison of the results based upon the parametric method with those based upon the non-parametric method shows that for the first method the required sample sizes are considerably smaller than for the latter. Moreover with the second method for the high percentage 98 % there is a large discrepancy between the requirements for the sample and those for the population (BQG). From tables 13.2 and 13.3 it becomes clear that the sensitivity for the high percentages quickly increases with sample size.

In BM-programmes, directed at evaluation of exposure and health risks for the **general population**, one can usually assume a (log) normal distribution, and so use a parametric method. In this case one can start with a small sample size e.g. n = 50. If the PbB values in this sample should appear high, the size can be extended. However, in case of **at risk groups** such an assumption is (often) not allowed; one has no idea about the type of distribution; one has to use a non-parametric method, and so large sample sizes. Also the expected higher PbB values, being closer to the BQG, in such groups urge for large samples. Even with large sample sizes, the uncertainty remains large for prediction of the absence of high (and from viewpoint of health more relevant) levels. So, one is forced to take very large samples on a combined set of levels, but on one level rarely to be exceeded, e.g. 95 % < 325 ppb or 98 % < 350 ppb.

14. SOCIO-MEDICAL ASPECTS

BM uses human beings as sampling units for providing information; so, BM could always be regarded as a **medical procedure**. BM-programmes have therefore to be carried out in a medical setting, the ultimate responsibility should be with a medical organization, even although the sampling and analytical methods might be outside the field of "normal" medicine.

In designing a BM-programme the following points should always be taken into account:

- Does the BM-programme really serve an objective of **interest to public health**, or has it merely a scientific interest ?
- Is a BM-programme **necessary** or highly desirable to achieve the objective ? Is the knowledge maybe already available, or can the objective be achieved by other means, e.g. by means of EM ?
- Is a specific BM-programme part of a **total public health approach**, or is it only an isolated undertaking, and are other factors determining health not looked for ?
- Is the **design valid**: do the data to be gained really promise to give an answer to the specific question asked for ? Are the methods valid, are the actual at risk groups chosen, are the groups adequately representative, is the sample size large enough ?
- Has the BM-programme been organized **efficiently**, so that the load to the human subjects is in proportion to the results that can be expected ? Did one its utmost to make inconvenience to the participants as small as possible ?
- Does the method employed carry any **health risk** ? There is always the difficulty in epidemiological studies in "healthy" subjects that one is much more limited in examination techniques than in examining hospital patients, whereas at the same time in "healthy" subjects the changes in biological parameters usually are much smaller, and so as such might demand a more sophisticated sampling and measuring technique with a possible risk to health, e.g. lumbar puncture, liver puncture, BSP. However, in BM-programmes the risk to health and well-being should be absent to minimal.
- A BM-programme should not induce undue **emotional unrest**. There should be good **information** to the public. The programme should be part of an established public health programme.
- Subjects have the right **to be informed** on their own **individual data**; these data should be regarded as **confidential** as is the case for all medical data. In case of abnormal results the general practitioner should be informed; because this physician may not always possess the necessary knowledge on how to deal with specific data, he should also be informed on this.
- The **group data** should be **made known** to the general public through the existing official channels. The individual data, as being medically confidential, should always be treated anonymously when entering group data.
- It will never be possible to make participation in BM-programmes **obligatory**; by means of open propaganda through diverse media subjects can be asked to participate voluntarily. However, only in case a large majority of elective subjects participate, a reasonable representativeness of the sample can be obtained. Discussion of **representativeness** of the sample should always precede the actual start of the programme.
- In accordance with local regulations and laws the matter of **legal responsibility** may have to be settled.

15. SUMMARY

Chapter 2:
- Immediate objective of BM: to provide estimate of exposure and of health risk
- Ultimate objective: protection of health of population
- BM based upon distribution of biological data in population groups, individual data only of interest insofar as contribution to group data; in health surveys individual data are of primary interest.

Chapter 3:
BM may have to be preferred over EM
- total external exposure integrated in body burden
- more linked with health protection
- pharmacokinetic variability taken into account
- other health parameters to be measured
- less expensive in manpower and budget.

Chapter 4:
Limitations of BM:
- inconvenience to subjects
- only for a limited number of compounds
  - no knowledge of exposure-internal load relationships available
  - no reliable methods
- compounds with short half life.

Chapter 5:
Classification of immediate objectives:
1. Occupational health versus public health
2.1. Estimation of recent exposure (short $t1/2$)
2.2. Estimation of exposure last months ($t1/2 \leq$ 1-2 mths)
2.3. Estimation of long-term exposure ($t1/2$ many mths)
2.4. Estimation of total life time exposure (persistent compounds)
3. Estimation of total exposure through one pathway, various sources
4. Estimation of graded exposure
5. Estimation of sequential exposure
So immediate objective has to be clearly specified.

Chapter 6:
Four concepts of exposure:
EE : external exposure in a general sense, i.e. concentration in sources, and T
EL : amount offered to body, and T
IL : internal load
ILE : internal load at effector site
Other concepts:
CC : critical concentration at cell level
COC : critical organ concentration
COR : criticial organ, i.e. that organ which first attains COC.

Chapter 7:
Exposure (dose)-response relationship, i.e. relationship between exposure (dose) and relative number of subjects with a specified intensity of a specified parameter.

Before starting a routine BM the relationship of EE $\rightarrow$ (EL) $\rightarrow$ IL $\rightarrow$ (ILE) $\rightarrow$ health risk should be known.

Chapter 8:
Possibilities of exposure can be classified as follows:
1. occupational exposure
    a. direct manmade
    b. indirect manmade
    c. natural presence
2. para-occupational domestic exposure
3. para-occupational exposure through leisure time activities
4. neighbourhood exposure
5. exposure through personal habits
6. true environmental exposure

Chapter 9:
BM may be directed at estimating exposure-health risk in
- general population
- at risk groups
  - increased exposure
  - different pharmacokinetics
  - different pharmacodynamics

An "average" human being does not exist.

Chapter 10:
Deviant subgroups at risk are of primary concern, so BM should bring forward the data from such groups. This cannot be done by averaging. Data in general population often are log-normally distributed; geometric average + standard deviation defines the distribution. Data in subgroups not necessarily follow a log-normal distribution. So, percentile distributions should be calculated, indicating the percentiles at risk.

Chapter 11:
Predictive validity of parameters as to the exposure (or health risk) to be estimated, should be evaluated, by means of calculating sensitivity and specificity.

In BM-programmes parameter and situation to be predicted should be exactly specified; the data should be in a percentile distribution; the methods should be exactly specified.

Chapter 12:
The distribution of biological data can be used to evaluate permissibility of exposure, and so as a biological quality guide (BQG) (or standard). The sequence of operation is as follows:
- determine relation between parameter and response
- determine acceptability of response, and so no-adverse level of parameter
- determine distribution of parameter in population groups
- determine BQG

If BQG is exceeded, then EM has to take place:
- determine contribution through various routes and sources
- take appropriate action as to that route and source which is mainly responsible for uptake.

Chapter 13:
The sample size should be large enough to assure with sufficient confidence that permissible limits set are not exceeded in the total population. In studying exposure of the general population one usually can use parametric methods; one could start with a small sample size (n=50); if levels in this sample appear high, the size has to be extended. In case of at risk groups one has to use non-parametric methods, and so large sample sizes. Even with large sample sizes, the uncertainty remains large for prediction of absence of high levels; by preference one should not base prediction on a combined set of levels, but at one level rarely to be exceeded.

Chapter 14:
Various socio-medical aspects have to be taken into account:
- is BM of interest to public health, and is it necessary
- is BM part of total public health programme
- is design valid

- is BM organized efficiently
- does BM have a health risk
- does BM induce emotional unrest
- are individual data treated confidentially
- are group data made known to the public
- does participation ensure representativeness
- has legal responsibility been taken into account.

BM should be regarded as a medical programme, and so should be carried out under medical authority.

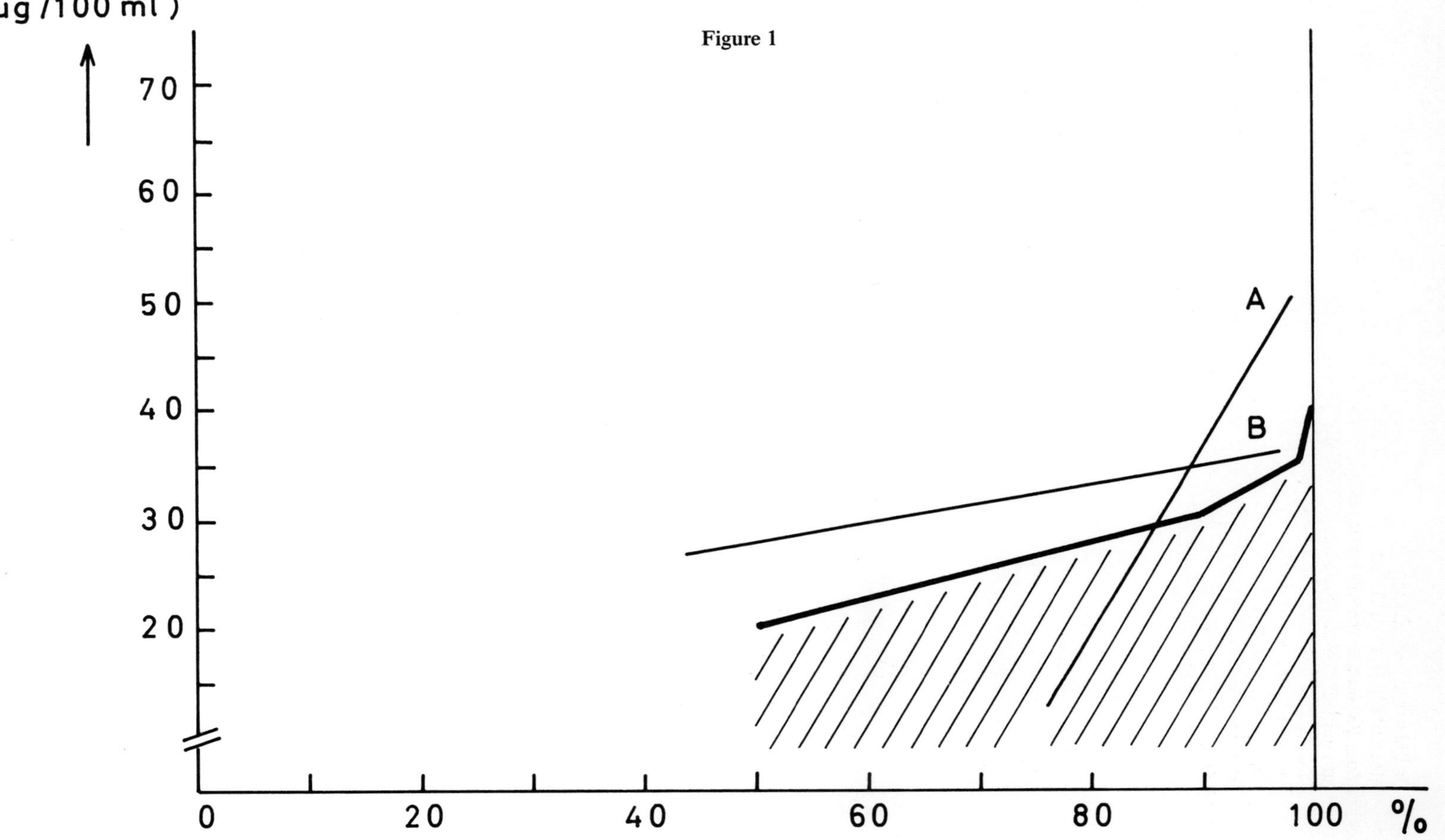

PbB
(µg /100 ml)
70
60
50
40
30
20
A
B
0
20
40
60
80
100
%
Figure 1
359

LIST OF PARTICIPANTS

BELGIUM

HUBLET P.
  Administration, Hygiène et
  Médecine du Travail
  53, rue Belliard
  1040 BRUXELLES

LAUWERYS R.
  Medical and Industrial Toxicology
  Unit - Univ. catholique de Louvain
  30, Clos Chapelle-aux-Champs
  1200 BRUXELLES

MERCIER M.
  Université catholique de Louvain
  Avenue Emmanuel Mounier 73
  1200 BRUXELLES

THIERS G.
  Institut d'Hygiène et d'Epidémio-
  logie - Rue Juliette Wytsman 14
  1050 BRUXELLES

BULGARIA

KALOYANOVA F.
  Institute of Hygiene and
  Occupational Diseases
  Centre of Hygiene
  Boul. D. Nestorov 15
  SOFIA 31

CZECHOSLOVAKIA

BARDODEJ Z.
  Department of Medical Chemistry
  Medical Faculty of Hygiene
  Sroborova 48
  100 42 PRAGUE 10

DENMARK

HANSEN J.
  Hygiejnisk Institut
  Aarhus Universitet
  Universitets Parken
  8000 AARHUS

FRANCE

BIGNON J.
  Université de Paris XII
  Service Hospitalo-Universitaire
  de Pneumologie
  Centre Hospitalier Intercommunal
  49, av. de Verdun
  94010 CRETEIL

RICHIER C.
  Institut d'Histopathologie Expérimentale
  Faculté de Médecine de Bordeaux
  33000 BORDEAUX

SEBASTIEN P.
  Lab. d'Etude des Particules Inhalées
  37, Bld St-Marcel
  75013 PARIS

FEDERAL REPUBLIC OF GERMANY

KORANSKY W.
Institut für Toxikologie und Pharmakologie der Philipps-Universität
Pilgrimstein 2
335 MARBURG/L

KORTE F.
Institute for Ecological Chemistry
Post Oberschleissheim
Ingolstädter Landstrasse 1
8042 NEUHERBERG

MUHS P.
Umweltbundesamt
Bismarckplatz 1
1000 BERLIN 33

SCHALLER K.-H.
Institut für Arbeits- u. Sozialmedizin
Universität Erlangen
Schillerstrasse 25-29
8520 ERLANGEN-NUERNBERG

SCHMIDT-BLEEK F.
Umweltbundesamt
Bismarckplatz 1
1000 BERLIN 33

STOEPPLER M.
Institut für Chemie der
Kernforschungsanlage Jülich GmbH
Angewandte Physikalische Chemie
517 JUELICH

VALENTIN H.
Institut für Arbeits- u. Sozialmedizin
Universität Erlangen
Schillerstrasse 25-29
8520 ERLANGEN-NUERNBERG

I R A N

FARVAR M.T.
Environmental Sciences and Eco-
development Cluster
BU-ALI SINA University
Box 211
HAMADAN

I R E L A N D

GRIMES H.
Department of Clinical Biochemistry
Western Health Board
GALWAY

I T A L Y

ALESSIO L.
Clinica del Lavoro
dell'Università di Milano
Via S. Barnaba 8
20122 MILANO

BURATTI M.
Clinica del Lavoro
dell'Università di Milano
Via S. Barnaba 8
20122 MILANO

FOA V.
Clinica del Lavoro
dell'università di Milano
Via S. Barnaba 8
20122 MILANO

PACCAGNELLA B.
Institute of Hygiene
University of Padova
Policlinic Borgo Roma
37100 VERONA

JAPAN

TSUCHIYA K.
  Department of Preventive Medicine
  and Public Health
  Keio University School of Medicine
  TOKYO 160

LUXEMBOURG

WENNIG R.
  Institut d'Hygiène et de
  Santé Publique
  1A, rue Auguste-Lumière
  LUXEMBOURG

MEXICO

ORDOÑEZ B.R.
  Secretariat of Public Health and Welfare
  Av. Chapultepeo 284
  Piso 13
  MEXICO CITY

NETHERLANDS

GREVE P.A.
  Laboratory for Toxicology
  National Institute for Public Health
  Antonie van Leewenhoeklaan 9
  Postbus 1
  2660 BILTHOVEN

ZIELHUIS R.L.
  University of Amsterdam
  Eerste Constantijn Huygensstraat 20
  AMSTERDAM

SWEDEN

NORDBERG G.
  Department of Environmental Hygiene
  Karolinska Institute
  104 01 STOCKHOLM 60

UNITED KINGDOM

BUXTON R.St.
  Department of Health and Social Security
  Hannibal House
  Elephant and Castle
  LONDON S.E.1

EGAN H.
  Laboratory of the Government Chemist
  Cornwall House
  Stamford Street
  LONDON SE1 9NQ

UNITED STATES OF AMERICA

ENGEL R.
U.S. Department of Agriculture
Animal and Plant Health Inspection Serv.
WASHINGTON D.C. 20250

GREENWOOD M.R.
Department of Radiation Biology
and Biophysics
University of Rochester
School of Medicine
ROCHESTER, New York

GINN R.L.
Ambassador of the
United States of America
LUXEMBOURG

HARLEY J.
Health and Safety Laboratory
U.S. Energy Research and
Development Administration
376 Hudson Street
NEW YORK N.Y. 10014

KNEIP T.
Institute of Environmental Medicine
New York University Medical Center
TUXEDO, New York 10987

LAFLEUR P.D.
Analytical Chemistry Division
National Bureau of Standards
WASHINGTON D.C. 20234

ROOK H.
Analytical Chemistry Division
National Bureau of Standards
WASHINGTON D.C. 20234

WOLFF A.H.
Environmental Health Sciences
School of Public Health
University of Illinois
Medical Center
P.O. Box 6998
CHICAGO, Illinois 60680

YUGOSLAVIA

WEBER O.
Institute for Medical Research
Yugoslav Academy of Sciences and Arts
P.O. Box 291
41001 ZAGREB

COMMISSION OF THE EUROPEAN COMMUNITIES

BERLIN A.
Health and Safety Directorate
Jean Monnet Building
LUXEMBOURG (G.D.)

BONINI A.
Health and Safety Directorate
Jean Monnet Building
LUXEMBOURG (G.D.)

FOSCHINI V.
Directorate-General
Internal Market and Industrial Affairs
Rond point Schuman
BRUSSELS (Belgium)

HORN W.
Health and Safety Directorate
Jean Monnet Building
LUXEMBOURG (G.D.)

HUNTER W.J.
Health and Safety Directorate
Jean Monnet Building
LUXEMBOURG (G.D.)

RECHT P.
Health and Safety Directorate
Jean Monnet Building
LUXEMBOURG (G.D.)

SMEETS J.
Environment and Consumer
Protection Service
200, rue de la Loi
1049 BRUSSELS (Belgium)

VAN DER VENNE M.Th.
Health and Safety Directorate
Jean Monnet Building
LUXEMBOURG (G.D.)

COUNCIL OF MINISTERS OF THE EUROPEAN COMMUNITIES

CORCELLE G.
Service Transport Environnement
170, rue de la Loi
1048 BRUSSELS

INTERNATIONAL ATOMIC ENERGY AGENCY

RYABUKHIN Y.
Kärntnerring 11-13
1010 WIEN

INTERNATIONAL UNION OF PURE AND APPLIED CHEMISTRY

EGAN H.
Laboratory of the Government Chemist
Cornwall House
Stamford Street
LONDON SE1 9NQ

EUROPEAN PARLIAMENT

ROLVERING H.
Commission de l'Environnement
Protection de la Santé et des
Consommateurs
LUXEMBOURG

VAN DER PERRE L.
Commission de l'Environnement
Protection de la Santé et des
Consommateurs
LUXEMBOURG

UNITED STATES ENVIRONMENTAL PROTECTION AGENCY

BARTH D.
Office of Research and Development
401 M Street
WASHINGTON D.C. 20460

GOLDSTEIN G.
Health Effects Research Center
RESEARCH TRIANGLE PARK
North Carolina 27711

HUETER G.F.
National Environmental Research Center
RESEARCH TRIANGLE PARK
North Carolina 27711

KUTZ F.W.
National Human Monitoring
WASHINGTON D.C. 20460

LOVING J.
Office of Research and Development
401 M Street
WASHINGTON D.C. 20460

WORLD HEALTH ORGANIZATION

BRAMAN S.
  Division of Environmental Health
  CH - 1211 GENEVA 27

HASEGAWA Y.
  Division of Environmental Health
  CH - 1211 GENEVA 27

JENKINS D.W.
  Pan American Health Organization
  Havre 30 - Piso 3
  MEXICO CITY 6 D.F. (Mexico)

MASIRONI R.
  Cardiovascular Diseases
  CH - 1211 GENEVA 27

VOUK V.B.
  Division of Environmental Health
  CH - 1211 GENEVA 27